3D Printing for the Radiologist

3D Printing for the Radiologist

NICOLE WAKE, PHD
Editor

Assistant Professor of Radiology, 3D Imaging Lab Director,
Department of Radiology, Montefiore Medical Center, Albert Einstein College of
Medicine, Bronx, NY, United States
Adjunct Instructor, Center for Advanced Imaging Innovation and Research (CAI^{2}R) and
Bernard and Irene, Schwartz Center for Biomedical Imaging, Department of Radiology,
NYU Langone Health, NYU Grossman School of Medicine, New York, NY, United States

ELSEVIER

Publisher: Cathleen Sether
Acquisitions Editor: Kayla Wolfe
Editorial Project Manager: Sam W. Young
Project Manager: Niranjan Bhaskaran
Cover Designer: Miles Hitchen

3251 Riverport Lane
St. Louis, Missouri 63043

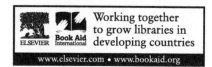

Working together
to grow libraries in
developing countries

www.elsevier.com • www.bookaid.org

List of Contributors

Amy E. Alexander, BME, MS
Senior Biomedical Engineer
Anatomic Modeling Unit
Department of Radiology
Mayo Clinic
Rochester, MN, United States

Alejandro Amor-Coarasa, PhD
Assistant Professor of Radiology (Nuclear Medicine)
Director Radiochemistry Lab
Department of Radiology
Montefiore Medical Center
Albert Einstein College of Medicine
Bronx, NY, United States

Louisa Bokacheva, PhD
Science Communications Specialist
Department of Radiology
NYU Langone Health
NYU Grossman School of Medicine
New York, NY, United States

Ryan Brown, PhD
Associate Professor
Center for Advanced Imaging
    Innovation and Research (CAI^{2}R)
Bernard and Irene Schwartz
    Center for Biomedical Imaging
Department of Radiology
NYU Langone Health
NYU Grossman School of Medicine
New York, NY, United States

Judah Burns, MD
Associate Professor
Department of Radiology
Montefiore Medical Center
Albert Einstein College of Medicine
Bronx, NY, United States

Jingyun Chen, PhD
Research Assistant Professor
Department of Neurology
NYU Langone Health
NYU Grossman School of Medicine
New York, NY, United States

Andy Christensen, BS, FSME
Adjunct Professor
Department of Radiology
University of Ottawa
Ottawa, ON, Canada

President
Somaden LLC
Littleton, CO, United States

Christopher M. Collins, PhD
Professor
Center for Advanced Imaging
    Innovation and Research (CAI^{2}R)
Bernard and Irene Schwartz
    Center for Biomedical Imaging
Department of Radiology
NYU Langone Health
NYU Grossman School of Medicine
New York, NY, United States

Pamela DuPré, MMP
Physicist
Department of Radiation Oncology
Inova Schar Cancer Institute
Fairfax, VA, United States

Lee Goddard, MPhys
Physicist
Department of Radiation Oncology
Montefiore Medical Center
Bronx, NY, United States

Yu-Hui Huang, MD, MS
Department of Radiology
University of Minnesota
Minneapolis, MN, United States

Carlotta Ianniello, MS
PhD Candidate
Center for Advanced Imaging
    Innovation and Research (CAI^{2}R)
Bernard and Irene Schwartz
    Center for Biomedical Imaging
Department of Radiology
NYU Langone Health
NYU Grossman School of Medicine
New York, NY, United States

Adam E. Jakus, PhD
Co-Founder & Chief Technology Officer
Dimension Inx Corp.
Chicago, IL, United States

Benjamin Johnson, BS
Director of Product Development
3D Systems Healthcare
Littleton, CO, United States

Shuai Leng, PhD, FAAPM
Professor
Division of Medical Physics
Department of Radiology
Mayo Clinic
Rochester, MN, United States

Peter Liacouras, PhD
Director of Services
3D Medical Applications Center
Department of Radiology
Walter Reed National Military Medical Center
Bethesda, MD, United States

Assistant Professor
Radiology and Radiological Services
Naval Postgraduate Dental School
Uniform Services University of the Health Sciences
Bethesda, MD, United States

Mohammad Mansouri, MD
Radiology Resident
Department of Radiology
Montefiore Medical Center
Albert Einstein College of Medicine
Bronx, NY, United States

Jane M. Matsumoto, MD
Staff Radiologist
Pediatric Radiology
Bioinformatics
Department of Radiology
Mayo Clinic
Rochester, MN, United States

Kiaran P. McGee, PhD
Consultant
Department of Radiology
Professor of Medical Physics
Assistant Professor of Biomedical Engineering
Mayo Clinic
Rochester, MN, United States

Jonathan M. Morris, MD
Assistant Professor of Neuroradiology
Director of Anatomic Modeling Lab
Department of Radiology
Mayo Clinic and Foundation
Mayo Clinic
Rochester, MN, United States

R. Ross Reichard, MD
Medical Director
Forensic Autopsy Services
Department of Anatomic Pathology
Mayo Clinic
Rochester, MN, United States

Sarah Rimini, BS, RT(R) (MR) (ARRT)
Program Director
Radiology 3D Lab
Geisinger Health
Danville, PA, United States

Fraser Robb, PhD
Chief Technology Leader
MRI Business
GE Healthcare, Inc
Aurora, OH, United States

Henry Rusinek, PhD
Professor
Department of Radiology
NYU Langone Health
NYU Grossman School of Medicine
New York, NY, United States

Jana Vincent, PhD
Senior RF Engineer
GE Healthcare, Inc
Aurora, OH, United States

Nicole Wake, PhD
Assistant Professor of Radiology
3D Imaging Lab Director
Department of Radiology
Montefiore Medical Center
Albert Einstein College of Medicine
Bronx, NY, United States

Adjunct Instructor,
Center for Advanced Imaging
    Innovation and Research (CAI^{2}R)
Bernard and Irene Schwartz
    Center for Biomedical Imaging
Department of Radiology
NYU Langone Health
NYU Grossman School of Medicine
New York, NY, United States

Kenneth C. Wang, MD, PhD
Staff Radiologist
Imaging Service
Baltimore VA Medical Center
Baltimore, MD, United States

Adjunct Assistant Professor
Department of Diagnostic Radiology and
    Nuclear Medicine
University of Maryland
School of Medicine
Baltimore, MD, United States

Kapil Wattamwar, MD
Resident Physician
Department of Radiology
Montefiore Medical Center
New York, NY, United States

Preface

Since the invention of three-dimensional (3D) printing in the 1980s, it has become a widely employed manufacturing technology used in many industries such as aerospace, automotive, consumer goods, industrial goods, and healthcare. As compared to traditional manufacturing technologies, 3D printing is a more efficient process that easily allows for the creation of customized products with greater design flexibility in a much reduced timeframe. Today, there are thousands of 3D printers operating around the world, and these include both low-cost desktop machines and high-end industrial machines.

At this time, 3D printed anatomic models derived from patient-specific volumetric medical imaging data are being created and used increasingly in medicine. These 3D printed models expand upon the current capabilities of traditional 3D medical image visualization on a two-dimensional (2D) screen by providing visuo-haptic feedback to enhance the understanding of complex anatomies. 3D printed anatomic models can be used for many applications in healthcare including surgical planning, intra-operative guidance, patient communication, and trainee education, ultimately leading to improved patient care.

The creation of 3D printed models from radiological imaging data is a complex process which involves manipulating the original imaging data into a volume that represents patient-specific anatomy. These select data are then optimized for 3D printing. As an extension of 3D printed anatomic models, anatomic guides may be created from these data to be used directly in the operating room. These same methods may also be used to create personalized implants; however, these will not be discussed in detail in this book due to regulatory concerns for printing high-risk devices in the hospital at the present time.

This book is targeted for the practicing radiologist interested in learning about current and future applications of 3D printing in radiology and medicine. Through this book, methods to create 3D printed anatomical models from medical images are described and clinical applications key to radiology are highlighted. It is important to note that the chapters in this book are focused on the 3D printing workflow to create medical models from imaging data. In addition, clinical areas such as interventional radiology, nuclear medicine, and radiation therapy which are important to radiologists are highlighted. The insights and explanations provided here are designed to be valuable to the reader for understanding the comprehensive workflow required to create medical models, identifying how 3D printing is used in radiology, and uncovering how these methods could shape the future of 3D printing in radiology and medicine.

Acknowledgments

Thanks to every author and contributor for helping me to make this book a reality. Also, special thanks to Samuel Young and Niranjan Bhaskaran, my Editorial and Production Project Managers, for their patience and assistance.

Contents

CHAPTER 1

An Abbreviated History of Medical 3D Printing

ANDY CHRISTENSEN, BS, FSME

INTRODUCTION

Three-dimensional (3D) printing technologies are now entering their fourth decade of use and many medical applications now are very well established and optimized. Despite this, many in the medical field are surprised to hear that 3D printing is not relatively new. This chapter is not an exhaustive look at every development along the timeline for medical 3D printing but instead meant to point out some major milestones which have led us to the state-of-the-art today.

The basis of much of the work done with 3D printing in medicine is surrounding personalization of surgery. This goes all the way back to the beginning and continues today. Personalization typically relies on use of volumetric medical imaging data, allowing the therapy to truly be personalized to the individual patient. Flexibility, complexity of design, and lot sizes of one make 3D printing a good fit for support of the tools, guides, models, and implants which make up the world of personalized surgery. If we consider the medical 3D printing technologies and applications as the toolbox, many pioneering engineers, surgeons, and others contributed to the creation of the tools in the toolbox. Over time the toolbox has continuously expanded by way of software tools, hardware tools, material tools, and workflows which combine these tools in specific ways to solve specific clinical problems. 3D printing has significantly altered several key areas of medicine including craniomaxillofacial surgery, orthopedic surgery, and beyond.

1980s—3D PRINTING PIONEERING WORK AND EARLIEST 3D PRINTING IN MEDICINE

The majority of the work for personalized surgery starts with a volumetric medical imaging study such as computed tomography (CT) or magnetic resonance imaging (MRI). With the advent of the CT scanner in 1967, volumes of data could be acquired, giving for the first time a sense of scale and position of different elements by density.[1] Traditional X-rays did not capture scale and compressed what was 3D data (the patient) into one very two-dimensional (2D) planar image. MRI was commercialized in the 1980s and led to the ability to image soft tissues with much more discretion than was allowed by CT. (Please refer to Chapter 2 for more information on medical imaging.)

In the early 1980s, inventors Hideo Kodama (Japan) and Chuck Hull (US) started independent work on the first 3D printing process which was later coined stereolithography. Hull's first US Patent was issued in 1987[2] and the first 3D printing company (3D Systems, Rock Hill, SC) was founded which focused on selling 3D printers, then referred to as the field of rapid prototyping. One might think that 1987 could be the start for 3D printing in medicine, but several very important building blocks, key to this field coming to fruition, actually stretch back to 1981.

In 1981, Dr. Jeffrey Marsh, a craniofacial surgeon, and Dr. Michael Vannier, a radiologist, both physicians at the Washington University School of Medicine (St. Louis, MO), worked with an engineer named James Warren (McDonnell Douglas, St. Louis, MO) on the concept of anatomic modeling. The goal was to take slice data from a CT scan and use it to replicate individual slices of materials that would form a 3D object when assembled. McDonnell Douglas was in the aerospace field and working with many high-performance materials including titanium. An image postprocessing technique called thresholding (Described in Chapter 3) was used to delineate the Hounsfield units (measure of grayscale intensity) for bone in the CT scan, creating individual slices of data just for the bone structure. This was first used to model a young boy with a large frontonasal encephalocele. The digital files from the segmented CT slices were transferred to a milling machine which traced these slices, which were of the same thickness as the CT scan slices, into titanium. When assembled and stacked up these slices formed, to scale, a model of the boy's bone structure which clearly illustrated the large bony perforation above his left orbit. This work continued into 1982 with less exotic materials, moving to acrylic sheets instead of titanium.[3,4] Due to lack of funding, the work ceased in 1982, but several of the models remain intact. Marsh and Vannier published a paper and a book on their pioneering efforts in 3D imaging in the early 1980s, but there was only a passing comment made in the paper regarding their physical modeling efforts (Fig. 1.1 and 1.2).[5,6]

Also in 1981, a physicist named F. Brix in Kiel, Germany, started work that used the external shape of the body, derived from a CT scan, milled from different materials, as radiation therapy compensators. This work led to others in Kiel, including Ulrich Kliegis, to start milling 3D shapes from solid blocks of foam, beginning with anatomic models.[7] Kliegis started a company called MEK/Endoplan (Kiel, Germany) to offer the service of anatomic modeling and later commercialized an anatomic modeling system that was even brought to the annual meeting of the Radiological Society of North

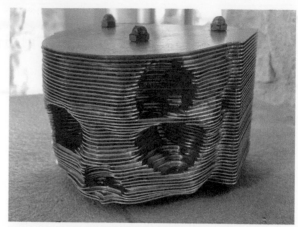

FIG. 1.2 A closer view of the model from 1981 which was constructed by milling individual layers of titanium to match the CT slices and stacking the individual layers to form the 3D model.

America (RSNA) in the mid-1980s. This concept was way ahead of its time and commercialization was slow, but work progressed in the 1980s and beyond for Kliegis and the group at Kiel. Many influential maxillofacial surgeons who in the 1980s trained at Kiel later took the concepts for anatomic modeling with them to Switzerland (Professor Dr. J. Thomas Lambrecht) and Austria (Professor Dr. Rolf Ewers) where the applications and technology continued to evolve and mature.[8,9] Lambrecht's book, published in 1996, contains clinical cases from the late 1980s to the early 1990s and is considered by many to be the authoritative work on early oral and maxillofacial surgery applications (Fig. 1.3).[8]

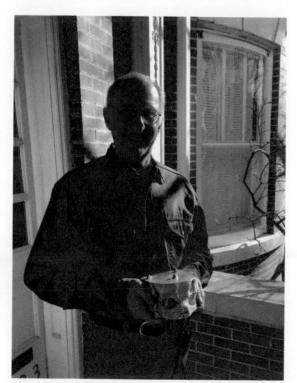

FIG. 1.1 Dr. Jeffrey Marsh is shown with the earliest known anatomic model created from medical imaging data. The model depicts a young patient with a large frontal encephalocele above the left orbit.

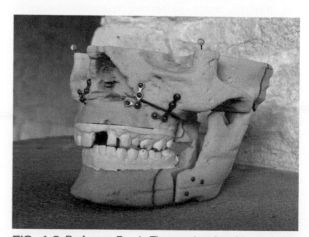

FIG. 1.3 Professor Dr. J. Thomas Lambrecht used this model which included integrated dental casts of the patient's teeth for planning orthognathic surgery. The model was milled from a lightweight foam material by Ulrich Kliegis in Kiel, Germany.

In the Department of Radiology at the University of California, Los Angeles (UCLA), in 1984, a physicist named Dr. Nicholas Mankovich was hard at work solving some of the same issues for anatomic modeling. He and his team used a similar approach to the St. Louis group for milling of individual slices of a CT scan from acrylic and stacking them to create life-sized 3D models of anatomy. The first clinical needs were for modeling the bone structure of patients with defects in their skull requiring cranial reconstruction.[10] The team created models that would allow for design and construction of patient-matched implants for the skull, called cranioplasties, working with legendary maxillofacial prosthodontist Dr. John Beumer. This work at UCLA continued until 1988 when Mankovich collaborated with Chuck Hull and Scott Turner at 3D Systems to create what was the very first 3D printed anatomic model, created with stereolithography.[11] Once the concept of stereolithography had been proven to work and showed the needed accuracy, the UCLA team abandoned the earlier stacked layer methods in favor of the more robust and accurate stereolithography process.

A US patent was issued to David White in 1982 for a technique surrounding anatomic modeling primarily for custom implant creation using subtractive, milling techniques.[12] CEMAX (Fremont, CA) licensed this patent in 1985 and used it to create a service business for anatomic modeling, servicing surgeons and medical device companies in need of these models to plan surgery or design patient-matched implants.[13] One such user of these anatomic models was Dr. William Binder and the company Implantech Associates (Ventura, CA).[14] Implantech has pioneered patient-matched silicone facial and body prostheses made using CT imaging.

Another competing method to the White method was being used at another California-based orthopedic implant company called Techmedica (Camarillo, CA) in the 1980s and into the early 1990s.[15] The model quality seems crude by today's standards, but the accuracy of the anatomic models met the clinical needs at that time. The models were created by tracing 1:1 CT scan images by a tracer into acrylic sheets which were then stacked together, smoothed along the outside contours with clay, and then used to cast sequential copies of the anatomy. The primary clinical focus for Techmedica was on large orthopedic tumor reconstruction cases, limb salvage cases, and complex joint revision cases. Techmedica was later sold to Intermedics Orthopedics (Austin, TX), but at least one product still exists from the Techmedica days, a patient-matched total joint replacement for the temporomandibular joint, now sold by TMJ Concepts (Ventura, CA).[16]

1990s—3D PRINTED ANATOMIC MODELS AND PERSONALIZED IMPLANTS

Fried Vancraen and his firm Materialise (Leuven, Belgium) play an important role in this industry starting in 1990, the same year that Materialise was founded. Vancraen was interested in the 3D printing of anatomic models with a newly acquired SLA-250, with serial number 32 (3D Systems, Rock Hill, SC), and his first anatomic model made by stereolithography was produced in November 1990.[17] Vancraen quickly learned that the software workflow for converting what were then proprietary file formats for each CT scanner was very difficult to utilize. In 1991, to help this workflow, the Materialise Interactive Medical Image Control System (Mimics) software was created; and it was commercialized in 1992.[18] This software paved the way in creating a service business for Materialise and for others to follow in their footsteps. Vancraen was instrumental in launching and leading the Phidias project in Europe to specifically study the clinical benefits of 3D printed anatomic models in comparison to static 3D virtual images. The Phidias Project, run by European radiologists, lasted from 1992 to 1995 with trailing data reports following.[19] This project was way ahead of its time in gathering data to support reimbursement for 3D printed anatomic models. One of the lasting and important contributions of the Phidias project was the creation of a first-of-its-kind material for stereolithography which allowed selective coloration by overcuring select regions of interest and biocompatibility. The material was developed by Materialise and Zeneca Specialties (London, United Kingdom) and allowed a second, red coloration to be used to highlight select anatomic structures within the otherwise clear anatomic model.[20] This material was commercialized by Zeneca and later sold to Huntsman (The Woodlands, TX). Huntsman was acquired by 3D Systems in 2011 and folded into their stereolithography materials portfolio. This material is still in active, worldwide use today.

3C Design (Founded by RW Christensen, DC Chase, and D Crook) was started in Dallas, TX, in 1992, to focus on aerospace, industrial, and medical uses for stereolithography. In 1995, the company folded and what would become Medical Modeling (Golden, CO) got its start with the same technology in Golden, Colorado. At first, the applications focused solely on preoperative anatomic models to assist with total joint replacement of the temporomandibular joint, but they quickly expanded to serve many surgical specialties and clinical needs. In 2000, Andy Christensen, employed with Medical Modeling since 1996, purchased the company and kept adding to its armamentarium of services and workflow development to support the medical applications of 3D printing.[21] This included anatomic modeling, design of personalized implants, virtual surgical planning, and eventually additive metals for implant production.

In 1994, on the other side of the globe, building on the work of Mankovich, Beumer, and others, the company Anatomics (Melbourne, Australia), led by neurosurgeon Dr. Paul D'Urso, was created with a focus on anatomic modeling and patient-matched cranioplasty implants. D'Urso and group later published a seminal paper on a prospective clinical trial for 3D printed anatomic models in 1999 which showed benefits to surgeon, patient, and hospital.[22]

Companies who sold 3D printers started to take notice of this emerging market; and, in 1996, there was major movement from Stratasys (Eden Prairie, MN), another major player in the 3D printer and material space. Scott Crump invented the technology called Fused Deposition Modeling (FDM) and cofounded Stratasys with his wife Lisa in 1989.[23] Lisa became quite interested in the anatomic modeling area and in 1996 led the effort for Stratasys to obtain the first (and possibly still the only) Food and Drug Administration (FDA) clearance of a 3D printer, the FDM MedModeller.[24] Stratasys commercialized the product and even exhibited at the RSNA annual meeting in Chicago in the late 1990s to try and market 3D printers to hospitals. The Materialise Mimics software was also FDA cleared at the same time to provide more of an end-to-end solution from CT scan to model.[25] A company was eventually spun-out of Stratasys to commercialize this idea, but eventually it was discontinued due to lack of traction. This concept was 20 years ahead of its time and the industry owes Lisa Crump a debt of gratitude for pushing point of care 3D printing first.

The very beginnings of virtual surgery also date back to the mid-1990s, with Dr. James Xia's work in Hong Kong. Xia's work dealt with manipulating, cutting, and moving objects in space related to oral and maxillofacial surgical procedures.[26] He relocated to Houston around 2000 and so began a long career with oral and maxillofacial surgeon Dr. Jaime Gateno first at University of Texas (Houston, TX) and later at Methodist Hospital (Houston, TX). The group's focus was on orthognathic surgery involving osteotomies of the mandible and maxilla. In the 2000s, this dynamic team had a singular focus on tackling each step of the virtual surgery and clinical transfer process step by step. Publishing each subsequent step along the way they established workflows and accuracy standards for this work in collaboration with clinical and industry collaborators.[27–29] Through work funded by several NIH grants, the team flushed out many of the key steps of the process along with collaborator Medical Modeling, who commercialized some of the workflow steps in its services for orthognathic surgical planning and guidance. At the core of these technologies was the ability to osteotomize bony segments in a virtual environment and then move these segments to desired, new, positions. Once the desired outcome was expressed digitally, a series of 3D printed templates or splints would be output to transfer the clinical plan from the computer to the operating room. This group went on to publish some of the most influential manuscripts in this space.[30,31]

2000s—DIGITAL DESIGN, ADDITIVE METALS, AND FOUNDATIONS FOR FUTURE VIRTUAL WORK

The first meaningful use of templates came with the launch of SurgiCase by Materialise in 2000. Building on previous software development and workflows, the SurgiCase software was initially targeted for dental implant simulation, translating the implant's position from the simulation to the patient, and it also included the creation of patient-specific, 3D printed dental drill guides.[32] In 2001, Materialise purchased Columbia Scientific (Columbia, MD), an industry leader for dental implant planning software (SimPlant), thereby combining their SurgiCase software product line with SimPlant. Another technological advance that helped push this application forward was the commercialization of Cone-Beam CT (CBCT), which allows for volumetric imaging studies to be performed in the oral surgeon's office and led to much wider use of CT in the craniomaxillofacial area.

Around 2000, computer-aided design (CAD) software programs started to become more advanced and products such as Freeform Modeling Systems 3D touch enabled haptic device systems for medical and dental modeling, product design, and digital content creation became available (Sensable Technologies, Woburn, MA). Dr. Richard Bibb in Cardiff, Wales, did pioneering work with these haptic devices and design software. Using the more artistic interface allowed for creation of patient-matched craniomaxillofacial implants; and for the first time these implants could be designed net shape, something very difficult previously with traditional CAD software. This work had an immense impact on the specific clinical application for patient-matched cranioplasty and changed how this work would be done in the future around the world.[33]

Meanwhile in Dallas, TX, in 2001, a craniofacial surgeon named Dr. Kenneth Salyer embarked on what would be a multiyear project to separate two twin boys born joined at the head (craniopagus twins). Using the latest anatomic modeling provided by Medical Modeling (Golden, CO), he and his team created 3D printed models of bone, skin, brains, venous and arterial systems, ventricles, and more that were integral to the successful separation which took place in 2003.[34] While not the first case where anatomic models were used by surgeons separating twins, this case garnered national attention and lead to a seminal paper on 3D printing for craniopagus cases and a 2004 3D Systems User Group SLA Excellence Award Grand Prize.[35] Earlier anatomic models for conjoined twins separation surgeries go back as far as 1995 with the Rainey twins who were separated at Wilford Hall Medical Center, Lackland Air Force Base in San Antonio, TX.[36] Medical Modeling's work for conjoined twins included modeling for 15 sets of twins by 2006.[37] Salyer is now retired from clinical practice but had used anatomic models to plan for more than 500 craniofacial surgeries during the 2000s (Fig. 1.4).

The work of Swedish metal additive manufacturing machine maker Arcam (Molndal, Sweden) came to the United States (US) in 2003 with the first machine being placed in an engineering lab at North Carolina State University (Raleigh, NC) with Dr. Ola Harryson (Industrial Engineering) and Dr. Denis Cormier (Materials Science). They quickly went to work qualifying titanium alloy (Ti6Al4V) using the electron beam melting (EBM) process, something that had not yet been accomplished.[38] This would be the start, in earnest, for the industry segment focused on using additive metals for implant production. The medical service bureau Medical Modeling built on this work and installed their first EBM machine in 2005 to focus on titanium implant production.[39] Harryson and Cormier went on to qualify many different materials for EBM along with spreading general knowledge about the application of additive metals to the manufacturing segment.

In the early 2000s, Walter Reed Army Medical Center (WRAMC, Washington, DC), under the leadership of Dr. Steven Rouse, was instrumental in establishing one of the first "point of care manufacturing" centers within WRAMC.[40] Rouse and colleagues including Dr. Peter Liacouras, the current 3D printing lab director, used 3D printing, originally in polymers, to help surgeons reconstruct all manner of traumatic injuries suffered by our soldiers in the gulf war. Hundreds of active duty military benefited from personalized implants, anatomic models, and more made by this

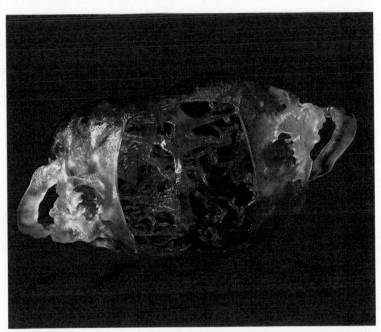

FIG. 1.4 A two-color stereolithography model of the Egyptian conjoined twin boys Ahmed and Mohammed Ibrahim, showing both bone and underlying vascular structures. Dr. Kenneth Salyer and team used this model and others to aid in preparation for the successful 38 h separation surgery.

lab. In 2011, WRAMC was combined with the Naval facility in Bethesda, MD, and saw the opening of a combined Walter Reed National Military Medical Center (WRNMMC) in Bethesda. Dr. Jerry Grant was head of this effort at WRNMMC in Bethesda for many years.[41]

Earlier discussion about virtual surgery and templating by Gateno, Xia, and the Materialise SurgiCase product was further expanded upon by orthopedic surgeon Dr. Steve Howell (Sacramento, CA) around 2005 for application to total joint arthroplasty.[42] Howell built a company called OtisMed (Hayward, CA) which focused on virtual planning for total knee arthroplasty (TKA) using his method of anatomic alignment. Using a CT scan to visualize the patient's bone structure, the specific size of a total knee replacement implant could be accurately predicted. Patient-matched cutting blocks were designed to transfer the position of the implants from the perfectly planned virtual session to the patient in surgery. Howell's method was agnostic to the manufacturer of the implant system, a concept that was definitely ahead of its time. While not originally 3D printed, the concept for TKA planning and guidance saw further growth with Stryker's acquisition of OtisMed in 2009 and companies such as Materialise, Biomet (now Zimmer Biomet, Warsaw, IN), Zimmer (now Zimmer Biomet, Warsaw, IN), DePuy Orthopaedics/Johnson & Johnson (Warsaw, IN), and Smith & Nephew (Nashville, TN) jumped in and continue to commercialize products and push this technology forward.[43] It is estimated that more than 100,000 TKA cases are performed annually using 3D printed surgical guides today.

Orthognathic surgery relates to the surgical procedures which correct dentofacial deformities of the face, most often involving the mandible and maxilla. Leveraging the research of Gateno and Xia, Medical Modeling launched products and trained surgeons in workflows aimed to turn what was a completely manual method for surgical planning of orthognathic surgeries into a mostly digital method. The old method, which was standard of care for 30 years, involved standard X-rays, tracing on acetate paper, taking impressions of teeth, mounting these impressions and then cutting and moving them around before finally producing by hand an acrylic bite wafer called a splint which would transfer this plan to surgery. Medical Modeling commercialized products for orthognathic surgical planning and templating in 2007 with a mostly digital workflow involving use of a CT or CBCT, digital dental models (then scanned from casts, today completely digital), and even digital measurements for how the patient

holds their head, the so-called Natural Head Position, which varies for each patient. These digital workflows offered an easier preparation for surgery (1 hr vs. 8 hrs) and a more predictable surgical experience because the surgeon was directly planning on the patient's anatomy.[44]

What Howell started for the orthopedic sector was taken to the head and neck region for tumor reconstruction by surgeons including Dr. Daniel Buchbinder (New York, NY), Dr. Evan Garfein (Bronx, NY), and Dr. David Hirsch (New York, NY) collaborating with companies such as Medical Modeling and Materialise.[45,46] Reconstruction of the mandible using a fibula free flap was routinely performed with limited ability to preoperatively plan prior to 2007. Following application of virtual surgery and templating, many of these procedures are now routinely carried out with 3D printed anatomic models, guides, and templates. The resection is planned and guided, the graft osteotomies are guided, and even the fixation is preplanned and either guided or personalized completely.[47]

Building on the novel ability to 3D print in biocompatible metals 3D printing was utilized to create the actual implanted part; and, in 2006, Professor Dr. Jules Poukens (Leuven, Belgium) implanted a titanium cranioplasty produced by EBM, perhaps the first known implanted 3D printed titanium part for craniomaxillofacial surgery.[48] The part was physically produced by Carl Fruth and FIT AG (Lupburg, Germany). Poukens later went on in 2011 to implant what was cited as the world's first 3D printed total jaw replacement, produced in conjunction with Xilloc (Sittard-Geleen, The Netherlands) and LayerWise (Leuven, Belgium, now part of 3D Systems).[49] In 2007, the company Enztec (Christchurch, New Zealand) worked with Medical Modeling and local orthopedic surgeon Dr. James Burn to produce patient-matched implants for complex total joint revision surgeries involving the hip and knee (Fig. 1.5).[50]

2010s—VIRTUAL SURGERY AND TEMPLATES, HOSPITAL-BASED 3D PRINTING, THE FDA, REIMBURSEMENT

Additive manufacturing in biocompatible metals such as titanium alloy and cobalt—chrome alloy had been around for five plus years already when in 2010 the first US FDA clearance for a product was issued in this space. Exactech (Gainesville, FL) gained clearance for their InteGrip acetabular implant line in 2010, partnered for production with Medical Modeling.[51] This was the first FDA clearance of any kind for a 3D printed metal

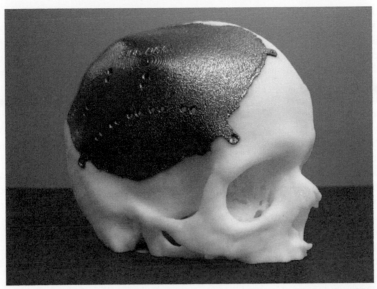

FIG. 1.5 Professor Dr. Jules Poukens implanted what may have been the world's first 3D printed titanium implant, a cranioplasty, in 2006. The electron beam melting process was used to produce this implant in titanium alloy.

implant. In 2011, the first spine implant, a fusion cage, was cleared through the FDA by 4Web Medical (Frisco, TX), again supported by Medical Modeling.[52] Interestingly, both of these FDA clearances were for off-the-shelf, non-personalized orthopedic implant components. The first FDA clearance for a polymeric 3D printed implant happened in 2013 with Oxford Performance Materials (South Windsor, CT) clearing their OsteoFab Patient-Specific Cranial Device.[53]

The FDA oversees all medical device marketing in the US and has been quite interested in 3D printing and its use for medical devices for a long time. In 2014, the FDA decided to convene an open forum meeting with industry, academia, and physicians invited to discuss the topic of additive manufacturing for medical devices.[54] Over two days about 500 attendees helped provide input to the FDA. This input was critical to the FDA's development of a technical guidance document for additive manufacturing of medical devices.[55] The FDA runs its own internal working group on additive manufacturing and continues to foster discussion regarding the safe and effective use of these technologies in the medical device space.

Around that time, along with the expiration of some of the original 3D printing patents held by Chuck Hull and Scott Crump, desktop 3D printers came into fruition and hospitals started to incorporate 3D printing. One of the first and largest initiatives was that by the Mayo Clinic (Rochester, MN), a world-leading medical center which has embraced 3D printing in a clinical environment since the mid-2000s. Centered in radiology, their efforts have been led by Dr. Jane Matsumoto (pediatric radiologist) and Dr. Jay Morris (interventional neuroradiologist).[56] In 2015, Mayo Clinic offered what was the first continuing medical education meeting to share their knowledge with the world related to 3D printing. Surgeons from a dozen surgical specialties, radiologists, and others in research shared their insights over three days in Scottsdale, Arizona.[57] This meeting was held annually for several years until being discontinued in 2019.

Another major step forward for hospital-based 3D printing happened in 2016 with the establishment of the RSNA 3D Printing Special Interest Group (SIG).[58] Dr. Frank Rybicki (University of Cincinnati) pioneered the establishment of the SIG and served as its first Chair. The first rotation of what would be elected positions in the leadership of the SIG were Dr. Jay Morris (Mayo Clinic), Dr. Jane Matsumoto (Mayo Clinic), Dr. William Weadock (University of Michigan), and Dr. Peter Liacouras (Walter Reed National Military Medical Center). This group focuses on education, creation of guidelines for appropriate clinical use of 3D printing, and the important topic of reimbursement for these tools when produced in a hospital environment.[59] To date the SIG has membership of over 500 individuals and RSNA has opened a 3D printing SIG membership category to all who are interested.[58]

The safety and accuracy of 3D printed medical models is of great concern to both hospitals and regulatory bodies such as the FDA. In 2017, the FDA and RSNA SIG held a joint meeting in specifically on anatomic models and the regulatory implications for production in hospitals.[60] Historically, production of anatomic models was accomplished by industry groups such as Materialise and Medical Modeling, but with the movement of these services inside of the hospital the regulatory environment has been changing. Several key points were clarified at this meeting including (1) clarification of what represents "diagnostic use," (2) the fact that image processing software has the most importance to the FDA, and (3) how industry could clear these products through FDA pathways, a slightly challenging process since the image processing software, 3D printing hardware, and even materials needed to be included. Following this meeting, in 2018, the first product to proceed through the "new" pathway to include indications for diagnostic use, 3D printed anatomic models was the Mimics InPrint product (Materialise).[61] Further considerations on this topic can be found in Chapter 9.

One more topic of conversation for the entire history of this field has been reimbursement for 3D printed anatomic models. A major step forward for this occurred in 2018 when the American Medical Association approved establishing first-ever Category III Current Procedural Terminology (CPT) Codes for anatomic models and anatomic guides.[62] The effort to establish these codes was led by the American College of Radiology (ACR) along with RSNA SIG leadership. Four Category III CPT Codes went "live" for use as reimbursement nomenclature in July of 2019. While payment for these Category III codes is voluntary, they open the door for future codes which have value associated with them and may be more widely reimbursed. In 2019, a registry for 3D printed anatomic models and guides was established by the RSNA and ACR.[63] The purpose of the registry, which is supported by 3D printing industry partners HP (Palo Alto, CA), Formlabs (Cambridge, MA), Materialise (Leuven, Belgium), and Stratasys (Eden Prairie, MN), is to gather data on hospital-based 3D printing in support of future reimbursement efforts. These data include the type of clinical indication, the effort put into the production of the model, the technology used, and the clinical feedback relating to the use of the model. The registry went "live" to accept new case submissions in 2020 and will continue for several years, furthering the evidence of 3D printed anatomic models and guides. More information on reimbursement and the RSNA-ACR 3D printing registry can be found in Chapter 8.

The previous sections provide some key milestones in the collective history of 3D printing in medicine. From the introduction and development of 3D printing technologies to their incorporation with medical imaging modalities, 3D printing has been utilized over the years to enhance patient care. With more and more hospitals utilizing the technologies along with rapid improvements in the technologies and possible reimbursement for models, it is expected that the use of 3D printing will become even more mainstream in the future. Furthermore, the combination of regenerative medicine technologies with medical imaging is expected to revolutionize personalized medicine. The next several years will be instrumental for medical 3D printing and it will be interesting to see which clinical applications are impacted the most.

REFERENCES

1. Beckmann EC. CT scanning the early days. *Br J Radiol.* 2006;79:5–8, 161.
2. Hull C. *Apparatus for Production of Three Dimensional Objects by Stereolithography.* US Patent 4575330. March 11, 1986.
3. Marsh JL (Personal Communication with Andy Christensen), St. Louis, MO, January 3, 2016.
4. Vannier MW, Marsh JL, Warren JO. Three dimensional CT reconstruction images for craniofacial surgical planning and evaluation. *Radiology.* 1984;150(1):179–184.
5. Marsh JL, Vannier MW. The "third" dimension in craniofacial surgery. *Plast Reconstr Surg.* June 1983:759–767.
6. Marsh JL, Vannier MW. *Comprehensive Care for Craniofacial Deformities.* Published by Mosby; 1985. ISBN: 978-0801631672.
7. Kliegis UG, Zeilhofer HF, Vitt KD, Sader R, Horch HH. Individuelle Operationsplanung als Instrument des Qualitätsmanagements in der Mund-, Kiefer- und Gesichtschirurgie [Individual surgical planning as a method of quality management in oromaxillofacial surgery]. *Biomed Tech.* 1997;42(Suppl):9–10.
8. Lambrecht JT. *3-D Modeling Technology in Oral and Maxillofacial Surgery.* Illinois: Quintessence Publishing Co; 1996.
9. Klug C, Schicho K, Ploder O, et al. Point-to-point computer-assisted navigation for precise transfer of planned zygoma osteotomies from the stereolithographic model into reality. *J Oral Maxillofac Surg.* 2006;64(3):550–559. https://doi.org/10.1016/j.joms.2005.11.024.
10. Mankovich NJ, Curtis D, Kugawa T, Beumer J. Comparison of computer-based fabrication of alloplastic cranial implants with conventional techniques. *J Prosthet Dent.* 1985;55(5):606–609.
11. Mankovich NJ, Cheeseman A, Stoker NG. The display of three-dimensional anatomy with stereolithographic models. *J Digit Imag.* 1990;3(3):200–203.
12. White DN. *Method of Forming Implantable Prostheses for Reconstructive Surgery.* US Patent 4436684. May 31, 1988.

13. Fisher LM. Advances in prosthetics: computers improve the fit of artificial joints. *NY Times*; April 1, 1987:D8. https://www.nytimes.com/1987/04/01/business/business-technology-advances-prosthetics-computers-improve-fit-artificial-joints.html. Accessed July 26, 2020.

14. Binder WJ, Kaye AH. Three-dimensional computer modeling. *Facial Plastic Surg Clin N Am*. 1994;2:357.

15. Goldstein A. Techmedica seeks edge in custom prostheses. *Los Angeles Times*; July 9, 1985. https://www.latimes.com/archives/la-xpm-1985-07-09-fi-8304-story.html. Accessed July 26, 2020.

16. Wolford LM, et al. Twenty-year follow-up study on a patient-fitted temporomandibular joint prosthesis: the Techmedica/TMJ concepts device. *J Oral Maxillofac Surg*. 2015;73(5):952–960.

17. VanCraen F. (Personal Communication with Andy Christensen), by Phone, December 10, 2015.

18. *Materialise, A History of Meaningful Innovations*. https://www.materialise.com/en/timeline. Accessed 26 July 2020.

19. Wouters K. Medical models, the ultimate representations of a patient-specific anatomy. In: McDonald, Ryall, Wimpenny, eds. *Rapid Prototyping Casebook*. published by John Wiley and Sons; 2001. ISBN 978-1-860-58076-5.

20. VanCraen F. *Building a Bionic Body? - Biomaterials Research for Healthcare*. https://ec.europa.eu/research/press/2000/pr2703-phidias.html. Accessed 26 July 2020.

21. Masters TE, Christensen AM, Perez RR. Effects of computerized axial tomography: technical factors and scanning techniques on the accuracy of anatomical biomodels. *Crit Rev Biomed Eng*. 2000;28(3–4):349–354.

22. D'Urso PS, Barker TM, Earwaker WJ, et al. Stereolithographic biomodelling in cranio-maxillofacial surgery: a prospective trial. *J Cranio-Maxillofacial Surg*. 1999;27(30).

23. Crump S. *Apparatus and Method for Creating Three-Dimensional Objects*. US Patent 5121329. June 9, 1992.

24. FDA. *510(k) Clearance Stratasys FDM MedModeller K971290*. https://www.accessdata.fda.gov/cdrh_docs/pdf/K971290.pdf. Accessed 26 July 2020.

25. FDA. *510(k) Clearance Materialise CT-Modeller System K970617*. https://www.accessdata.fda.gov/cdrh_docs/pdf/K970617.pdf. Accessed 26 July 2020.

26. Xia J, Samman N, Yeung RW, et al. Three-dimensional virtual reality surgical planning and simulation workbench for orthognathic surgery. *Int J Adult Orthod Orthognath Surg*. 2000;15(4):265–282.

27. Gateno J, Teichgraeber J, Xia J. Three-dimensional surgical planning for maxillary and midface distraction osteogenesis. *J Craniofac Surg*. 2003;14:833.

28. Gateno J, Teichgraeber J, Hultgren B. The precision of computer-generated surgical splints. *J Oral Maxillofac Surg*. 2003;61:817.

29. Xia JJ, Gateno J, Teichgraeber JF, et al. Accuracy of the computer-aided surgical simulation (CASS) system in the treatment of complex cranio-maxillofacial deformities: a pilot study. *J Oral Maxillofac Surg*. 2007;65(2):248–254.

30. Xia JJ, Phillips CV, Gateno J, et al. Cost-effectiveness analysis for computer-aided surgical simulation in complex cranio-maxillofacial surgery. *J Oral Maxillofac Surg*. 2006;64:1780–1784.

31. Gateno J, Xia J, Teichgraeber J, et al. Clinical feasibility of computer-aided surgical simulation in the treatment of complex cranio-maxillofacial deformities. *J Oral Maxillofac Surg*. 2007;65:728–734.

32. FDA. *510(k) Clearance for Materialise SImplant System K033849*. https://www.accessdata.fda.gov/cdrh_docs/pdf3/k033849.pdf. Accessed 26 July 2020.

33. Bibb R, Eggbeer D, Paterson A. *Medical Modelling: The Application of Advanced Design and Development Techniques in Medicine*. Woodhead Publishing.; 2006. ISBN 9781845691387.

34. CNN. *Twins Joined at Head Are Separated*; October 13, 2003. https://www.cnn.com/2003/HEALTH/10/12/egyptian.twins/index.html. Accessed July 26, 2020.

35. Christensen A, Humphries S, Goh K, Swift D. Advanced "tactile" imaging for separation surgeries of conjoined twins. *Childs Nerv Syst*. 2004;20:547–553.

36. Doski JJ, Heiman HS, Solenberger RI, et al. Successful separation of ischiopagus tripus conjoined twins with comparative analysis of methods for abdominal wall closure and use of the tripus limb. *J Pediatr Surg*. 1997;32(12):1761–1766. https://doi.org/10.1016/s0022-3468(97)90529-7.

37. Christensen AM, Humphries SM, Vermilye TL. *A Review of Tactile Imaging Technology Supporting Separation Surgeries of 15 Sets of Conjoined Twins. CARS 2006 Computer Assisted Radiology and Surgery*. Osaka, Japan; Joint Congress of CAR/ISCAS/CMI/CAD, June 28 – July 1, 2006

38. Harrysson OLA, Cansizoglu O, Marcellin-Little DJ, Cormier DR, West HA. Direct metal fabrication of titanium implants with tailored materials and mechanical properties using electron beam melting technology. *Mater Sci Eng C*. 2008;28(3):366–373. ISSN 0928-493.

39. Christensen A, Kircher R, Lippincott A. *Qualification of Electron Beam Melted (EBM) Ti6Al4V-ELI for Orthopaedic Applications (Conference Presentation)*. CA, USA: ASM MPMD (American Society for Materials/Materials and Processes for Medical Devices) Meeting, Desert Springs; September 23, 2007.

40. Sabol JV, Grant GT, Liacouras P, Rouse S. Digital image capture and rapid prototyping of the maxillofacial defect. *J Prosthodont*. 2011;20(4):310–314. https://doi.org/10.1111/j.1532-849X.2011.00701.x.

41. Taft RM, Kondor S, Grant GT. Accuracy of rapid prototype models for head and neck reconstruction. *J Prosthet Dent*. 2011;106(6):399–408. https://doi.org/10.1016/S0022-3913(11)60154-6.

42. Howell SM, Kuznik K, Hull ML, et al. Results of an initial experience with custom-fit positioning total knee arthroplasty in a series of 48 patients. *Orthopedics*. 2008;31(9):857–863.

43. De Vloo R, Pellikaan P, Dhollander A, Vander Sloten J. Three-dimensional analysis of accuracy of component positioning in total knee arthroplasty with patient specific and conventional instruments: a randomized controlled trial. *Knee*. 2017;24(6):1469–1477. https://doi.org/10.1016/j.knee.2017.08.059.

44. McCormick SU, Drew SJ. Virtual model surgery for efficient planning and surgical performance. *J Oral Maxillofac Surg*. 2011;69(3):638–644. https://doi.org/10.1016/j.joms.2010.10.047.

45. Okay DJ, Buchbinder D, Urken M, Jacobson A, Lazarus C, Persky M. Computer-assisted implant rehabilitation of maxillomandibular defects reconstructed with vascularized bone free flaps. *JAMA Otolaryngol Head Neck Surg*. 2013;139(4):371–381. https://doi.org/10.1001/jamaoto.2013.83 [Published correction appears in JAMA Otolaryngol Head Neck Surg. 2013 Aug 1;139(8):771].

46. Hirsch DL, Garfein ES, Christensen AM, Weimer KA, Saddeh PB, Levine JP. Use of computer-aided design and computer aided manufacturing to produce orthognathically ideal surgical outcomes: a paradigm shift in head and neck reconstruction. *J Oral Maxillofac Surg*. 2009;67:2115–2122.

47. Roser SM, Ramachandra S, Blair H, et al. The accuracy of virtual surgical planning in free fibula mandibular reconstruction: comparison of planned and final results. *J Oral Maxillofac Surg*. 2010;68:2824–2832.

48. Poukens J, Laeven P, Beerens M, et al. Custom surgical implants using additive manufacturing. *Digital Dental News*. 2010;4:30–33.

49. Xilloc. *The world's first 3D printed total jaw reconstruction*. https://www.xilloc.com/patients/stories/total-mandibular-implant/. Accessed 28 July 2020.

50. D'Alessio J, Christensen A. 3D printing for commercial orthopaedic applications: advances and challenges. In: DiPaola M, Wodajo F, eds. *3D Printing in Orthopaedics*. Elsevier; 2018. ISBN 9780323662116.

51. FDA. *Exactech 510(k) K102975 Exactech Novation Crown Cup with InteGrip Acetabular Shell*. https://www.accessdata.fda.gov/cdrh_docs/pdf10/K102975.pdf. Accessed 26 July 2020.

52. FDA. *4Web Medical 510(k) K112316 ALIF Spinal Truss System Interbody Fusion*. https://www.accessdata.fda.gov/cdrh_docs/pdf11/K112316.pdf. Accessed 26 July 2020.

53. FDA. *Oxford Performance Materials 510(k) K121818 OsteoFab™ Patient-Specific Cranial Device*. https://www.accessdata.fda.gov/cdrh_docs/pdf12/K121818.pdf. Accessed 26 July 2020.

54. FDA. *Public Workshop: Additive Manufacturing of Medical Devices*; October 8–9, 2014. https://www.federalregister.gov/documents/2014/05/19/2014-11513/additive-manufacturing-of-medical-devices-an-interactive-discussion-on-the-technical-considerations. Accessed July 26, 2020.

55. FDA. *Technical Considerations for Additive Manufactured Medical Devices*. Issued December 5, 2017. https://www.fda.gov/media/97633/download. Accessed 7.26.20.

56. Thompson JL, Zarroug AE, Matsumoto JM, Moir CR. Anatomy of successfully separated thoracopagus-omphalopagus conjoined twins. *Clin Anat*. 2007;20(7):814–818. https://doi.org/10.1002/ca.20514.

57. Mayo Clinic. *Collaborative 3D Printing in Medical Practice 2015*. https://ce.mayo.edu/radiology/content/collaborative-3d-printing-medical-practice-2015. Accessed 26 July 2020.

58. RSNA. *RSNA 3D Printing Special Interest Group*. https://www.rsna.org/en/membership/involvement-opportunities/3d-printing-special-interest-group. Accessed 26 July 2020.

59. Chepelev L, Wake N, Ryan J, et al. Radiological Society of North America (RSNA) 3D printing Special Interest Group (SIG): guidelines for medical 3D printing and appropriateness for clinical scenarios. *3D Print Med*. 2018;4(1):11. https://doi.org/10.1186/s41205-018-0030-y. Published 2018 Nov 21.

60. FDA. *FDA/CDRH RSNA SIG Joint Meeting on 3D Printed, Patient-specific Anatomic Models*; August 31, 2017. https://www.fda.gov/medical-devices/workshops-conferences-medical-devices/fdacdrh-rsna-sig-joint-meeting-3d-printed-patient-specific-anatomic-models-august-31-2017. Accessed July 26, 2020.

61. Davies S. Materialise received 510k clearance for Mimics inPrint software. *TCT Magazine*; March 26, 2018. https://www.tctmagazine.com/additive-manufacturing-3d-printing-news/materialise-fda-clearance-mimics-inprint-software/. Accessed July 26, 2020.

62. ACR. *New ACR-Sponsored CPT Codes Approved by the AMA*. https://www.acr.org/Advocacy-and-Economics/Advocacy-News/Advocacy-News-Issues/In-the-November-2-2018-Issue/New-ACR-Sponsored-CPT-Codes-Approved-by-the-AMA. Accessed 26 July 2020.

63. ACR. *3D Printing Registry*. https://www.acr.org/Practice-Management-Quality-Informatics/Registries/3D-Printing-Registry. Accessed 26 July 2020.

CHAPTER 2

Medical Imaging Technologies and Imaging Considerations for 3D Printed Anatomic Models

NICOLE WAKE, PHD • JANA VINCENT, PHD • FRASER ROBB, PHD

Medical imaging technologies, which allow us to "see into" and understand living systems, play a significant role in biology and medicine. The X-ray has paved the way for many high-tech medical imaging technologies that are used today including computed tomography (CT), magnetic resonance imaging (MRI), ultrasound, and positron emission tomography (PET). It is possible a number of scientists inadvertently produced X-rays including William Morgan[1] and Nicola Tesla.[2] However, the real discovery and understanding of the X-ray was by Wilhelm Röntgen in late 1895 when he realized X-rays could pass through opaque objects and could be used to generate an image. Röntgen was the first to document this phenomenon using a recording of a photograph of the bones in his wife's hand, and he coined the term "X-ray."[2]

X-rays are a penetrating form of electromagnetic radiation carried by photons, with a wavelength ranging from 0.01 to 10 nm that places them into an ionizing radiation category. They are produced in an X-ray tube when a beam of high-energy electrons strikes a high-density target, resulting in production of energy in the form of both heat and these high-energy photons. X-rays have a shorter wavelength and higher frequency than that of visible light.

Not long after X-rays were discovered, the first use of X-rays under clinical conditions was by John Hall-Edwards in Birmingham, England, in 1896 when he radiographed a needle stuck in the hand of an associate.[3] On February 5, 1896, J. T. Bottomley, Lord Blythswood, and John Macintyre gave a presentation to the Philosophical Society of Glasgow on X-rays. Soon after, in March 1896, Mcintyre obtained the permission of the managers of Glasgow Royal Infirmary to set up an X-ray department, which was the first one to be established in the world.[2]

Since the development of the X-ray, there have been many major advancements in medical imaging, and the use of volumetric medical imaging including CT and MRI have played a critical role in the development of medical 3D printing over the years with advancements in both fields being closely intertwined over the decades (Fig. 2.1).

Today, volumetric medical imaging is the backbone of 3D printing in medicine since imaging data are used to create patient-specific, 3D printed anatomic models and guides. Anatomic models may be created from any volumetric dataset, with sufficient contrast and spatial resolution to separate structures, using dedicated image post-processing software (discussed in Chapter 3). When a 3D model is requested prior to an imaging study, the image acquisition and reconstruction techniques should be tailored so that the anatomy in the intended 3D model can be effectively visualized, with the optimal imaging modality, imaging protocol, and image reconstruction depending on the anatomy being imaged.

CT is the most common clinical technique adopted to generate 3D printed anatomic models due to the fact that CT uses X-rays; accordingly, there is only one contrast mechanism, making image post-processing of CT data relatively simple.[4] MRI, which provides exquisite soft tissue contrast without using ionizing radiation, and 3D ultrasound data may also be used. However, implementation is challenging and time-consuming for MRI (due in part to intrinsically low signal-to-noise ratio (SNR) and image artifacts resulting in nonanatomical signal variation); and implementation is even more difficult for ultrasound data due to the non-tomographic nature of ultrasound acquisition. This chapter will review the imaging systems that are typically used to create 3D printed anatomic models

3D Printing for the Radiologist. https://doi.org/10.1016/B978-0-323-77573-1.00005-1

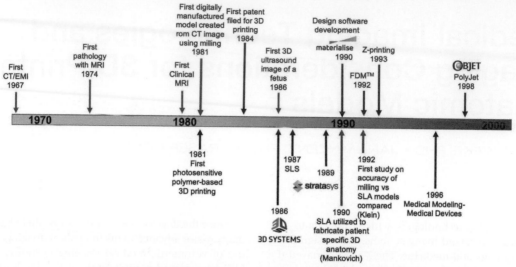

FIG. 2.1 Major early development in medical imaging and 3D printing.

including CT, MRI, and ultrasound. Nuclear medicine imaging modalities and utilization of 3D printing will be discussed in Chapter 12.

COMPUTED TOMOGRAPHY

The history of CT dates back to 1917 with the invention of the Radon transform by Johann Radon, an Austrian mathematician, who showed that a function could be reconstructed from an infinite set of its projections.[5] A comprehensive review of the mathematics is available in many texts including Epstein et al.[6] In short, the transformation that takes one-dimensional (1D) projections of a two-dimensional (2D) object over many angles is called the 2D Radon transform. For a fixed angle theta (*q*), *g(l,q)*, is called a projection; and for all *l* and *q*, *g(l,q)*, is the 2D Radon transform of *f(x,y)*. In order to represent an image, the Radon transform takes multiple, parallel-beam projections of an image from different angles by rotating the source around the center of an image at a specified rotation angle.

$$R_\theta(x') = \int_{-\infty}^{\infty} f(x'\cos\theta - y'\sin\theta, x'\sin\theta + y'\cos\theta)dy'$$

where

$$\begin{bmatrix} x' \\ y' \end{bmatrix} = \begin{bmatrix} \cos\theta & \sin\theta \\ -\sin\theta & \cos\theta \end{bmatrix} \begin{bmatrix} x \\ y \end{bmatrix}$$

The projection of an object results from the tomographic measurement process at any given angle, θ, and is made up of a set of line integrals (Fig. 2.2). The set of projections of a single slice is called a sinogram.

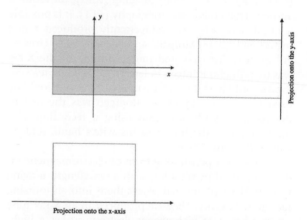

FIG. 2.2 Horizontal and vertical projections for a simple two-dimensional function.

In general, the Radon transform of *f(x,y)* is the line integral of *f* parallel to the y'-axis:

The first CT scanner was created in 1967 by Sir Godfrey Hounsfield who, while working at Electrical and Musical Industries (EMI) Central Research Laboratories, used X-rays applied at various angles to create an image of an object. Hounsfield was working on the pattern recognition of letters and was trying to reconstruct a 3D representation of the contents of a box when he realized that it was easier to reconstruct the volume by considering it as a series of slices.[7] Once Hounsfield had verified this principle, he proceeded to construct a testing rig built on the bed of an old lathe that he had from a prior project. This test unit, now known as the

"Lathe bed model," used Americium 95 as its gamma source and had a photon counter as the detector. Initially, it took 9 days to acquire the images and 2.5 h to reconstruct them with an International Computers Limited mainframe computer system.[7]

The first EMI CT scanner was installed in 1971 at the Atkinson Morley Hospital in England and the first human patient brain exam was performed.[7] CT scanners were introduced in the United States (US) a couple of years later with the first clinical scan performed at the Mayo Clinic in 1973.[8] In 1975, EMI marketed the first body scanner which was inaugurally installed at Northwick Park Hospital in London. Shortly after, the first body scanner in the US was installed at the Mallinckrodt Institute at the Washington University School of Medicine in St. Louis, Missouri. By 1976, approximately 17 distinct companies were offering CT scanners and over 475 were sold worldwide.[9] In 1979, Sir Godfrey Hounsfield and Allan McLeod Cormack were both awarded the Nobel Prize in medicine for their pioneering work in the development of CT.[10]

The standard method of reconstructing CT slices is the "backprojection" method which originates from the fact that a 1D projection needs to be filtered by a 1D Radon kernel (backprojected) in order to obtain a 2D signal. The backprojection method starts from a projection value and backprojects a ray of equal pixel values that would sum to the same value (Fig. 2.3). Structures in a complete image can only be restored if a sufficient number of projection angles are collected; however, blurring of the computed image can result if this relatively simple method is employed. Therefore, it is more common to use a filtered backprojection method where a stabilized and discretized version of the inverse Radon transform is typically used.

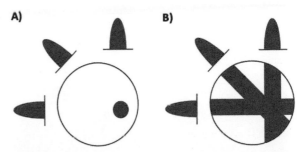

FIG. 2.3 **(A)** Projections of point object from three directions and **(B)** Backprojection onto reconstruction plane.

Since the invention of CT, there have been substantial improvements in speed, slice count, radiation dose, and image quality. The important phases in CT development are single-slice CT, helical CT, multiple detector row CT (MDCT) also known as multislice CT, and spectral CT imaging. Single-slice CT systems have 1D detector arrays, thereby acquiring data in a single section plane and reconstructing only one plane per rotation. Helical CT systems perform acquisitions by continually rotating the source and detectors around the patient as the table is moved along the axis of the scanner, enabling the scan to be performed rapidly (Fig. 2.4).[11]

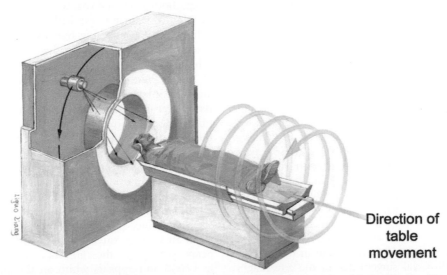

Direction of table movement

FIG. 2.4 Illustration of helical CT scanning. (Courtesy of Liguo Liang, Montefiore Medical Center, Bronx, NY.)

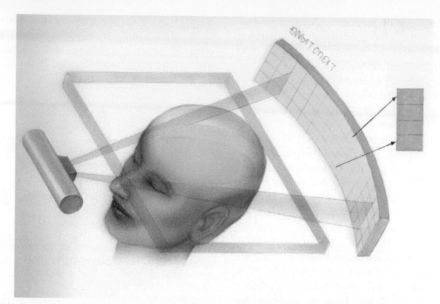

FIG. 2.5 Illustration of MDCT scanning. (Courtesy of Liguo Liang, Montefiore Medical Center, Bronx, NY.)

The speed of the table is important for exams such as CT angiography where table motions oscillate at several cm/second.[12]

MDCT, introduced in 1992, combines multiple rows of detectors and fast gantry rotation speeds to rapidly gather a cone of X-ray data. MDCT scanners have rapidly evolved from four detector row systems (Fig. 2.5) to systems with 256-slice and 320 detector rows.[13] In comparison to single-row detector CT, MDCT scanners have the advantages of shorter scan durations, longer scan ranges, and thinner slice sections which are especially useful for 3D rendering.[14]

Spectral CT imaging uses different energy levels to capture images, which allows elements in the body to be differentiated based on their material density or atomic number.[15] The energy of the reconstructed image can be altered on a sliding scale and can be processed to create many advantages over conventional CT such as the creation of virtual unenhanced images and amplification/removal of iodine or calcium suppressed images. A comprehensive review by Erik Fredenberg lists the many advantages of this acquisition type including improved soft-tissue and contrast agent—based contrast-to-noise ratio (CNR) and better detection of lesions and plaque characterization.[16]

Cone beam computed tomography (or CBCT), a variant type of CT, uses a cone-shaped X-ray beam and 2D detectors instead of a fan-shaped X-ray beam and 1D detectors.[17] CBCT is important in the field of oral and maxillofacial surgery due to the advantages over conventional 2D X-ray methods, such as ease of

imaging in a seated or standing position with a rotation of the gantry around the head.[17] With the availability of the equipment in dentist offices, this method is also used in orthodontics and endodontics. Additionally, image-guided radiation therapy often utilizes this method.[18]

CT images are comprised of grayscale pixels, also known as picture elements. The physical size of a pixel depends on the image resolution which is set in the image acquisition. Similar to a pixel, a voxel represents an array of elements of a volume that constitute a 3D image. Both pixels and voxels typically do not have their position/coordinates explicitly encoded with their values. Instead, rendering systems infer the position of pixels and voxels based on their position relative to other pixels/voxels.

In CT, there is only one contrast mechanism; the grayscale intensity of the image is proportional to the tissue density with the grayscale value seen in each pixel reflecting how the amount of the X-ray beam the tissue attenuated as it passed through the patient. The Hounsfield unit (HU) scale, named after Sir Godfrey N. Hounsfield, used in these images is a linear transformation of the original linear attenuation coefficient mechanism, and it provides information regarding what type of tissue types may be present (i.e., air, bone, soft tissue, blood, etc.). On the HU scale, air is represented by a value of −1000 and appears black on the grayscale image and bone is +1000 and appears white on the grayscale image (Fig. 2.6).

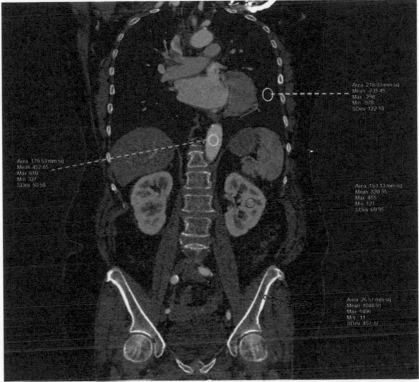

FIG. 2.6 Example coronal CT image of the chest, abdomen, and pelvis with Hounsfield Units (HUs) for certain tissues shown including the lungs (air) with a mean HU = −735.45, aorta (blood pool) with a mean HU = 452.65, kidney with a mean HU = 320.35, and pelvis (bone) with a mean HU = 1048.91.

MAGNETIC RESONANCE IMAGING

MRI is a dynamic and flexible noninvasive imaging technology that operates at the radiofrequency (RF) range and produces detailed anatomic images without ionizing radiation exposure. MRI was originally called NMRI (nuclear magnetic resonance imaging) after the nuclear magnetic resonance (NMR) phenomenon, first described by Isidor Isaac Rabi in 1938. By passing a particle beam of lithium chloride molecules through a vacuum chamber and manipulating the beam with different magnetic fields, Rabi demonstrated how the magnetic moments of nuclei could be induced to flip their principal magnetic orientation. Rabi won the Nobel Prize in Physics for this discovery in 1944.[19] With the NMR foundation in hand, Felix Bloch at Stanford and Edward Mills Purcell at Harvard measured the precession of spins around a magnetic field in condensed matter, using a concept which is known today as continuous-wave NMR.[20,21] Bloch and Purcell were awarded the 1952 Nobel Prize for Physics for their development of new approaches and methods for nuclear magnetic precession measurements.[22]

The physical basis of NMR centers around the concept of a nuclear spin, which gives a nucleus a magnetic moment related to its angular momentum by

$$\mu = \gamma s,$$

where μ is the magnetic moment, γ is the gyromagnetic ratio (a nucleus-dependent property), and s is the spin angular momentum. The NMR effect can only be observed for nuclei with odd numbered protons or neutrons such as ^1H (protons), ^{11}Na, ^{13}C, ^{19}F, or ^{31}P. Since hydrogen atoms (^1H), with a nucleus consisting of a single proton, are most prevalent in human tissue, most MRI techniques focus only on the resonance effects of these protons. For ^1H, the gyromagnetic ratio is 42.58 MHz/T.

To measure nuclear resonance, a sample is placed in a static magnetic field, B_0. In this field, the magnetic moment vectors of individual nuclei align with the direction of the field, and the protons precess at a well-defined frequency based on the field strength, called the Larmor frequency (ω_0) which is proportional to B_0 and is defined as

$$\omega_0 = \gamma B_0$$

At rest, nuclei precess about B_0, but since they are all randomly oriented with respect to each other, there is no detectable signal. When external energy in the form of a RF magnetic field is applied at the Larmor frequency, resonance, a natural phenomenon characterized by an oscillating response occurs. The ^1H nuclei are excited out of their equilibrium state into a state of alignment tipped away from the direction of B_0; however, they still precess about B_0, and their precessional motion results in their net nuclear magnetic fields inducing RF currents in nearby conductors, or RF coils, emitting a detectable signal. In the human body, signals vary depending on the tissue type with greater proton density yielding to a higher signal and vice versa. Depending on the surrounding molecules (i.e., tissue type), ^1H nuclei within the magnetic field return to a state of equilibrium at different rates. If the spins aligned with B_0 are added together, they result in a net magnetization vector (Fig. 2.7).

In NMR, free induction decay (FID), first performed by Erwin Hahn, is defined as the observable NMR signal generated by non-equilibrium nuclear spin magnetization precessing around B_0.[23] In FID, following RF excitation, the magnetization relaxes and the protons undergo dephasing which attenuates the transverse component of the magnetization and causes the signal to decay and energy loss which causes the longitudinal component of the magnetization to recover its equilibrium value. The magnitude of a FID signal is dependent upon a number of parameters such as the sample size and composition, the strength of the magnetic field, and the flip angle (FA). The FA, also known as the tip angle, is the amount of rotation the net magnetization (M) experiences during the application of an RF pulse (Fig. 2.8).

In MRI, after excitation, each tissue returns to its equilibrium state. Longitudinal or spin-lattice relaxation describes the loss of energy from the spins to their environment, causing recovery of the longitudinal component of the equilibrium value M_0, with time constant T_1. Transverse or spin–spin relaxation is the irreversible dephasing among spins due to microscopic interactions between molecules and nuclei in the transverse direction; it occurs with time constant T_2. The choice of echo time (TE: the time between the initial excitation pulse and the time at which signal is acquired) and repetition time (TR: the time between successive acquisitions, equivalent to the time between successive excitations) determines the signal contrast. If a short TR is chosen, tissues with long T_1 do not fully recover to equilibrium between successive excitations, thus they produce a weak signal. Alternatively, tissues with short T_1 recover more quickly and produce a relatively strong signal. Table 2.1 shows relaxation times at 3T for some sample tissues.[24] Different pulse sequences may be exploited to produce signal contrast in MRI and these MRI techniques may be adapted to optimize conspicuity of certain structures or pathologies.

The concept of pulse sequences was first introduced by Erwin Hahn who demonstrated that the NMR effect could also be observed with a modified experimental method based on finite RF pulses.[25] Hahn also discovered the spin echo which results from two successive RF pulses, a 180 degree pulse following a 90 degree pulse, representing regeneration of spin phase information lost during the decay of the FID.[26] In a conventional spin echo pulse sequence, one line of imaging data is collected within each TR period and the pulse sequence

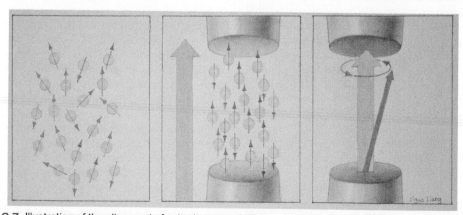

FIG. 2.7 Illustration of the alignment of spins in magnetic field and precession. Schematic representation of a group of microscopic magnetic moments (Left), Alignment of magnetic moments in the presence of an external magnetic field (Middle), Net magnetization vector (Right). (Courtesy of Liguo Liang, Montefiore Medical Center, Bronx, NY.)

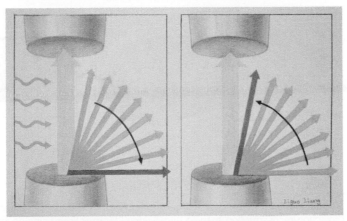

FIG. 2.8 Illustration showing the effect of an RF pulse (Left) and subsequent recovery after RF pulse is turned off (Right). (Courtesy of Liguo Liang, Montefiore Medical Center, Bronx, NY.)

TABLE 2.1

T_1 and T_2 Relaxation Times for Select Tissues at 3T.

	T_1 (ms)	T_2 (ms)
Kidney cortex	1142 ± 154	76 ± 7
Kidney medulla	1545 ± 142	81 ± 8
Spleen	1328 ± 31	61 ± 9
Paravertebral muscle	898 ± 33	29 ± 4
Subcutaneous fat	382 ± 13	68 ± 4
Prostate	1597 ± 42	74 ± 9
Pancreas	725 ± 71	43 ± 7
Cervix	1616 ± 61	83 ± 7

Derived from de Bazelaire CM, Duhamel GD, Rofsky NM, Alsop DC. MR imaging relaxation times of abdominal and pelvic tissues measured in vivo at 3.0 T: preliminary results. *Radiology.* 2004;230(3): 652–659.

is repeated for multiple TR periods until all phase-encoding steps are collected. By altering the echo times, MRI pulse sequences may be tailored to test how fast these protons return to equilibrium, which influences the overall appearance of the signal, thus highlighting certain anatomy. Though this is an excellent method to produce soft tissue contrast, it does not present a singular contrast mechanism, like CT, which can affect post-processing protocols.

Magnetic resonance spectroscopy was proposed as a means of differentiating tumor and healthy tissues for the first time in 1964 by John Mallard.[27] Subsequently, Raymond Damadian discovered that there was a marked difference in the T_1 and T_2 times between normal and abnormal tissues, suggesting that NMR relaxation times could be used to distinguish cancer from healthy tissue. This work was published in 1971.[28] In 1973, Paul Lauterbur was the first to demonstrate that it was possible to use NMR to create an image using linear gradient fields to distinguish between NMR signals originating from different locations and combined this with a form of reconstruction.[29] That same year, Sir Peter Mansfield published his method for the determination of spatial structures in solids by NMR which formed the basis of slice selection used routinely until today.[30] In 1974, James Hutchison, from the University of Aberdeen, likely showed the first pathology with MRI using projection reconstruction—the image was colored using pencils but clearly showed the rat's cause of death—cervical dislocation (see Fig. 2.9).[31]

The echo-planar imaging (EPI) technique which allowed multiple lines of imaging data to be acquired after a single RF excitation was developed by Mansfield in 1975. Similar to conventional spin echo, spin echo EPI starts out with a 90 degree pulse followed by a 180 degree pulse. Following the 180 degree pulse, the frequency-encoding gradient oscillates rapidly from a positive to a negative amplitude, forming a train of gradient echoes. By using a resonant gradient system, images could be acquired in 100 ms or less during the rapid oscillation of a magnetic field gradient. Using this technique, Mansfield produced the first MR image of live human anatomy.[32]

In the late 1970s and early 1980s, the University of Aberdeen team worked to make MRI useable and robust by combining the concepts of slice selection, frequency encoding, and phase encoding in the Spin Warp Imaging sequence which became the foundation of MRI sequences and enabled the widespread adoption and

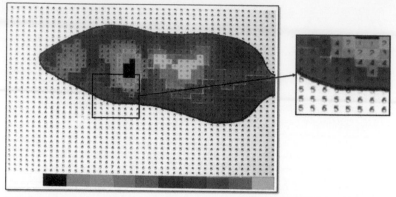

FIG. 2.9 This is likely the first MRI image demonstrating pathology. A dead mouse was imaged on a 0.06T MRI scanner with projection-reconstruction imaging based upon 25 projections using an inversion recovery sequence which generated a T_1 image. The array of numbers was colored by hand. Blood pooling around the neck injury is colored in black. (Used by kind permission of David Lurie, University of Aberdeen.)

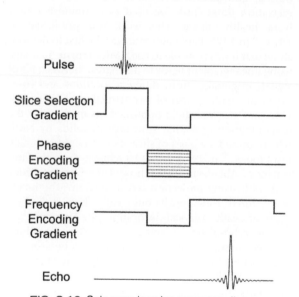

FIG. 2.10 Spin warp imaging sequence diagram.

industrialization of MRI for the decades to come (Fig. 2.10).[33] The phrase "Spin Warp" actually was conceived by Jim Hutchison's wife Margaret Foster (a highly respected scientist in her own right) who was an avid fan of Star Trek.[34] Together, Sir Peter Mansfield and Paul Lauterbur were awarded the 2003 Nobel Prize in Physiology and Medicine for their "discoveries concerning MRI."[35]

Following Aberdeen's success, the first commercial MR imaging systems were introduced in the early 1980s.[36] These systems had limited options for pulse sequences, typically having only basic spin-echo and

gradient-echo techniques allowing for T_1- and T_2-weighted imaging. Over the past 40 years, there have been significant advancements in hardware, pulse sequences, and image reconstruction algorithms, ultimately allowing for better and faster MR imaging. The use of superconducting magnets has enabled imaging at high field strengths; today, 1.5 and 3T magnets are routinely used for clinical imaging. Improved speed and resolution of MRI examination have also been achieved with use of phased array coil detection,[37] parallel imaging,[38] and sensitivity encoding.[39] More recently, MRI has moved from being a tool for seeing pure morphology to one of understanding basic physiology.[40]

Current MRI Systems

In modern-day MRI, a slice can be prescribed in any plane and with any slice thickness. Thin slices are generally prescribed in 2D imaging, but for 3D imaging thick slabs are typically utilized. The center frequency of the RF pulse controls the location of the imaging plane along the direction of the slice select gradient. For a slice at isocenter, the scanner applies an RF pulse at the center frequency. If slices far away from isocenter need to be collected, an RF pulse with a frequency offset must be applied. An RF pulse of finite duration will have a band of frequencies, called the bandwidth (BW). The slice thickness Δz can be described in terms of the RF pulse BW and an applied gradient in z-direction G_z,

$$\Delta z = BW/\gamma G_z.$$

Image reconstruction techniques in MRI are dependent on how the spatial information (frequency and phase) is encoded. The basic principal of frequency encoding is that an applied gradient causes nuclear spins at different locations in the direction of that gradient to precess at different frequencies as the signal is acquired. The phase-encoding gradient is a magnetic field gradient that allows the encoding of a spatial signal location. The frequency and phase of the signal are encoded by the modulation of gradient fields in space and time; and this relationship can be determined by the Fourier transform.

For the purposes of MRI, the 1D Fourier transform plays a very important role in allowing a signal to be decomposed into its frequency components written as

$$S(k_x) = \int_{-\infty}^{\infty} I(x)e^{-i2\pi k_x x}\, dx$$

where S is the detected signal at one point in time, I is the amplitude of the signal source (which is a function of the relaxation times T_1, and T_2 and proton density at each location in space as well as on TR and TE of the pulse sequence and numerous other parameters), x is location in space, and k_x is the immediate location in k-space, which is a function of the duration and strength of the field gradient orientated in x.

The use of a Fourier transform to process these signals would appear as a single projection through the excited slice of the object in question. Simple backprojections could then be used to produce an image as shown by Lauterbur, but other CT-type Radon Transform reconstruction techniques could also be utilized. It is much more common though to acquire all the data in the multidimensional spatial frequency-domain "k-space" and generate an image by performing a multidimensional Fourier transform. K-space is therefore the mathematical space representing the Fourier transform of a spatial function.

K-space data that are sampled rectilinearly can more easily be reconstructed with Fourier transformation in all orthogonal spatial dimensions without any prior weighting or interpolation. Rectilinear data acquisition uses phase encoding in combination with frequency encoding to resolve the locations of the spins in both in-plane directions (Fig. 2.11A). Phase-encoding gradients, which are applied for finite durations, produce a unique phase in the signal which is a linear function of position in the direction that is conventionally orthogonal to that used for frequency encoding. Sampling of k-space may also be performed radially, with frequency-encoding gradients applied sequentially in many different directions as described above (Fig. 2.11B). For radial acquisitions, a 2D Fourier transform can only produce a 2D image of the slice after special interpolation or weighting of the data

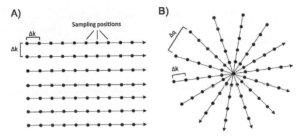

FIG. 2.11 Illustration of the **(A)** Cartesian sampling scheme **(B)** and radial scheme.

points is done due to their uneven distribution in k-space.

ULTRASOUND

Ultrasound is a noninvasive imaging modality which uses high-frequency sound waves (2–15 MHz) to produce images of human anatomy. Ultrasound waves are longitudinal, mechanical waves that propagate through a medium. When the wave is created, it has the highest energy, and as it interacts with the neighboring molecules of the medium, energy is gradually lost. Four important parameters describing the wave include wavelength, frequency, propagation velocity, and amplitude (Table 2.2).

As a technique, ultrasound is ubiquitously known as a preferred means of fetal imaging and for imaging of the cardiovascular system. Austrian psychiatrist and neurologist Karl Dussik first proposed ultrasound for diagnostic use in 1942 and, subsequently, used this method for imaging the brain.[41,42] The use of ultrasound flourished with the pioneering work of John Wild who, in 1950, worked to detect cerebral tumors by ultrasonic pulses[43] and, in 1952, detected the first 2D breast tumors.[44,45] The first ultrasound of the heart (echocardiogram) was performed in 1954 by Inge Edler and engineer Carl Hellmuth Hertz.[46] Several years later, Ian Donald from the University of Glasgow demonstrated it as a tool for fetal imaging in 1958[47]; and ultrasound rapidly became a ubiquitous imaging method around the world.

A basic ultrasound system includes a transducer, associated electronics, and a display (Fig. 2.12). Ultrasound systems generate and detect ultrasound waves via the transducer, which acts as the transmitter and receiver using piezoelectric elements. Ultrasound images are based on the reflection and scattering of the ultrasound waves by body tissues, which have different acoustic impedances (Table 2.3).[48]

All clinical ultrasound systems assume a propagation velocity of 1540 m/s, the average for soft tissues,

TABLE 2.2
Four Basic Ultrasound Wave Parameters.

Parameter	Definition	What it is Determined by
Frequency (f)	The number of compression or rarefaction cycles that occur per time, measured in hertz (Hz).	The wave source.
Wavelength (λ)	The physical distance from one peak compression to the next peak compression, defined by the equation λ = c/f.	The wave source and properties of the medium.
Propagation velocity (c)	The rate at which the wave travels through the medium.	Properties of the medium.
Amplitude	The strength, volume, or size of the wave.	Wave source (initially), changes as wave propagates.

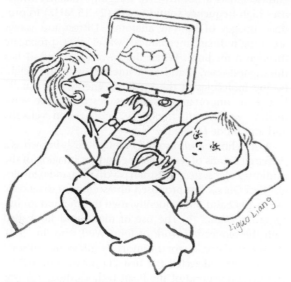

FIG. 2.12 An illustration of a basic ultrasound unit showing a sonographer performing an ultrasound on a child's abdomen. (Courtesy of Liguo Liang, Montefiore Medical Center, Bronx, NY.)

TABLE 2.3
Acoustic Properties of Various Materials.

Material	Density, $\rho[kg/m^3]$	Propagation Velocity [m/s]
Air (STP)	1.2	330
Water (25°C)	1000	1495
Fat	920	1450
Brain	1030	1510
Liver	1060	1570
Kidney	1040	1560
Muscle	1070	1570
Blood	1060	1570
Bone	1300–1810	4080
Soft tissue (average)	~1000	1540

Derived from Prince J, Links J. *Medical Imaging Signals and Systems.* 2nd ed. Pearson Education, Inc.; 2006.

to determine depth of structures. Depth can be calculated by measuring the time between the transmit event and the returning echoes. The distance to a reflector is determined from the arrival time of its echo, defined by the range equation:

$$d = cT/2,$$

where d is the depth of the interface, T is the echo arrival time, and c is the propagation velocity. The reflected echoes are converted to an electrical signal and presented

as a grayscale image of the human anatomy on the display. Each point in the image corresponds to the anatomic location of an echo generating tissue and the brightness displayed corresponds to the echo strength.

Ultrasound imaging can be divided into four major scanning techniques: A-mode, B-mode, C-mode, and M-mode. A-mode signal, or amplitude-mode signal, is a 1D display portraying echo signals and their amplitudes along a single line. B-mode, or brightness-mode, images are created by scanning the transducer beam in a plane. As the sound beams are swept over a region,

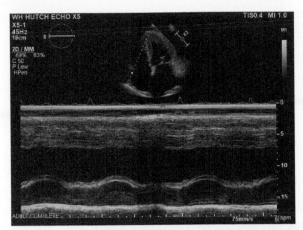

FIG. 2.13 Example of M-Mode ultrasound image of right atrial motion over time.

the echo signals are registered on a 2D matrix in a position that corresponds to the anatomic location. The brightness displayed corresponds to the echo strength. In C-mode, or constant depth mode, the distance equation is used to turn the receiver elements on and off as it listens to echoes returning from a certain depth. Pulsed-wave (PW) Doppler is the most common application of C-mode. In PW Doppler, the sample volume can be moved or positioned at the specific depth of interest at which the system electronics detect the signal. For M-mode, or motion-mode, imaging, a single acoustic line is repeatedly transmitted in the same direction and the returning echo amplitudes are converted to brightness along the depth. This mode is most often used to image the motion of the heart and cardiac valves (Fig. 2.13). Traditional 2D ultrasound imaging is dependent on probe positioning and lacks cardinal orientation—transverse, sagittal, and coronal planes which are standard in CT and MRI.

IMAGING CONSIDERATIONS FOR 3D PRINTED ANATOMIC MODELS

When image acquisition is performed after a model has been requested, the image acquisition and reconstruction can be tailored to ensure that the appropriate anatomic structures are well visualized and to simplify the medical modeling process. Considerations pertinent to creating 3D printed anatomic models including volumetric data acquisition, spatial resolution and slice thickness, SNR and CNR, and image artifact are described below.

Volumetric Data

A typical 3D dataset is comprised of a stack of 2D imaging slices, data of a finite thickness which are acquired at increments usually along the axis of an object being scanned. This approach is always used in CT and often used in MRI. In CT, slice thickness is largely determined by the detector size but this is not true of MRI, where slice thicknesses are defined by the amplitude of the slice select gradient, G_z, and the RF pulse BW. In MRI, the slice thickness is often much greater than the 2D resolution of the resultant image. In MRI, volumetric imaging may also be accomplished by acquiring data from a 3D volume before performing a Fourier transform in each of the three orthogonal spatial directions, rather than a series of single tomographic slices of finite thickness. Volumetric images can take much longer to acquire but they have inherently much higher SNR than 2D image slices. For MRI, it more typical to excite a thick slab of tissue with an RF pulse rather of single slice. Fundamentally, spatial encoding is performed in 3D by using additional phase encoding in the direction perpendicular to the selected slab, and a 3D Fourier transform is applied after every combination of the two-phase—encoding gradients is acquired.

Spatial Resolution and Slice Thickness

To create accurate 3D models, it is important to avoid looking overly digitized in the slice direction, and this requires that the slice thickness is sufficiently narrow in the direction of the slices to allow the preservation of important details. For 3D modeling purposes, images with a small slice thickness, 1 mm or less, are recommended. A choice of large slice thicknesses can result in stair-step boundaries which can be visible on the segmented model unless we use postprocessing to smooth out the image (Fig. 2.14).

Image acquisition should also be optimized in order to maximize the signal in the tissue of interest and the spatial resolution should be chosen to accurately represent the anatomy to be modeled. In the simplest terms, the spatial resolution of an image refers to the smallest resolvable distance between two different objects or two different features of the same object. Low spatial resolution techniques will be unable to differentiate two adjacent structures that have similar tissue properties. In MRI, voxels are specified in terms of matrix size, the field of view, and the slice thickness. Such voxels may be isotropic or rectangular solids in nature solids and the resolution may be different in the three dimensions. The broader the coverage we have in k-space, the better the MR spatial resolution and finer details resolved. It is important to ensure that the slice thickness chosen for an image, which obviously has an influence on the spatial resolution and image noise, can also be optimized depending on the intended application.

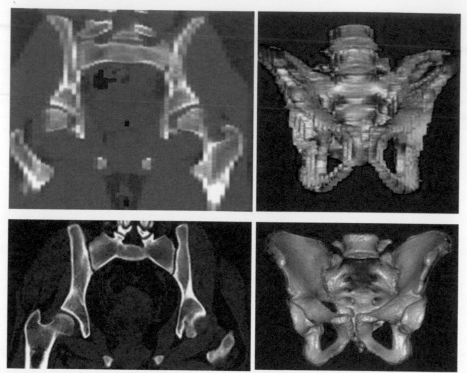

FIG. 2.14 Coronal CT images acquired with 5 mm slice thickness (top) and 1 mm slice thickness (bottom) with corresponding 3D reconstructions.

In CT, since the tube voltage (kV) is directly proportional to the energy of the X-rays produced, we can adjust the tube current (mA) to improve the image quality. Together with slice distance, consideration may be given regarding the thickness of the X-ray beam (collimation) and overlap. In most cases, the slice distance and collimation are the same. However, in the circumstance where the slice distance is actually smaller than the collimation, an overlap would result which could lead to improved results. The appearance of specific anatomical structures may also be affected by the reconstruction parameters selected. The reconstruction kernel, also known as the image filter, is similar to slice thickness, in that it impacts both the spatial resolution and image noise, and they must be balanced based on the application. Typically, filters or kernel options range from "smooth" to "sharp." Smoothing filters not only reduce noise content in images but also decrease edge sharpness. Conversely sharpening filters increase edge sharpness at a cost of increasing noise. For larger, low contrast models, a smooth kernel is more appropriate but for models with fine structures, such as the temporal bone, a sharp kernel is preferred (Fig. 2.15).[49]

Signal-to-Noise Ratio and Contrast-to-Noise Ratio

The SNR specifies the signal quality and is defined as the ratio of the signal power to the noise power. To calculate the SNR, the main value of the signal is divided by the noise. A higher SNR implies a better imaging situation and more trustworthy data. Another measure used to determine image quality, the CNR, is the relationship of the signal intensity differences between two regions, scaled to image noise.

For two tissues which are labeled A and B with signals S_A and S_B, their signal difference can be defined as contrast:

$$C_{AB} = S_A - S_B.$$

The CNR is defined as

$$CNR_{AB} = (C_{AB})/\sigma_0$$

where σ_0 is the standard deviation of the image noise. Improving CNR increases the perception of differences between two different regions of interest. High contrast between various organs in the body is an important feature of medical imaging and is necessary to delineate structures for 3D printing.

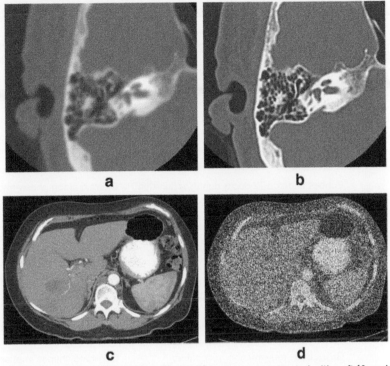

FIG. 2.15 Temporal bone **(A** and **B)** and liver **(C** and **D)** images reconstructed with soft **(A** and **C)** and sharp kernels **(B** and **D)**. (Reproduced with open access permission from Leng S, McGee K, Morris J, et al. Anatomic modeling using 3D printing: quality assurance and optimization. *3D Print Med.* 2017;3(1):6.)

Image Artifacts

Image artifacts can be considered image inaccuracies and can be defined as any feature which appears in an image which is not present in the original imaged object. Sources of artifact may be due to the improper operation of the scanning equipment or could be a consequence of natural processes or properties of the human body. Image artifacts in any modality can have minor or major consequences for a physician's interpretation of pathology. In addition, image artifacts would, by definition, affect the accuracy of any future 3D printed model with some affecting the quality of final model more than others. The seriousness of the artifact will affect whether the examination will need to be repeated or not and this would likely be at the judgment of staff operating the imaging equipment.

In MRI, artifacts can be due to nonuniformity in the static magnetic field (B_0), gradient field artifacts (B_1) inhomogeneity, RF inhomogeneities, or MR encoding errors.[50] Some examples of major MRI artifacts are summarized in Table 2.4.[50–52] For MRI, 3T MRI continues to gain wider acceptance in the general clinical community, and many artifacts are more prominent at 3T due to increase in the SNR.[52] Since image intensity nonuniformities and artifacts can severely degrade the quality of the data, it is important to be able to recognize artifacts, so that they can be prevented or, alternatively, one can use the information content of an artifact to contribute to diagnostic content.[50] Nonuniformity correction is an active area of research; and corrections may be performed prospectively or retrospectively (see Chapter 3.2).[53]

CT has its own unique types of artifacts which may be hardware-based resulting from imperfections in scanner function, physics-based resulting from the physical processes involved with image acquisition, or patient-based resulting from patient movement or metal (Table 2.5).[54]

Identification and the mitigation of artifacts in CT is always a subject of research and investigation.[55] Iterative reconstruction techniques may be applied to reduce noise in data associated with conventional filtered back-projection reconstruction techniques may be used to reduce beam hardening and scatter.[55,56] Partial volume effects may be avoided by using thin acquisition section

TABLE 2.4
List of Common MRI Artifacts, Causes, and Appearance.

Artifact Type	Cause	Appearance
Aliasing	Corruption in the spatial encoding of objects outside the field of view (FOV) which cannot be distinguished from objects inside the FOV.	Image with overlapping of objects outside the FOV on the opposite side of the image. May appear as swirling.
Banding	Undesired phase shifts, usually seen in balanced steady-state free precession imaging.	Band-like signal loss in areas of increased B_0 nonuniformity.
Chemical shift	Magnetic field nonuniformity due to spatial misregistration of fat and water molecules.	Black and white bands on anatomic part in the frequency-encoding direction.
Direct current (DC)	A constant signal in the receiver.	A bright spot in the center of the image.
Echo train blurring	Echoes undergo T2 decay during acquisition.	Blurring along phase-encoding direction.
Eddy current	Residual currents generate in cryostat from gradient switching.	Ghosting.
Fast spin-echo cusp	Gradient nonlinearity from spins near the edge of the magnet.	A "featherlike" appearance. Seen along the phase-encoding direction in sagittal or coronal fast spin-echo images.
FID signal artifact	Mixture of issues including poor slice profile, B_1 inhomogeneity issues, and problems with spoiler gradients.	Line across the center of the image.
Flow displacement	Spins moving between frequency and phase-encoding gradients.	Confusing misregistration of pixel locations.
Ghosting	Gross body movement or respiratory/cardiac/bowel motion.	Duplicate shapes in phase-encoding direction.
Gibbs ringing	Lack of frequency and phase-encoding steps in images with abrupt tissues interfaces.	Series of lines in an image.
Gradient nonlinearity	Imperfect gradients.	Spatial distortion at image corners.
India Ink (black boundary)	Occurs when water and fat spins are out of phase and cancel each other out.	Artificial black line located at fat–water interfaces.
Metal	Large magnetic susceptibility effects.	Strong image distortion/complete regional blow out of image.
Motion	Corruption of k-space data during acquisition.	Blurring, ghosting, or signal loss.
Off resonance effects	Due to disturbance of magnetic field due to metallic materials.	As above—strong localized distortion of the image.
Partial volume	Averaging of mixed tissues within thick slices.	Smearing of image data.
Pulsatile flow	Due to frequency-modulated spectral sidebands.	Light and dark ghosting structures close to small arteries.
Quadrature imbalance	Constructive and destructive interference from RF standing waves.	Regions of nonuniformity with increased or decreased signals.
Stimulated echo	Slice interference due to short time between slice acquisition.	Line artifact in frequency-encoding direction—light and dark pixels.
Venetian blind	Saturation effect of inflowing blood.	Loss of signal of flowing blood.
Zipper	Extraneous RF noise from poor RF shielding or from other spurious noise sources.	Bands of spurious signal through the center of the image.

Derived from Graves MJ, Mitchell DG. Body MRI artifacts in clinical practice: a physicist's and radiologist's perspective. *J Magn Reson Imaging*. 2013;38(2):269–287; Morelli JN, Runge VM, Ai F, et al. An image-based approach to understanding the physics of MR artifacts. *Radiographics*. 2011;31(3):849–866; Bernstein MA, Huston J, 3rd, Ward HA. Imaging artifacts at 3.0T. J Magn Reson Imaging. 2006;24(4):735–746.

TABLE 2.5
List of Common CT Artifacts, Causes, and Appearance.

Artifact Type	Cause of Artifact	Appearance
Aliasing (undersampling)	An error in the accuracy proponent of analog to digital converter (ADC) during image digitization.	Fine stripes appear to be radiating from the edge of, but at a distance from, a dense structure.
Beam hardening	Mean energy of X-ray beam increases as lower energy photons absorbed more rapidly.	Streaking—light or dark bands across the image.
Compton scatter	Produced when a high-energy photon collides with a valence electron causing ionization and produces a secondary lower-energy photon that may strike the detector and falsely increase the photon count.	Streaking.
Cone beam effect	X-ray beams become cone shaped instead of fan shaped, causing undersampling.	Noise and streaks, particularly at edges.
Metal	Metallic objects, particularly those with high atomic numbers.	Streaking.
Motion	Patient, cardiac, respiratory, bowel.	Blurring, double imaging, and/or streaking.
Out of field	Suboptimal reconstruction algorithm.	Bright pixels at the edge of the FOV.
Partial volume	Tissues with widely different absorption encompassed in the same CT voxel producing a beam attenuation proportional to the average value of these tissues.	Blurring.
Photon starvation	Due to high attenuation, insufficient photons reach the detector and noise is magnified.	Streaking.
Poisson noise	Due to the statistical error of low photon count.	Random thin bright and dark streaks that appear preferentially along the direction of greatest attenuation.
Ring	Miscalibrated or defective detectors.	Circular artifacts/dark void in image if a central detector is affected.
Stair-step	Wide collimations and nonoverlapping reconstruction intervals.	Serrations on coronal or sagittal reformats.
Tube arcing	A short-circuit in the X-ray tube.	Near-parallel streaking.
Windmill	A high contrast edge between two detector rows, causing an error in the interpolated value.	Smooth periodic dark and light streaks originating from high contrast edges.
Zebra	Helical interpolation process leading to noise inhomogeneity along the z axis.	Periodic stripes of more or less noise at the image periphery seen on coronal or sagittal reformats.

Derived from Barrett JF, Keat N. Artifacts in CT: recognition and avoidance. *Radiographics*. 2004;24(6):1679–1691 and Boas FE, Fleischmann, D. CT artifacts: causes and reduction techniques. *Imag Med*. 2012;4(2).

widths and out of field artifacts can be reduced by improving the reconstruction algorithm.[55] Finally, metal artifact reduction algorithms have been the subject of investigation over the decades.[57–59] Early techniques determined the boundaries of metal implants and used linear interpolation to fill in the missing projections.[58] More recent techniques include the Metal Deletion Technique which reduce artifacts due to photon starvation, beam hardening, and motion; selective algebraic reconstruction; and projection-based metal artifact reduction algorithms.[60] Many CT scanners now have built-in metal artifact reduction techniques incorporated and these methods may be combined with beam hardening correction software in order to further minimize metallic artifacts due to beam hardening.[54]

Image Storage

Digital Imaging and Communications in Medicine (DICOM) is the international standard for storing and transmitting medical images that was developed in the 1980s by the American College of Radiology (ACR) and the National Electrical Manufacturers Association. DICOM enables the integration of medical imaging devices with picture archiving and communication systems (PACS) from multiple manufacturers. DICOM includes protocols for image exchange, image compression, 3D visualization, image presentation, and results reporting. DICOM differs from other image formats because information is grouped into datasets. A DICOM file consists of a header and image datasets packed into a single file. The information within the header (i.e., name, patient identifier, date of birth, study date, etc.) is organized as a constant and standardized series of tags. Currently, DICOM images cannot be directly sent to a 3D printer for printing, so medical images are segmented and converted to a file type such as the stereolithography (STL) file that is recognized by 3D printers.

Recently, DICOM Working Group (WG)-17 helped to establish the "DICOM 2018b" standard in which 3D file information in an STL format is contained within a DICOM Information Object.[61] At the current time this functionality is being implemented by both printer and PACS vendors, allowing 3D files, in the form of STLs, to be stored in a patient's medical record and directly used for 3D printing purposes. This integration will allow for STL files to be traceable and properly integrated into a patient's medical record. DICOM WG-17 is also working to extend and promote the use of DICOM for the creation, storage, and management of virtual reality (VR) and augmented reality (AR) technologies.[61]

DISCUSSION

Volumetric medical imaging has played a crucial role in the development of medical 3D printing over the years. CT is often considered the imaging modality of choice for certain cases, especially for imaging of bones and is often used to produce 3D anatomical models of hard tissue structures. However, with the advent of MRI and the successful improvement in MRI hardware and software, the enhanced visualization of soft tissues and organs is now possible. As both advanced volumetric imaging technologies and 3D printing technologies become more accessible, accurate, and reproducible, it is expected that 3D printing of anatomical structures will become more widespread. For MRI, growth in unique areas like MR neurography, for visualization of nerves,[62] is also likely to be benefited from medical 3D printed methods. In addition, expansion of the use of 3D printing from other imaging modalities such as ultrasound, nuclear imaging, and optical imaging techniques is also expected in the future. Coregistration of multiple image datasets (e.g., CT and MRI, MR-PET) as well as incorporating functional quantitative information (e.g., functional MRI, diffusion MRI) can also increase the value of 3D printed models. Additionally, with the strong interest in metabolic imaging, models could be created based upon Hyperpolarized ^{13}C for oncologic imaging in diseases such as prostate and pancreatic cancer.[63]

To date, 3D printed anatomic models are typically created to facilitate with surgical planning and to provide intraoperative guidance for complex cases. Even though radiologists and surgeons are adept in the interpretation of 2D medical images, there may be errors in interpretation, and mentally reconstructing and translating 2D imaged into 3D is complicated.[64–66] It is expected that having an improved comprehension of anatomy will lead to improved surgical planning and ultimately will improve patient outcomes.[65,67] In regard to the impact of 3D printing in patient care, quantitative surgical metrics including operating times, length of hospital stay, blood loss, and positive tumor margins may be quantitatively measured, and it could be shown through these measures how 3D printing positively influences patient outcomes.

Although Category III current procedural terminology (CPT) codes for 3D printed anatomic models and guides were established in July 2019,[68] at this time clinical indications for when a 3D printed model should be utilized have not been determined. Recently the Radiological Society of North America (RSNA) 3D Printing Special Interest Group published guidelines for medical 3D printing and appropriateness for use which lists the maturity of 3D printing for several different medical conditions on a rating scale of 1–9 with a rating scale of 1–3 being rarely appropriate, 4–6 being may be appropriate, and 7–9 on usually appropriate.[69,70] Furthermore, in conjunction with the recently established CPT III codes, the RSNA and ACR worked together to establish a 3D printing registry to gain evidence for the widespread use 3D printed anatomic models and guides as well as to determine in which case types 3D printing is utilized the most and for which cases 3D printing has the largest impact on patient care.[71] Considerations for documentation and reimbursement are discussed in Chapter 8.

Another topic of utmost importance for medical 3D printing is quality assurance and the accuracy of 3D printed medical models. It is imperative that 3D printed anatomic models and guides created from medical images are highly accurate and steps should be taken during all steps of the modeling process, from ensuring that the image acquisition is of optimal quality and free of all major artifacts to delivery of the final printed part, to certify that there are no errors in the final model (see Chapter 7).[49,72] Phantom development to assess hardware performance and image acquisition parameters is also ripe for improvement with more realistic 3D anthropomorphic phantoms being created using 3D printing technologies and more options for material printing choices (see Chapter 14).

In addition to 3D printed anatomic models, VR and AR are other methods of advanced imaging visualization which may be used to enhance patient care. As compared to 3D printing, AR and VR may be advantageous due to the decreased upfront cost and decreased time require to generate anatomic models from medical imaging data. In addition, AR and VR techniques can display temporal information as well as geometrical information making them more suitable platforms for visualizing certain data such as cardiac anatomy which fluctuates over the cardiac cycle as the heart beats (Fig. 2.16). AR, since by nature it allows for the virtual and real environment to be visualized simultaneously, can also provide real-time intraoperative guidance by overlaying pertinent anatomic structures over the patient during surgical procedures.

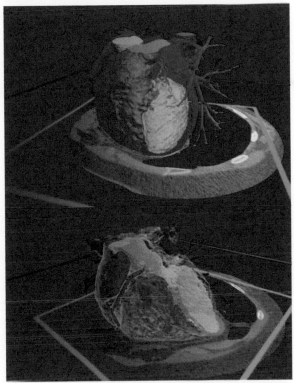

FIG. 2.16 Example images of VR heart models overlaid onto CT data. (Images courtesy of Realize Medical Inc., Ottawa, CA.)

Evidently, we are at the cusp of a 3D visualization revolution which has the capacity to transform the concept of personalized patient care. Combining improved medical imaging techniques with 3D printing technologies truly has important implications for the treatment and diagnosis of disease. Although costs and production times of 3D printed models remain a major concern, it is believed that the fields of both medical imaging and 3D printing will continue to leverage each other to fill the gaps in the clinical application as we move from 2D visualization to physical, hand-held 3D printed models.

REFERENCES

1. Anderson JG. William Morgan and X-rays. *Trans Faculty Actuaries.* 1945;17:219–221.
2. Thomas AMK, Banerjee AK. *The History of Radiology.* Oxford Medical Histories; 2013.
3. Meggit G. *Taming the Rays: A History of Radiation and Protection.* Pitchpole Books; 2018.

4. Bibb RWJ. A review of the issues surrounding three-dimensional computed tomography for medical modelling using rapid prototyping techniques. *Radiography*. 2010;16:78—83.

5. Radon J. Ber die Bestimmung von Funktionen durch ihre Integralwerte Langs Gewisser Mannigfaltigkeiten (English translation: on the determination of functions from their integrals along certain manifolds). *Ber Saechsische Akad Wiss*. 1917;29:262.

6. Epstein CL. *Introduction to the Mathematics of Medical Imaging*. Second edition. Society for Industrial and Applied Mathematics; 2007.

7. Beckmann EC. CT scanning the early days. *Br J Radiol*. 2006;79(937):5—8.

8. Baker Jr HL, Campbell JK, Houser OW, Reese DF. Early experience with the EMI scanner for study of the brain. *Radiology*. 1975;116(02):327—333.

9. Hodgkinson GP, Starbuck W. *The Oxford Handbook of Organizational Decision Making*. Oxford University Press; 2008.

10. *The Nobel Prize in Physiology or Medicine 1979*. Nobel Media AB; 2014. http://www.nobelprize.org/nobel_prizes/medicine/laureates/1979/. Accessed May 27, 2018.

11. Zeman RK, Fox SH, Silverman PM, et al. Helical (spiral) CT of the abdomen. *AJR Am J Roentgenol*. 1993;160(4):719—725.

12. Fukuda A, Lin PJ, Matsubara K, Miyati T. Measurement of table feed speed in modern CT. *J Appl Clin Med Phys*. 2014;15(3):275—281.

13. Hsieh J. *Computed Tomography: Principles, Design, Artifacts, and Recent Advances*. 3rd ed. vol PM259. The International Society for Optics and Photonics; 2015.

14. Hammerstingl RM, Vogl TJ. Abdominal MDCT: protocols and contrast considerations. *Eur Radiol*. 2005;15(Suppl 5):E78—E90.

15. McCollough CH, Leng S, Yu L, Fletcher JG. Dual- and multi-energy CT: principles, technical approaches, and clinical applications. *Radiology*. 2015;276(3):637—653.

16. Fredenberg E. Spectral and dual-energy X-ray imaging for medical applications. *Nucl Instrum Methods Phys Res A Accel Spectrom Detect Assoc Equip*. 2018;878:74—87.

17. De Vos W, Casselman J, Swennen GR. Cone-beam computerized tomography (CBCT) imaging of the oral and maxillofacial region: a systematic review of the literature. *Int J Oral Maxillofac Surg*. 2009;38(6):609—625.

18. Jaffray DA, Drake DG, Moreau M, Martinez AA, Wong JW. A radiographic and tomographic imaging system integrated into a medical linear accelerator for localization of bone and soft-tissue targets. *Int J Radiat Oncol Biol Phys*. 1999;45(3):773—789.

19. *The Nobel Prize in Physics 1944*. Nobel Media AB; 2014.

20. Bloch FHW, Packard M. Nuclear induction. *Phys Rev*. 1946;69:127.

21. Purcell EMTH, Pound RV. Resonance absorption by nuclear magnetic moments in a solid. *Phys Rev*. 1946;69:37—38.

22. *The Nobel Prize in Physics*. Nobel Media AB.Web; 1952.

23. Hahn EL. An accurate nuclear magnetic resonance method for measuring spin-lattice relaxation times. *Phys Rev*. 1949;74:145—146.

24. de Bazelaire CM, Duhamel GD, Rofsky NM, Alsop DC. MR imaging relaxation times of abdominal and pelvic tissues measured in vivo at 3.0 T: preliminary results. *Radiology*. 2004;230(3):652—659.

25. EL H. Nuclear induction due to free larmor precession. *Phys Rev*. 1950;77:297—298.

26. Hahn EL. Spin echoes. *Phys Rev*. 1950;80(4):580.

27. Mallard JR, Kent M. Differences observed between electron spin resonance signals from surviving tumour tissues and from their corresponding normal tissues. *Nature*. 1964;204(4964), 1192-1192.

28. Damadian R. Tumor detection by nuclear magnetic resonance. *Science*. 1971;171(3976):1151—1153.

29. Lauterbur PC. Image formation by induced local interactions - examples employing nuclear magnetic-resonance. *Nature*. 1973;242(5394):190—191.

30. Mansfield P, Grannell PK. Nmr diffraction in solids. *J Phys C Solid State*. 1973;6(22):L422—L426.

31. Hutchison JMS, Mallard JR, Goll CC. In-vivo imaging of body structures using proton resonance. In: *Proceedings of 18th Ampère Congress. Magnetic Resonance and Related Phenomena. Nottingham 9—14 September*. Amsterdam, Oxford: North-Holland Publishing Company; 1974: 283—284.

32. Mansfield P, Maudsley AA. Medical imaging by Nmr. *Brit J Radiol*. 1977;50(591):188—194.

33. Edelstein WA, Hutchison JM, Johnson G, Redpath T. Spin warp NMR imaging and applications to human whole-body imaging. *Phys Med Biol*. 1980;25(4):751—756.

34. Page R. *Mark-1 the World's First Whole Body MRI Scanner*; 2017. https://vimeo.com/210578984. Accessed August 18, 2020.

35. *The Nobel Prize in Physiology or Medicine 2003*. Nobel Media AB; 2003.

36. Edelman RR. The history of MR imaging as seen through the pages of Radiology. *Radiology*. 2014;273(2s):S181—S200.

37. Roemer PB, Edelstein WA, Hayes CE, Souza SP, Mueller OM. The NMR phased array. *Magn Reson Med*. 1990;16(2):192—225.

38. Sodickson DK, Manning WJ. Simultaneous acquisition of spatial harmonics (SMASH): fast imaging with radiofrequency coil arrays. *Magn Reson Med*. 1997;38(4):591—603.

39. Pruessmann KP, Weiger M, Scheidegger MB, Boesiger P. SENSE: sensitivity encoding for fast MRI. *Magn Reson Med*. 1999;42(5):952—962.

40. Nelson SJ, Kurhanewicz J, Vigneron DB, et al. Metabolic imaging of patients with prostate cancer using hyperpolarized [1-(1)(3)C]pyruvate. *Sci Transl Med*. 2013;5(198):198ra108.

41. Dussik KT. On the possibility of using ultrasound waves as a diagnostic aid. *Neurol Psychiat*. 1942;174:153—168.

42. Dussik K. Ultrasound application in the diagnosis and therapy of diseases of the central nervous system. In:

Matthes K, Rech W, eds. *Ultrasound in Medicine*. Zurich: Hirzel; 1949:179–182.

43. French LA, Wild JJ, Neal D. Detection of cerebral tumors by ultrasonic pulses; pilot studies on postmortem material. *Cancer*. 1950;3(4):705–708.

44. Wild JJ, Reid JM. Further pilot echographic studies on the histologic structure of tumors of the living intact human breast. *Am J Pathol*. 1952;28(5):839–861.

45. Wild JJ. The use of ultrasonic pulses for the measurement of biologic tissues and the detection of tissue density changes. *Surgery*. 1950;27(2):183–188.

46. Edler I, Hertz CH. The use of ultrasonic reflectoscope for the continuous recording of the movements of heart walls. *Clin Physiol Funct Imag*. 2004;24(3):118–136.

47. Donald I, Macvicar J, Brown TG. Investigation of abdominal masses by pulsed ultrasound. *Lancet*. 1958;1(7032): 1188–1195.

48. Prince J, Links J. *Medical Imaging Signals and Systems*. Pearson Education, Inc.; 2006.

49. Leng S, McGee K, Morris J, et al. Anatomic modeling using 3D printing: quality assurance and optimization. *3D Print Med*. 2017;3(1):6.

50. Graves MJ, Mitchell DG. Body MRI artifacts in clinical practice: a physicist's and radiologist's perspective. *J Magn Reson Imag*. 2013;38(2):269–287.

51. Morelli JN, Runge VM, Ai F, et al. An image-based approach to understanding the physics of MR artifacts. *Radiographics*. 2011;31(3):849–866.

52. Bernstein MA, Huston 3rd J, Ward HA. Imaging artifacts at 3.0T. *J Magn Reson Imag*. 2006;24(4):735–746.

53. Belaroussi B, Milles J, Carme S, Zhu YM, Benoit-Cattin H. Intensity non-uniformity correction in MRI: existing methods and their validation. *Med Image Anal*. 2006;10(2):234–246.

54. Barrett JF, Keat N. Artifacts in CT: recognition and avoidance. *Radiographics*. 2004;24(6):1679–1691.

55. Boas FE, Fleischmann D. CT artifacts: causes and reduction techniques. *Imag Med*. 2012;4(2).

56. Singh S, Kalra MK, Hsieh J, et al. Abdominal CT: comparison of adaptive statistical iterative and filtered back projection reconstruction techniques. *Radiology*. 2010; 257(2):373–383.

57. Glover GH, Pelc NJ. An algorithm for the reduction of metal clip artifacts in CT reconstructions. *Med Phys*. 1981;8(6):799–807.

58. Kalender WA, Hebel R, Ebersberger J. Reduction of CT artifacts caused by metallic implants. *Radiology*. 1987; 164(2):576–577.

59. Katsura M, Sato J, Akahane M, Kunimatsu A, Abe O. Current and novel techniques for metal artifact reduction at CT: practical guide for radiologists. *Radiographics*. 2018; 38(2):450–461.

60. Boas FE, Fleischmann D. Evaluation of two iterative techniques for reducing metal artifacts in computed tomography. *Radiology*. 2011;259(3):894–902.

61. DICOM. WG-17 3D. https://www.dicomstandard.org/wgs/wg-17. Accessed 18 August 2020.

62. Sneag DB, Queler S. Technological advancements in magnetic resonance neurography. *Curr Neurol Neurosci Rep*. 2019;19(10):75.

63. Kurhanewicz J, Vigneron DB, Ardenkjaer-Larsen JH, et al. Hyperpolarized (13)C MRI: path to clinical translation in oncology. *Neoplasia*. 2019;21(1):1–16.

64. Itri JN, Tappouni RR, McEachern RO, Pesch AJ, Patel SH. Fundamentals of diagnostic error in imaging. *Radiographics*. 2018;38(6):1845–1865.

65. Wake N, Wysock JS, Bjurlin MA, Chandarana H, Huang WC. "Pin the tumor on the kidney:" an evaluation of how surgeons translate CT and MRI data to 3D models. *Urology*. 2019;131:255–261.

66. Parag P, Hardcastle TC. Interpretation of emergency CT scans in polytrauma: trauma surgeon vs radiologist. *Afr J Emerg Med*. 2020;10(2):90–94.

67. Wake N, Rude T, Kang SK, et al. 3D printed renal cancer models derived from MRI data: application in presurgical planning. *Abdom Radiol (NY)*. 2017;42(5): 1501–1509.

68. Centers_for_Medicare_and_Medicaid_Services_Medical_Learning_Network
. *Update of the hospital outpatient prospective payment system (OPPS)*. MLN Matters; 2019. https://www.cms.gov/Outreach-and-Education/Medicare-Learning-Network-MLN/MLNMattersArticles/downloads/MM11318.pdf. Accessed June 1, 2020.

69. Chepelev L, Wake N, Ryan J, et al. Special interest Group for 3D printing. Radiological Society of North America (RSNA) 3D printing special interest Group (SIG): guidelines for medical 3D printing and appropriateness for clinical scenarios. *3D Print Med*. 2018;4(11):1–38.

70. Ballard DH, Wake N, Witowski J, et al. Radiological Society of North America (RSNA) 3D Printing Special Interest Group (SIG) clinical situations for which 3D printing is considered an appropriate representation or extension of data contained in a medical imaging examination: abdominal, hepatobiliary, and gastrointestinal conditions. *3D Print Med*. 2020;6(1):13.

71. Radiologic Society of North America and American College of Radiology. *3D Printing Registry*; 2020. https://nrdr.acr.org/Portal/3DP. Accessed 2/5 August 2020.

72. George E, Liacouras P, Rybicki FJ, Mitsouras D. Measuring and establishing the accuracy and reproducibility of 3D printed medical models. *Radiographics*. 2017;37(5): 1424–1450.

CHAPTER 3

Image Segmentation and Nonuniformity Correction Methods

JINGYUN CHEN, PHD • LOUISA BOKACHEVA, PHD • HENRY RUSINEK, PHD

INTRODUCTION

In medical imaging, a three-dimensional (3D) image, or volume, is often acquired by stacking up a series of two-dimensional (2D) slice images. Just as 2D images are made up of pixels, 3D volumes such as computed tomography (CT) or magnetic resonance imaging (MRI) scans consist of voxels as the basic elements. The printing of a specific object (bone, tissue, etc.) from a medical image usually involves the following steps (Fig. 3.1):

1. The raw volumetric image dataset containing the target object is acquired.
2. Voxels belonging to the target object are marked on the stack of 3D images.
3. A 3D surface is reconstructed from the cluster of voxels forming the target object.
4. The 3D surface is smoothed and fixed for any topological defects.
5. The polished 3D surface is exported for printing.

The procedure of marking a target object on an image is known as segmentation. Segmentation can be performed manually slice by slice on the image stack, using software with a paintbrush or a lasso tool. However, this approach can be extremely time-consuming, as modern medical images often contain hundreds of slices. One way to accelerate the procedure is to perform manual segmentation only on selected slices (e.g., alternate slices or every third slice), with interpolation in between. Some software packages, such as Mimics (Materialise, Leuven, Belgium), support 3D interpolation between orthogonal slices (axial, coronal, or sagittal). However, when processing a large number of medical images, manual segmentation is still limited in efficiency and consistency. To solve this problem, various automated segmentation algorithms have been developed.

Most automated segmentation algorithms rely on the signal intensity of voxels (abbreviated as voxel intensities, or just intensities). The voxel intensities not only reflect the characteristics of the imaged tissue (e.g., proton density in MRI, radiodensity in CT) but are also affected by the setup parameters of the scanner (e.g., echo time and repetition time in MRI). In general, the image segmentation algorithms can be categorized into region-based (3.1.1), boundary-based (3.1.2), atlas-based (3.1.3), and classification-based (3.1.4). Accurate segmentation of medical images often depends on the intensity features of the target object, or the intensity difference between target and background. However, undesirable artifacts may be introduced during the imaging procedure, such as noise, nonuniformity, partial volume effect, etc. These artifacts may cause geometric distortion and missegmentation of the target object. Therefore,

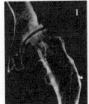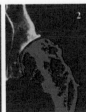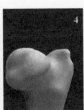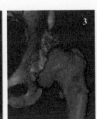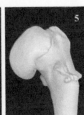

FIG. 3.1 Illustration of the medical 3D printing workflow. From left to right: (1) Raw image; (2) Segmented target object (red); (3) Reconstructed 3D surface (red); (4) Smoothed 3D surface (pink); (5) Printed object (white).

3D Printing for the Radiologist. https://doi.org/10.1016/B978-0-323-77573-1.00014-2

preprocessing is often necessary in order to improve the segmentation accuracy (see Section Nonuniformity Correction for Accurate MRI Segmentation).

Region-Based Segmentation

In region-based segmentation, the algorithms are based on the intensity homogeneity within the target object and/or the background. The simplest example of a region-based algorithm is intensity thresholding, where the input 3D image is divided into foreground (i.e., target object) and background, by comparing the intensity of each voxel to a constant value (threshold). The output of thresholding is usually a binary image of the same dimension as the input image, called a mask. Let $I(x,y,z)$ be the voxel intensity at coordinate (x,y,z), then the voxel intensity of mask M is defined as

$$M(x,y,z) = \begin{cases} 0 & \text{if } I(x,y,z) < T \\ 1 & \text{otherwise} \end{cases} \tag{3.1}$$

where T is a constant. In some cases, the constant threshold T is set manually based on prior knowledge. Automated algorithms have also been developed to identify a threshold, such as Otsu's method.[1]

Another commonly used region-based algorithm is region growing.[2] First, a seed region containing one or more voxels is defined on the 3D image, either manually or by automated computational tools. The seed region is then extended to its neighboring voxels, until it reaches certain preset constraints, such as the similarity of all neighbors. The final form of the region is used as the target object. A common example of region growing is the watershed algorithm. Consider a simple case of a 2D image. The image is treated as an elevation map, with voxel intensity representing the voxel's altitude. The watershed method uses one of two strategies to decompose the image into subregions, or watersheds: 1) flooding or immersion and 2) rainfall.[3] For both strategies, the process begins with identifying and tagging all local minima. In watershed by flooding, water sources are placed in each local minimum. The water level is systematically increased, creating a set of barriers. The

process terminates when different water regions merge.[4] In watershed by rainfall, for each voxel, the algorithm finds the direction in which a raindrop would flow if it fell on this voxel. The neighboring voxel is found at the flow direction. The voxel and its neighbor are then merged, and the process continues until the local minimum is reached.[5]

Instead of region growing, sometimes region peeling is necessary in order to reduce the size of the segmented region, or separate two target regions touching each other. The mathematical morphology[6] provides an elegant framework for both region growing and region peeling. For binary morphology, a binary mask (named a structuring element) B is set, which defines the connected components (or neighborhood) for any voxel z in the image. Common 2D examples of B are illustrated in Fig. 3.2. Note that the radius of B is conventionally an odd number. The 3D version of B can be obtained by extending the 5×5 matrices in Fig. 3.2 to $5 \times 5 \times 5$ matrices, while maintaining the same binary profiles.

Let A be the input image. Then for any given voxel z in A, a set of connected voxels (denoted B_z) can be obtained by shifting the center of the structuring element B to the coordinates of z and including all the voxels covered by B. The four basic morphological operations —erosion $E(A,B)$, dilation $D(A,B)$, opening $O(A,B)$, and closing $C(A,B)$— can then be defined as

$$\begin{aligned} E(A,B) &= \{z | B_z \subseteq A\} \\ D(A,B) &= \{z | B_z \cap A \neq \varnothing\} \\ C(A,B) &= E(D(A,B),B) \\ O(A,B) &= D(E(A,B),B) \end{aligned} \tag{3.2}$$

In other words, the erosion of image A by element B is the set of all voxels z such that B_z is contained in A, while the dilation of A by B is the set of all voxels z such that B_z overlaps with A by at least one voxel.[7] The closing operation, which consists of dilation followed by erosion, is particularly useful for 3D printing, as it can fill small holes in the segmented regions before 3D reconstruction and printing.

Square						Diamond						Cross				
1	1	1	1	1		0	0	1	0	0		0	0	1	0	0
1	1	1	1	1		0	1	1	1	0		0	0	1	0	0
1	1	1	1	1		1	1	1	1	1		1	1	1	1	1
1	1	1	1	1		0	1	1	1	0		0	0	1	0	0
1	1	1	1	1		0	0	1	0	0		0	0	1	0	0

FIG. 3.2 Three common types of structuring elements with radius = 3.

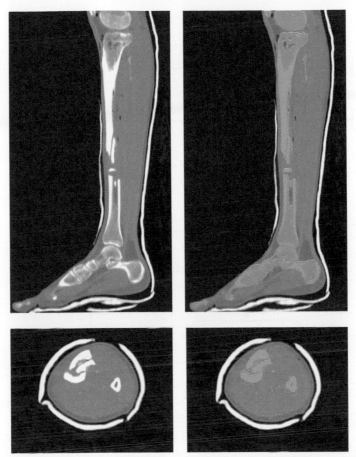

FIG. 3.3 Thresholding followed by connectivity to segment the bone from a CT exam of the bone fracture. The left column contains the original images. Segmentation results are showed in cyan in the right column of images.

In practice, different region-based algorithms can be combined to achieve more accurate segmentation. For example, in orthopedic imaging, thresholding and morphological operations can be jointly applied to separate gypsum cast from the bone on CT scans (Fig. 3.3).

Boundary-Based Segmentation

In boundary-based segmentation, the algorithms locate the tissue boundary (i.e., the edge) by evaluating local changes (known as gradients) of voxel intensity. For example, the Canny edge detector[8] measures the intensity gradient within a moving window called a kernel. The active contours algorithm[9] converts intensity change into the energy functions, and locates the boundary via optimization searches.

A boundary-based algorithm can also be combined with other algorithm types to achieve a more sophisticated segmentation. One such example is the EdgeWave algorithm in FireVoxel[10], which combines boundary detection with thresholding and morphology, or the shape characteristics of an image (Fig. 3.4). In FireVoxel, the EdgeWave algorithm is used for several key processing workflows, such as measuring body fat composition on abdominal CT images. The EdgeWave algorithm contains the following main steps:

1. The original image is resampled, as needed.
2. Thresholding by image intensity is applied to roughly delineate the region that needs to be segmented, called the Core Set. The Core Set must enclose the segmentation target, otherwise the segmentation will fail.

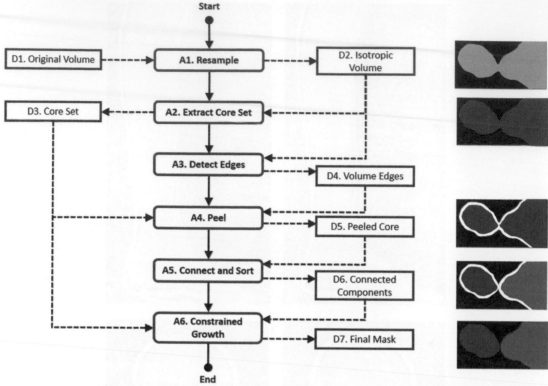

FIG. 3.4 Schematic of the Edge Wave algorithm. The red boxes contain the six main steps (A1–A6). The drawings on the right represent the outputs (D2–D7) of the corresponding algorithm steps.

3. Edges detection is performed and the locations of the Core Set where image intensity changes abruptly are defined.
4. The boundary of the Core Set is eroded, or peeled. The Peel operation removes all voxels within a certain distance from the boundary using rules applied to each voxel and its neighbors. Peeling enlarges the gaps between different regions of the image, removes small details, and breaks "bridges" between weakly connected areas. The thickness of the region to be removed is controlled by the *peel distance*, measured in voxels or millimeters.
5. The algorithm breaks up the peeled Core Set into blobs, or connected components. It then determines which connected components are to be retained and which ones should be discarded.
6. The selected connected components are subjected to constrained growth, or dilation. The Grow operation adds voxels within a given distance of the region of interest (ROI) boundary. Any recovered voxels must

still belong to the Core Set. The thickness of the recovered region is controlled by the *grow distance*, which should be larger than the *peel distance*.

Atlas-Based Segmentation

In atlas-based segmentation, ROIs are first segmented (usually manually) on a reference image called a template. This reference segmentation is commonly known as the atlas. To perform segmentation on a new image, the template image is first warped to the target image through image registration. The same transformation computed during the registration step is then applied to the preexisting atlas to propagate the ROIs on the target image.[11] Fig. 3.5 illustrates this procedure with brain image samples. To reduce the impact of intersubject variability, multiple reference images can be registered to the same target image, with different reference segmentations propagated and merged into a final segmentation. This approach is called multi-atlas segmentation.[12]

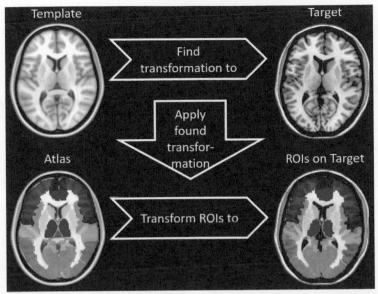

FIG. 3.5 Schematic of atlas-based segmentation. First, a transformation is found that best aligns the template (upper left) with the target (upper right) brain. The same transformation is then applied to the regions of interest (ROIs, shown in color) defined on the template brain (i.e., brain atlas, bottom left) to propagate ROIs onto the target brain (bottom right).

Classification-Based Segmentation

In classification-based algorithms, the segmentation is achieved by classifying certain image features. Classifications can be grouped into supervised and unsupervised types. Unsupervised classifications, such as K-means clustering,[13] are achieved without prelabeled training data. Supervised classifications, on the other hand, rely on prior knowledge of target objects imported from the training dataset. For example, the Markov random field algorithm[14] treats the segmentation labels as random variables with a certain probability distribution, where conditional probabilities and the Bayesian theorem relate class probabilities and voxel values.[15] A new family of classification methods has emerged from the recent developments in deep learning, based on convolutional neural network (CNN) models. In CNN models, raw intensity features derived from the image go through successive layers of processing to become high-level abstract features, before weighing into the final classification.[16] One of the most successful CNN models in biomedical image segmentation is the U-net model, whose layers consist of downsampling followed by upsampling (thus forming a U-shape model architecture).[17]

NONUNIFORMITY CORRECTION FOR ACCURATE MRI SEGMENTATION

Image intensity nonuniformity is a common MRI artifact, manifested by the variation of signal intensity across the image even within the same tissue. This artifact is also referred to as shading, bias field, or image inhomogeneity. Nonuniformity may be caused by RF field inhomogeneity, inhomogeneous receiver coil sensitivity, and patient's influence on the magnetic and electric fields.[18] While smoothly varying nonuniformity does not appear to affect visual radiologic diagnosis, it is detrimental to tissue quantification, including image segmentation. Medical image segmentation methods require that a given tissue be represented by constant signal intensity throughout the field of view. Thus, correcting for nonuniformity artifact is a crucial step. Several nonuniformity correction approaches have been developed for a variety of applications.

Prospective Approaches

Prospective nonuniformity correction methods acquire information to infer the spatial pattern of nonuniformity. The earliest attempts, inspired by the methods employed to calibrate scintillation detectors in nuclear medicine,[19] used images of a uniform phantom[20] acquired using the same sequence as the one used for patient imaging. Such efforts have been mostly abandoned due to the realization that this approach ignores the significant influence of the electromagnetic properties of the object being imaged and their interaction with magnetic field.[21]

More recent methods acquire additional calibration information by imaging the patient using different sequences. Their goal is to estimate the sources of the

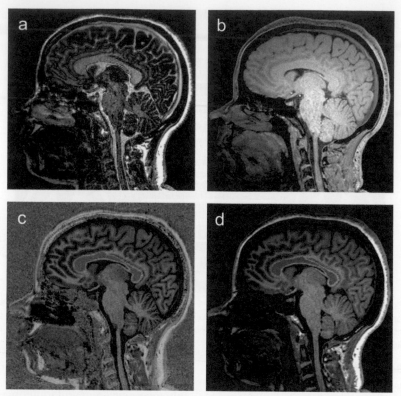

FIG. 3.6 Improvement in the uniformity of T1-weighted brain MRI can be achieved using the dual inversion MP2RAGE sequence. **(A)** Image at first inversion; **(B)** image at second inversion; **(C)** the two inversions are combined to eliminate the main sources of nonuniformity at the cost of a longer acquisition time; **(D)** image of the same person and approximately the same sagittal section obtained using a conventional single inversion MPRAGE. One aspect of signal uniformity can be measured using the coefficient of variability (CV) in a presumably homogenous region, such as corpus callosum (highlighted in red). Here CV = 4.1% for MP2RAGE versus 9.0% for MPRAGE.

nonuniformity artifact, such as the flip angle variation. An important example of this approach is the MP2RAGE sequence, which aims to improve on a well-known MPRAGE (Magnetization-Prepared RApid Gradient Echo) sequence.[22] Developed in the early 1990s, MPRAGE remains the most popular sequence for high-resolution T1-weighted brain imaging. The sequence begins with a nonselective 180-degree inversion pulse that inverts the magnetization. The magnetization then recovers over an inversion time interval (TI), which is typically 700–1000 ms at 3T. This recovery interval is followed by a series of gradient echo samplings characterized by a short (about 3 ms) echo time and small (about 10 degree) flip angles.

MPRAGE images are often corrupted by gradient field inhomogeneities, susceptibility, and eddy current effects. The MP2RAGE sequence has been developed

to correct for these shortcomings.[23] MP2RAGE introduces a second inversion time, TI2 (with the typical value of 2500 ms at 3T), in order to acquire a second readout with predominantly spin density-weighted contrast. By combining image data from the first and second readouts, the T2* and B1 inhomogeneity effects can be largely canceled out, generating a new and more uniform T1-weighted image at the cost of a longer acquisition time (Fig. 3.6).

Retrospective Approaches

Retrospective nonuniformity correction methods estimate the nonuniformities directly, with no additional specialized imaging, thus shortening the acquisition time. They promise to be more versatile than prospective techniques. Retrospective approaches entail estimating a bias field $B(r)$, where $r = (x,y,z)$, to correct

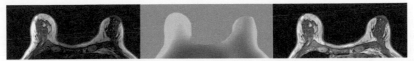

FIG. 3.7 General scheme of the retrospective nonuniformity correction entails estimating a smooth bias field $B(r)$ (middle panel) from the original image (left panel), without acquiring additional sequences. The corrected image (right panel) is then computed as the voxel-wise ratio of the original image and $B(r)$. Note that $B(r)$ is best estimated after excluding the background air portion of the imaging field.

the image (Fig. 3.7). If we ignore image noise, the acquired image $I_a(r)$ can be represented as a product of the bias field $B(r)$ and the corrected image $I_c(r)$:

$$I_a(r) = I_c(r)B(r). \qquad (3.3)$$

The goal of the reverse transformation, from $I_a(r)$ to $I_c(r)$, is to preserve the relative signal contrast across tissue while removing the variation within each tissue. This is clearly an ill-posed (underdetermined) problem, since both $I_c(r)$ and $B(r)$ are unknown. To deal with this problem, several practical solutions have been proposed. These approximations postulate additional constraints, such as smoothness of $B(r)$.

For most methods, a logarithmic function is applied to the three images in the above equation. This transformation conveniently changes the multiplication operator to addition, but it also requires care when dealing with background (air) signal values that are expected to have values near zero, where the logarithm is undefined. The air region provides little information about $B(r)$, and therefore it is appropriate to exclude it from the analysis.

N3/N4 Algorithm

The most widely used MRI nonuniformity correction algorithm is the Nonparametric Nonuniformity Normalization, or N3.[24] The term "nonparametric" refers to the fact that $B(r)$ is not prescribed analytically and the number of tissue classes is arbitrary. N3 is incorporated in several popular brain segmentation packages.[25,26] A more recent variant, known as N4 or N4ITK, has been developed within the open source Insight Toolkit of the National Institutes of Health. N4 includes an improved B-spline approximation and several other refinements.[27]

The N3/N4 technique, rather than dealing directly with the bias field $B(r)$, operates in the domain of the probability density. In the context of discrete images, this translates to operating on the histogram of signal intensities. The basic assumption of the N3/N4 method is that $h(B)$, the histogram associated with B, is a zero-centered Gaussian distribution. The Gaussianity assumption helps to significantly simplify the search for $B(r)$ by collapsing the search space to a single

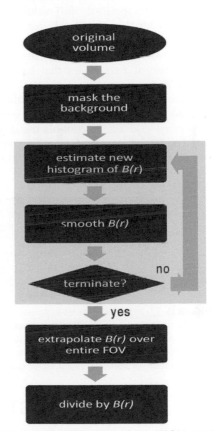

FIG. 3.8 Simplified flowchart of the N3/N4 method. The shaded block indicates operations done in logarithmic transform space and after excluding the background.

dimension—the width σ of the histogram. As demonstrated on several clinical head MRI datasets,[24] this assumption appears to be valid.

The N3/N4 algorithm estimates the bias field $B(r)$ in an iterative fashion (Fig. 3.8). Each iteration consists of three steps:
1. A new estimate of the histogram of $B(r)$ is made that results in <u>sharpening</u> of the current estimate of $I_c(r)$.
2. The bias field $B(r)$ is <u>smoothed</u>.

3. The <u>termination</u> criterion is computed and tested against a specified threshold.

All computations within the iterative block (the shaded part of Fig. 3.8) are done in the logarithmic transform space. Thus, before the start of this block, logarithms are applied to images $I_a(r)$ and $B(r)$. The exponential function is applied at the exit.

In step 1, the image is <u>sharpened</u> by subjecting the image histogram to Wiener deconvolution.[28] A Gaussian filter of specified full-width at half-maximum σ is used in this step. The Wiener deconvolution filtering attenuates the frequencies according to their signal-to-noise ratio: it minimizes the impact of deconvolved noise at frequencies that have a poor signal-to-noise ratio.

In step 2, the bias field is <u>smoothed</u> by fitting to the current estimate a cubic B-spline field of a 3D grid size d. The user-specified grid size d controls the degree of smoothing. For images acquired using a body or a head coil, d is typically about 200 mm. However, smaller values of d may be needed to correct images acquired using localized surface coils.

In the final step 3, the <u>termination</u> criterion used in the N3/N4 is derived from the changes in $B(r)$ and $I_c(r)$ between two successive iterations. In practical applications, it is often difficult to estimate the termination threshold. Instead, the program is usually controlled by the number of iterations specified by the user.

Although the N3/N4 algorithm is titled "nonparametric," its performance strongly depends on three key parameters that need to be selected by the user. The parameter σ controls the full-width at the half-maximum of the deconvolution kernel (step 1); the B-spline grid size d controls the degree of smoothing (step 2); and the number of iterations (step 3) provides the compromise between the execution time and improvement in signal uniformity.

Figs. 3.9 and 3.10 show the effect of the N4 correction on T1-weighted MRI of the breast, illustrating an improved uniformity of the fibroglandular tissue (FGT).

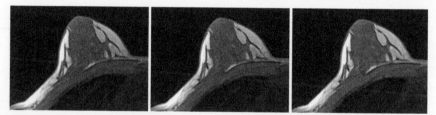

FIG. 3.9 T1-weighted non-fat-suppressed breast MRI acquired using a dedicated breast coil: original (left) and N4-corrected with five iterations (middle) and 50 iterations (right). The fibroglandular tissue (FGT) is the gray area in the central portion of the breast. The volume fraction of FGT is used to measure the breast density. Note a strong nonuniformity in the acquired image and the improvement (with preserved tissue contrast) in the N4-corrected version. See Fig. 3.10 for quantitative evidence of improvement.

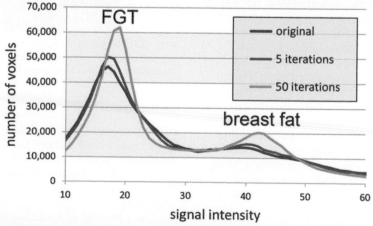

FIG. 3.10 Signal histograms for the three images from Fig. 3.9 (voxel counts vs. signal intensity). Note the improvement in separation of the fibroglandular tissue (FGT) peak from the breast fat. The uniformity correction translates into more accurate tissue segmentation.

The volume fraction of FGT correlates with mammographic breast density, which has been associated with the risk of developing breast cancer.[29,30] As a result, there is a growing interest in the automated segmentation and quantitative estimates of FGT from breast MRI. However, accurate FGT segmentation is challenging, primarily because of the poor signal uniformity of breast coils (Fig. 3.9).

BiCal Algorithm

The N3/N4 method may not perform well in challenging imaging situations such as abdominal, ultrahigh field or accelerated MRI. The BiCal method, implemented by Artem Mikheev and available in FireVoxel[10], aims to overcome these limitations. In BiCal, $B(r)$ is estimated directly as a linear combination of smooth 3D basic functions such as direct cosines or 3D Legendre polynomials. After preprocessing to remove sharp edges and the air region, the partial derivatives of $I_a(r)$ are identified as partial derivatives of $B(r)$.[31] The resulting overdetermined system of linear equations allows for the direct computation of the basis functions expansion. As in N3/N4, the estimation of $B(r)$ is done after applying the logarithmic transform.

If we assume that $B(r)$, $r = (x,y,z)$ is expanded in the 3D Legendre polynomials $P_i(x)$, then the l-th degree approximation takes the form

$$B^l(r) = \sum_{i=0}^{l} \sum_{j=0}^{l-i} \sum_{k=0}^{l-i-j} a_{ijk} P_i(x) P_j(y) P_k(z) \quad \text{(3.4)}$$

The coefficients a_{ijk} are estimated by matching the partial derivatives:

$$\frac{dB^l(r)}{dx} = \frac{dI_a(r)}{dx}, \quad \frac{dB^l(r)}{dy} = \frac{dI_a(r)}{dy}, \quad \frac{dB^l(r)}{dz} = \frac{dI_a(r)}{dz} \quad \text{(3.5)}$$

Note that Eq. (3.5) is a valid source of approximation of the bias field only for voxels r located away from the tissue edges (Fig. 3.11).

We compared the performance of BiCal to that of N4 (Table 3.1) in three challenging applications: abdominal MRI acquired at 3T using an accelerated radial Golden-angle RAdial Sparse Parallel MRI (GRASP) sequence, a 3T breast imaging using a dedicated breast coil, and a 7T head imaging. Patient datasets were randomly selected from previous research studies.[32,33] The studied datasets were as follows:

A. Abdominal images with individual frames extracted from dynamic studies obtained using GRASP (3D stack-of-star radial FLASH sequence, TR/TE = 3.6/1.7 msec, FA = 12 degrees, voxel size = $1.5 \times 1.5 \times 3$ mm^3) and acquired on a 3T Siemens Aera or Magnetom system.

B. Breast images were acquired with an axial non-fat-suppressed T1-weighted sequence (TR/TE = 4.74/1.79 ms, FA = 10 degrees, 448 × 358 x 116 matrix) on a 3T Siemens Trio using a seven-element surface breast coil (Sentinelle, Invivo, Gainesville, FL, USA).

C. Magnetization Prepared Rapid Acquisition Gradient Echo (MPRAGE) head images (TR/TE/TI = 2.6/2600/1100 msec, FA = 6 degrees, 144 acquired slices, isotropic 0.6 mm^3 voxels, 346 × 323 × 248 matrix) were acquired on a 7T Siemens Magnetom system with a volume-transmit 24-element receive coil array (Nova Medical, Boston, Mass).

In order to assess nonuniformity for each image set, we defined two sets of regions, delineated by expert observers in areas of known, uniform tissue (A: fat and muscle, B: fat and FGT, C: white matter and gray matter) throughout the imaged organ. To quantify the nonuniformity before and after correction, we used the

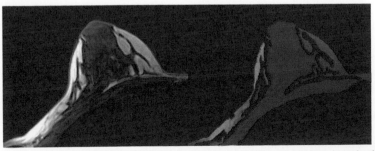

FIG. 3.11 The initial preprocessing step of BiCal is to identify the region, shown here in red, where Eq. (3.5) is applicable. Note that the background air region and the transitions between tissues are eliminated from processed area. The transitions are identified using an image edge-detection filter. In the remaining voxels, the partial derivatives of the image in the x, y, and z directions are identified as the partial derivatives of the bias field $B(r)$.

TABLE 3.1
Quantitative Comparison of N4 and BiCal Nonuniformity Correction.

Measure	A. Abdomen	B. Breast	C. 7T Brain
Original CJV	4.926 ± 3.324	0.558 ± 0.180	1.236 ± 0.187
CJV after N4	1.826 ± 0.682	0.270 ± 0.122	0.672 ± 0.097
CJV after BiCal	0.634 ± 0.095	0.255 ± 0.062	0.375 ± 0.070
P-value: N4 versus BiCal	0.007	0.64	0.0002

CJV data are mean $\pm$ standard deviation.

coefficient of joint variation (CJV), defined as $(\sigma_1+\sigma_2)/|\mu_1-\mu_2|$, where μ and σ are the mean and standard deviation of the intensity of the two regions. CJV both quantifies the intensity variability in each set and controls for the potential undesirable loss of tissue contrast by the algorithm. Both N4 and BiCal were optimized on the training datasets, selected as random subsets of the studied images. The optimal parameters were selected to minimize the CJV of corrected images on the training sets and then used to process the test cases.

The abdominal dataset (A) showed the highest nonuniformity, i.e., the largest CJV values before nonuniformity corrections. The breast images (B) were the most uniform, and the 7T brain MRIs (C) were in the intermediate position (Table 3.1). For each of the three datasets, both N4 and BiCal significantly reduced the nonuniformity measured by CJV relative to the original, uncorrected images ($P < .05$ for (A), $P < .001$ for (B) and (C)). For abdominal and brain images (A and C), but not for the breast images (B), BiCal showed a significant advantage over N4.

In summary, both prospective and retrospective, postprocessing approaches to MR image nonuniformity correction are being actively developed and are routinely used in image segmentation. However, there is no consensus regarding the measures of performance enabling meaningful comparison of different correction methods. The average coefficient of variability, post-correction segmentation accuracy, and other metrics have been suggested as such measures. In spite of its limitations to account for just two tissues, CJV appears to be the most appropriate method to evaluate the performance of correction techniques.

The lack of agreement about the most appropriate uniformity-correction method is also due to the requirement for tedious algorithm optimization needed to fine-tune multiple parameters separately for a particular clinical situation. The development of sensitive

performance measures and robust parameter optimization procedures is an area of much needed research to advance this important field of medical image analysis.

SEGMENTATION SOFTWARE
Software for medical 3D printing and advanced 3D visualization, including augmented reality and virtual reality applications, is considered a Class II medical device and should be reviewed and regulated through the 510(k) pathway when models are being created for diagnostic use. Some commercial 3D software packages have gone through FDA clearance for medical 3D printing (Table 3.2) and many others for advanced 3D visualization of medical images (Table 3.3). Most of these systems have generalized segmentation tools that can be used for any anatomy, and some also have specialized modules for specific target tissues. The current recommendation for clinical use of 3D printing in hospitals is to employ 510(k) approved software. However, many software tools are highly valuable for research applications despite the lack of FDA clearance. (Table 3.4). Many of them are open source freeware, with a large online community of active users.

AFTER SEGMENTATION
Following the segmentation, geometric refinement such as smoothing, filling, trimming, and sculpting, is often necessary. The smoothing of object surface (e.g., Gaussian smoothing[34]) can reduce the effort of physical polishing of printed object. The filling of holes can fix topological flaws of the segmented object and ensure the structural robustness of the printed object. This fix can be achieved by the morphological operation "close."[35] When automated software over segments the object and causes leakage from object surface, trimming is performed. One common way to conduct trimming is via

TABLE 3.2

Medical Image Processing Software with FDA Clearance to Produce "Diagnostic Use" 3D Printed Anatomic Models.

Product	Company	Website	Relative Cost
D2P	3D Systems	https://www.3dsystems.com/dicom-to-print	$$$
Mimics inPrint	Materialise	https://www.materialise.com/en/medical/software/materialise-mimics-inprint	$$$
Mimics	Materialise	https://www.materialise.com/en/medical/mimics-innovation-suite/mimics	$$$
Mimics Enlight	Materialise	https://www.materialise.com/en/medical/software/materialise-mimics-enlight	$$$

TABLE 3.3

Medical Image Processing Software with FDA Clearance to be Used for Advanced Visualization of Medical Images in 3D (on Screen, Not 3D Printed).

Product	Company	Website	Relative Cost
3D Doctor	Able Software Corp.	http://www.ablesw.com/3d-doctor/3ddoctor.html	$
Amira	Thermo Fisher Scientific	www.fei.com/software/amira-3d-for-life-sciences	$$$
AW	GE	https://www.gehealthcare.com/en/products/advanced-visualization	$$$
Dolphin 3D Surgery	Dolphin/Patterson Dental	www.dolphinimaging.com	$$
F.A.S.T.	Fovia	www.fovia.com	$$
IntelliSpace Portal	Philips	https://www.usa.philips.com/healthcare/product/HC881102/intellispace-portal-10-advanced-visualization	$$$
iNtuition	TeraRecon	www.terarecon.com	$$$
Medical Design Studio	Anatomage	https://www.anatomage.com/medical-design-studio/	$$
OsiriX MD	Pixmeo	www.osirix-viewer.com	$
Simpleware ScanIP Medical	Synopsys	https://www.synopsys.com/content/dam/synopsys/simpleware/datasheet/simpleware-scanip-medical_mar2019.pdf	$$$
Synapse 3D	Fuji	https://www.fujifilmusa.com/products/medical/medical-informatics/radiology/3D/	$$$
Syngo.Via Frontier	Siemens	https://www.siemens-healthineers.com/en-us/medical-imaging-it/advanced-visualization-solutions/syngo-via-frontier	$$$
Visage 7	Visage Imaging	https://visageimaging.com/platform/	$$$
Vitrea	Vital Images/Canon	www.vitalimages.com/product-information/3d-printing	$$$

TABLE 3.4
Medical Image Processing Software Without FDA Clearance, for Research/Other Purposes.

Product	Company/Institution	Website	Relative Cost
FireVoxel	Department of Radiology, NYU Langone Health	https://firevoxel.org/	$
3D Slicer	Brigham and Women's Hospital	www.slicer.org	$
Analyze Analyze Pro	Analyze Direct	www.analyzedirect.com	$/$$
AnatomicsRx	Anatomics	https://www.anatomics.com/au/applications/software.html	$$
Itk-SNAP	Collaboration between University of Utah and University of Pennsylvania	www.itksnap.org/pmwiki/pmwiki.php	$
MeVisLab	Mevis Medical Solutions AG	www.mevislab.de	$
NemoFAB	Nemotec	www.nemotec.com/en/software/fabsoftware	$$
OsiriX Lite	Pixmeo	www.osirix-viewer.com	$
Ossa 3D	Conceptualiz	www.conceptualiz.com/products_ossa.html	$
Rhino3D Medical	Mirrakoi	https://mirrakoi.com/rhino3d-medical/	$
Seg3D Biomesh3D	University of Utah	www.sci.utah.edu/cibc-software/seg3d.html	$
Sliceomatic 5.0	Tomovision	http://www.tomovision.com/products/sliceomatic.html	$
SPM	Wellcome Centre for Human Neuroimaging, University College London	www.fil.ion.ucl.ac.uk/spm	$
FSL	Wellcome Centre for Integrative Neuroimaging, Oxford University	www.fmrib.ox.ac.uk/fsl	$
Freesurfer	Athinoula A. Martinos Center for Biomedical Imaging	http://surfer.nmr.mgh.harvard.edu	$

the morphological operation "erosion."[35] The morphological operations are described in detail in Section Region-Based Segmentation. Finally, manual correction (sculpting) is sometimes required to remove the residual errors from the automated segmentation results. Many segmentation software packages, such as D2P and Mimics, Freesurfer, and FSL, offer 3D visualization modules where users can review and revise the segmentation results. Manipulations may also be performed following segmentation using computer-aided design software. These considerations are described in the following chapter.

REFERENCES

1. Otsu N. A threshold selection method from gray-level histograms. *IEEE Trans Syst Man Cybern.* 1979;9(1):62–66.
2. Pal NR, Pal SK. A review on image segmentation techniques. *Pattern Recogn.* 1993;26(9):1277–1294.
3. Romero-Zaliz R, Reinoso-Gordo JF. An updated review on watershed algorithms. In: *Soft Computing for Sustainability Science.* Springer International Publishing AG; 2018.
4. Beucher S. The morphological approach to segmentation : the watershed transformation. *Math Morphol Image Process.* 1993:433–482.
5. Cousty J, et al. Watershed cuts: minimum spanning forests and the drop of water principle. *IEEE Trans Pattern Anal Mach Intell.* 2009;31(8):1362–1374.
6. Serra J. *Image Analysis and Mathematical Morphology.* Academic Press, Inc; 1983.
7. Gonzalez RC, Woods RE. *Digital Image Processing.* Addison-Wesley Longman Publishing Co., Inc; 2001.
8. Canny J. *A Computational Approach to Edge Detection.* PAMI-8. IEEE Transactions on Pattern Analysis and Machine Intelligence; 1986:679–698.

9. Kass M, Witkin A, Terzopoulos D. Snakes: active contour models. *Int J Comput Vis.* 1988;1(4):321–331.

10. Mikheev A, et al. Fully automatic segmentation of the brain from T1-weighted MRI using Bridge Burner algorithm. *J Magn Reson Imaging.* 2008;27(6):1235–1241.

11. Cardenas CE, et al. Advances in auto-segmentation. *Semin Radiat Oncol.* 2019;29(3):185–197.

12. Iglesias JE, Sabuncu MR. Multi-atlas segmentation of biomedical images: a survey. *Med Image Anal.* 2015; 24(1):205–219.

13. Lloyd S. Least squares quantization in PCM. *IEEE Trans Inf Theor.* 1982;28(2):129–137.

14. Li S. *Markov Random Field Modeling in Image Analysis.* Springer; 2001.

15. Wang L, et al. Principles and methods for automatic and semi-automatic tissue segmentation in MRI data. *Magma.* 2016;29(2):95–110.

16. Litjens G, et al. A survey on deep learning in medical image analysis. *Med Image Anal.* 2017;42:60–88.

17. Ronneberger O, Fischer P, Brox T. U-Net: convolutional networks for biomedical image segmentation. In: *Medical Image Computing and Computer-Assisted Intervention – MICCAI 2015.* Cham: Springer International Publishing; 2015.

18. Belaroussi B, et al. Intensity non-uniformity correction in MRI: existing methods and their validation. *Med Image Anal.* 2006;10(2):234–246.

19. Zanzonico P. Routine quality control of clinical nuclear medicine instrumentation: a brief review. *J Nucl Med.* 2008;49(7):1114–1131. Official Publication, Society of Nuclear Medicine

20. Axel L, Costantini J, Listerud J. Intensity correction in surface-coil MR imaging. *AJR Am J Roentgenol.* 1987; 148(2):418–420.

21. Wells WM, et al. Adaptive segmentation of MRI data. *IEEE Trans Med Imag.* 1996;15(4):429–442.

22. Mugler 3rd JP, Brookeman JR. Rapid three-dimensional T1-weighted MR imaging with the MP-RAGE sequence. *J Magn Reson Imag.* 1991;1(5):561–567.

23. Marques JP, et al. MP2RAGE, a self bias-field corrected sequence for improved segmentation and T1-mapping at high field. *Neuroimage.* 2010;49(2):1271–1281.

24. Sled JG, Zijdenbos AP, Evans AC. A nonparametric method for automatic correction of intensity nonuniformity in MRI data. *IEEE Trans Med Imaging.* 1998;17(1):87–97.

25. Arnold JB, et al. Qualitative and quantitative evaluation of six algorithms for correcting intensity nonuniformity effects. *Neuroimage.* 2001;13(5):931–943.

26. Boyes RG, et al. Intensity non-uniformity correction using N3 on 3-T scanners with multichannel phased array coils. *Neuroimage.* 2008;39(4):1752–1762.

27. Tustison NJ, et al. N4ITK: improved N3 bias correction. *IEEE Trans Med Imag.* 2010;29(6):1310–1320.

28. Gonzalez RC, Woods RE, Eddins SL. *Digital Image Processing Using MATLAB.* Upper Saddle River, NJ: Pearson/Prentice Hall; 2004.

29. McCormack VA, dos Santos Silva I. Breast density and parenchymal patterns as markers of breast cancer risk: a meta-analysis. *Cancer Epidemiol Biomark Prev.* 2006;15(6): 1159–1169.

30. Dontchos BN, et al. Are qualitative assessments of background parenchymal enhancement, amount of fibroglandular tissue on MR images, and mammographic density associated with breast cancer risk? *Radiology.* 2015; 276(2):371–380.

31. Vokurka EA, Thacker NA, Jackson A. A fast model independent method for automatic correction of intensity nonuniformity in MRI data. *J Magn Reson Imag.* 1999;10(4): 550–562.

32. Pujara AC, et al. Clinical applicability and relevance of fibroglandular tissue segmentation on routine T1 weighted breast MRI. *Clin Imag.* 2017;42:119–125.

33. Fujimoto K, et al. GRASP with motion compensation for DCE-MRI of the abdomen. *Proc. Intl. Soc. Mag. Reson. Med.* 2017;25. Program No. 2009.

34. Haddad RA, Akansu AN. A class of fast Gaussian binomial filters for speech and image processing. *IEEE Trans Signal Process.* 1991;39(3):723–727.

35. Batchelor BG, Waltz FM. Morphological image processing. In: Batchelor BG, ed. *Machine Vision Handbook.* London: Springer London; 2012:801–870.

CHAPTER 4

Computer-Aided Design Principles for Anatomic Modeling

SARAH RIMINI, BS, RT(R) (MR) (ARRT) • JANA VINCENT, PHD • NICOLE WAKE, PHD

INTRODUCTION

The process of creating a physical three-dimensional (3D) printed model from medical imaging data is complicated and involves numerous steps. In order for a patient-specific anatomic model to be suitable for 3D printing, segmented anatomical regions of interest must be designed, prepped, and then converted into 3D file types that are recognized by vendor-specific 3D printing slicing software. Common, vendor neutral file formats for printing represent 3D geometry by a triangulated polygon mesh surface with node and vector data and include standard tessellation language or stereolithography (STL), alias wavefront object (OBJ), virtual reality modeling language (VRML), ZPR (a file format created by ZCorp), additive manufacturing (AMF), and 3D manufacturing format (3MF).

The STL file format, invented by the Albert Consulting Group for 3D Systems commercial printers in 1987, has been the predominant file format choice for years. There are two types of STL files: *binary* STL files that describe a single part and *ASCII* STL files that contain multiple independent parts. No color or texture is specified in the STL file format. A binary STL can be printed with a single material property, thus is ideal for printing a single component such as an organ, implant, or surgical guide. Multiple binary STL files can be combined or an ASCII STL file can be used to produce multicolored or multimaterial anatomical models such as a kidney and tumor (e.g., two different colors) or an aorta with calcification (e.g., a soft material for the aorta and hard material for the calcification). Since STL files do not encode color or material properties, those are selected using 3D printer-specific software.

In 2011, an initial effort was made to move away from STL files and the AMF was created. However, this file format was never fully adopted by the industry and 3D printer manufacturers. More recently, in 2015, an industrial effort led to the creation of the 3MF file format. This file format reduces the file size and enables the file to carry other data, such as units, color, lattices, and textures. Similar color and texture information is also incorporated in VRML files.

Regardless of the file format, in the preparation phase, minor changes may be necessary to make the model more suitable for printing or major modifications to the model might be needed to facilitate intervention planning.[1] Additionally, model analysis, digital planning, and surgical simulations may be performed in computer-aided design (CAD) software and personalized surgical guides, templates, and molds may be designed. In this chapter, CAD principles and common tools/operations used for medical models will be discussed and clinical examples will be provided. Understanding these tools and methods is critical for any radiologist overseeing the creation of 3D printed models in a hospital setting and can help radiologists to work with surgeons to optimize treatment plans and execute surgeries.

CAD PRINCIPLES

In medicine, CAD systems allow for the visualization and manipulation of 3D anatomical and associated structures as defined by geometrical parameters. There are many CAD programs where objects can be constructed and editing performed (Table 4.1).

The majority of the CAD software uses solid modeling principles to create 3D representations of objects of interest. Apart from solid modeling, other techniques for the creation of objects include surface modeling (described below), parametric modeling (where a variety of parameters such as dimensions, features, and material properties are input to derive the required geometry), and 3D surface scanning.

3D Printing for the Radiologist. https://doi.org/10.1016/B978-0-323-77573-1.00010-5

TABLE 4.1
List of Some Common CAD Programs Utilized in Hospitals.

Program	Company
3-matic and Magics	Materialise (Leuven, Belgium)
3ds Max, Fusion 360, Inventor, Maya, Meshmixer	Autodesk (San Rafael, CA)
Blender	Blender Foundation
Geomagic Freeform	3D Systems (Rock Hill, SC)
Meshlab	CNR, distributed under the GPL 3.0 Licensing Scheme
Rhinoceros	Robert McNeel and Associates (Seattle, WA)
Solidworks, CATIA	Dassault Systèmes (Waltham, MA)

Constructive solid geometry (CSG) and boundary representation are the two main methods used in solid modeling. CSG uses Boolean operations (merge, subtract, etc.) to create complex objects from instances of simpler forms such as cylinders, rods, and cubes. Two-dimensional (2D) representations may be swept along a plane or other trajectory to form more complex solid objects and then manipulated against other primitives.

Sweeping operations are also a feature of boundary representation modeling which connects faces, edges, and vertices with geometric surfaces, curves, and points. This technique offers a powerful method to create solid models of unusual shapes. Some well-known boundary representation systems are ROMULUS, Parasolid, and ACIS. The features of these systems form the basis, or are incorporated, into other CAD products.[2]

Solid objects created using 3D modeling techniques can be combined with 3D models rendered from medical imaging, as well as STL files, to form composite images. In addition, 3D and four-dimensional (4D) data visualization, processing, and analysis software can produce additional objects, typically using surface mesh modeling where the surface of the object is represented by a simple surface mesh of vertices and edges. Image segmentation software, introduced in Chapter 3, along with associated modules can be used to create the integrated forms. This software can also post process medical image data using the following mesh modeling techniques. Once a segmented anatomical region of interest has been defined from volumetric medical images, there are two commonly used approaches to model parts by surface mesh modeling, tessellation and the marching cubes algorithm. The most widely used method is the marching cubes algorithm, where the extracted polygonal mesh of an isosurface from 3D voxels is divided into a discrete set of cubes from the input volume associated with that part. This was developed by William Lorensen and Harvey E. Cline as a result of their research at General Electric.[3] The approach uses information from the original 3D imaging slices to derive interslice connectivity, surface locations, and surface gradient information with the resulting triangle model being displayed on conventional graphics display systems using standard rendering algorithms.

A second approach to CAD modeling is tessellation where the polygonal data are converted into a number of triangles proportional to the total surface area of a specific part in question. A higher number of triangles can more accurately represent the part, whereas a smaller number of triangles would decrease the surface detail, resulting in a less accurate representation of that part (Fig. 4.1). Higher triangle counts need more computer processing power to render and are saved as larger

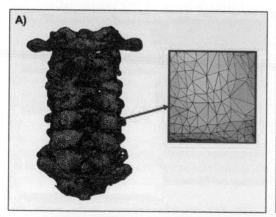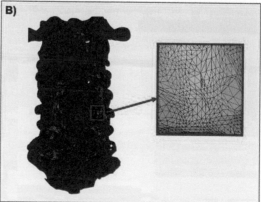

FIG. 4.1 Posterior cervical spine model with **(A)** 95,000 triangles and **(B)** 325,000 triangles.

file sizes due to the information stored from each triangle's vertices; therefore, a balance of surface quality and file size needs to be taken into account when selecting an appropriate number of triangles of a given part. Cut planes, to reduce the size of the model and surface connectivity, can also play a role in reducing the file size while still maintaining a higher level of surface quality. Decimation can be used, as well, to reduce the triangle count of a part. This allows users to select an amount of reduction of triangles in a specific part in order to reduce its size while still maintaining an appropriate number of triangles to represent the part.

DESIGN OPERATIONS

Anatomic Models

Once a 3D file has been generated from medical imaging data, further postprocessing of the mesh models may be necessary to ensure that the geometry is suitable for printing. A 3D triangular mesh file consists of three vertices stored in a counterclockwise fashion with a unit normal that defines the outer edge of a triangle. To be suitable for printing, each triangle in the file must be shared with the edge of an adjacent triangle and their surface must be facing the proper direction. Diagnostic testing can be performed to assess errors in triangulation and, in some cases with equipped software, the errors can automatically be repaired.

Some operations may be performed to ensure that the files sent to specific slicing software prior to printing have a decrease in common errors that will potentially make these anatomic models print at a higher success rate. Commonly used design operations include smoothing, wrapping, Boolean operations, labeling, hole filling, mirroring, hollowing, and adding shells. These tasks do not make significant changes to the anatomy but allow the user to refine the final parts for proper printing.[1]

Smoothing, which helps to rectify jagged or unrefined areas, may be performed to reduce the pixelated appearance of a model. It is important to note that higher levels of smoothness can change the part's volume and dimensions and more smoothing can decrease the ability to differentiate nearby structures (Fig. 4.2).

Missing triangles result in holes that are not acceptable for printing since the model will not be "watertight" causing errors due to the gaps in geometry. If there are holes in the mesh, then they must be filled using tools such as hole filling or face extruding to close the gaps. Wrapping operations will create a wrapping surface of the selected entities and can be used to filter small inclusions or close small holes. Wrapping the mesh model generates a watertight STL model around complex tiles, making these files suitable for 3D printing. If a single anatomical model is composed of multiple STL files, then a Boolean subtraction must be performed before printing so that the printer does not try to print two overlapping parts. Note that triangles with an inverted normal direction may look similar to missing triangles (Fig. 4.3). Since both errors will show you similar defects, it is important to identify whether the triangles are inverted or missing prior to choosing a unification method.

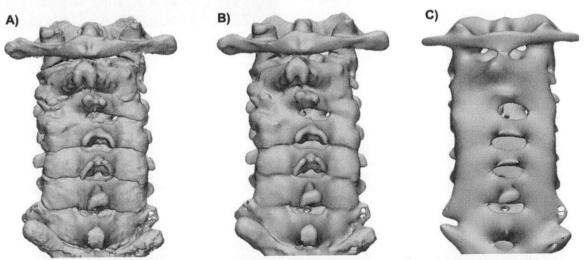

FIG. 4.2 Posterior cervical spine model with **(A)** no smoothing, **(B)** minor smoothing, and **(C)** major smoothing showing loss of structures and merging of bones.

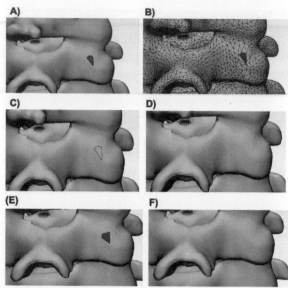

FIG. 4.3 Missing triangles shown with **(A)** smooth shaded display; with the inside triangles on the opposite side of the model (shown in red). **(B)** A wireframe mesh showing the inside triangles. **(C)** Missing triangles were fixed using a hole filling tool and **(D)** shown with the surfaced merged together as one. **(E)** Inverted normal direction of some triangles and **(F)** fixed triangles. The triangles that were facing the wrong direction were selected and inverted in order to fix this error.

Some anatomic models may be composed of multiple anatomic structures. For example, multiple bones or different heart structures may be delineated in order to demonstrate their relationship to one another. Bones may need to be connected to one another (Fig. 4.4) or the heart may be split and printed in two halves to better show the internal structures (Figs. 6.8 and 6.9). In these cases, support structures such as cylinders, that extrude on one piece and intrude on the other, or slots, where small magnets are placed, can be created to hold the parts together. Note that these additional parts do not change the design of the anatomic structure, but aid in the model's clinical utility.

Although these operations are imperative in most cases, some can be misused or overused to the point that the mesh is no longer accurate when compared to the original dataset. Users must educate themselves on these operations and the correct order in which they should be performed so they can associate how these actions influence the mesh file in order to use them safely. If significant postprocessing, such as smoothing, is made to the model, it is important to verify that the

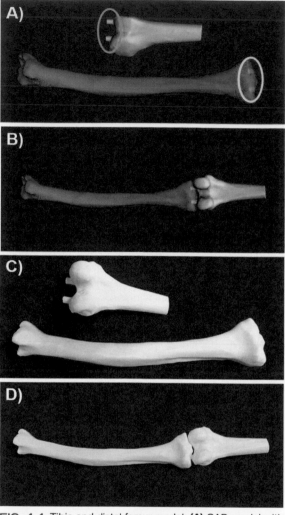

FIG. 4.4 Tibia and distal femur model: **(A)** CAD model with cylinders added to the distal femur (*blue circle*) and subtracted from the tibia (*yellow circle*), **(B)** CAD model with parts placed together in the correct anatomic position. **(C)** Separate 3D printed parts and **(D)** assembled printed parts. The model was printed with material extrusion (Ultimaker S5, Ultimaker, Utrecht, Netherlands).

model is still an accurate representation of the anatomy of interest. In order to verify this, the contours of the STL file can and should be routinely checked against the source data. In the example below, it is also important to ensure that no translations or rotations of the models are made, so that the data can be accurately registered (Fig. 4.5).

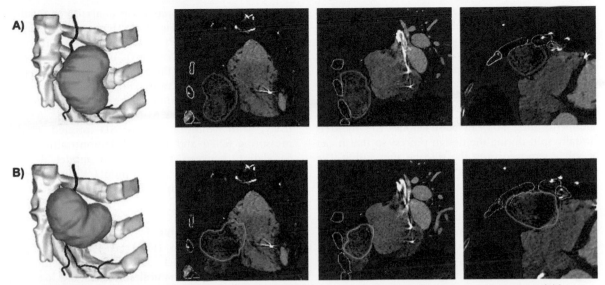

FIG. 4.5 Mesh, Coronal, Sagittal, and Axial images of the segmented and designed chest wall mass overlaid onto the original DICOM data (left to right) **(A)** with contours properly aligned and **(B)** with misalignment of the mass after rotation has been performed in CAD software.

To facilitate intervention planning, major modifications to 3D anatomic models may be necessary. Major modifications significantly alter the anatomy as derived from the medical imaging data and can include mirroring, subtraction of a device/implant, or addition of a graft or implant template[1] (Fig. 4.6).

Anatomic Guides and Molds

Once an anatomic part has been designed, CAD can be used to create 3D printed anatomic guides, molds, and patient-specific devices that can also aid in the patient's care without needing to print a model of that bone or organ. Patient-specific anatomic cutting and drilling guides can be designed to aid in an operative procedure by projecting the surgical plan made in the CAD software to the patient's anatomy. Considerations for designing these are discussed in Chapter 6 along with some illustrative case examples. For these guides, it is imperative that the requesting surgeon, skilled engineer, and radiologist are all involved in the planning and design so that anatomy and/or margins of a mass are represented correctly and the designed guide will be printed successfully and strong enough for its use case. Information on print material, postprocessing, biocompatibility, and sterilization verification testing and validation is essential to understand and produce prior to diving deeper into surgical guides.

Due to the limitations of most printers and their inability to produce realistic tissues tailored to specific

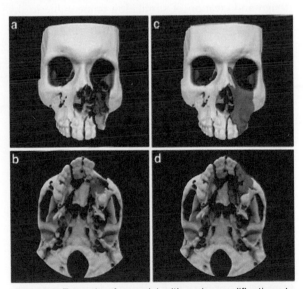

FIG. 4.6 Example of a model with major modifications to the original patient anatomy with **(A)** and **(B)** Patient after trauma to the maxilla showing large osseous defect including teeth and **(C)** and **(D)** Model demonstrating design of a suitable graft to facilitate surgical reconstruction. Missing bone is designed using the contralateral anatomy and output as a separate file for 3D printing a template (purple). (Reprinted with permission – creative commons from Christensen A, Rybicki FJ. Maintaining safety and efficacy for 3D printing in medicine. *3D Print Med*. 2017;3(1):1.)

organs or vessels, molds can be printed and injected with specific silicones and/or epoxies instead of printing the anatomic parts. CAD modeling of the mold includes the modeling of the specific anatomical structure. A shell is then designed around the anatomic structure which is subtracted from a solid body to form the negative space that serves as the printable mold. Fill and exhaust holes are then designed by adding cylinders and performing Boolean subtractions. The mold is virtually split during the design process so that it can be safely removed from the silicone after curing. The number of splitting surfaces along the mold and part assembly pieces/layers is dictated by the sophistication of the part and how difficult it will be to demold the part post cure. Simple models might only need a two-part mold, whereas a complex model might require a multi-part/multilayer mold. Molds can also be designed for specific layers of anatomy such as muscle, fat, and skin, all of which require different densities of silicone to achieve a realistic part (Fig. 4.7). The innermost layer of the mold is poured, cured, and removed before it is nested in the next layer's mold. This process is repeated until the last, or outermost part, is poured and cured. Molding can be quite cost-effective, especially in the design and creation of simulation trainers due to the reusability of the 3D printed mold with just the additional costs of silicone for each, rather than the costs of printing the model each time.

3D printed molds fabricated from patient's preoperative, cross-sectional, magnetic resonance imaging (MRI) data have also been utilized to correlate imaging findings with pathology.[4,5] Pathology specimens are sectioned in the same plane as the imaging acquisition and allow for excellent radiologic–pathologic correlation (Fig. 4.8).

MODEL ANALYSIS AND SIMULATION THROUGH CAD

CAD is not only used for model creation but also for analysis and simulation. Through specialized software, parts can be run through specific simulations as if they were already printed. This could reduce the amount of print iterations prior to finalizing a design. These simulations can also be applied to anatomical parts, as well, to simulate bone density, vessel flow patterns,

or to perform part comparison analysis for Quality Assurance programs (Fig. 4.9). Herein, a 3D printed prostate cancer model was scanned with a Micro-CT system (Bruker, Billerica, MA), image segmentation of the model including the prostate and lesion was performed, and the parts were compared to the original segmentation. The volume of the original segmented prostate and lesion was 61.04 and 1.28 cm^3, respectively, with volumes of the 3D printed model measuring 62.76 and 1.34 cm^3 demonstrating good correlation between the intended model derived from the MRI and the printed model. Virtual procedure planning with templates may also be performed in CAD platforms.

Finite Element Analysis

Finite element analysis (FEA) takes the virtual part along with inputs such as material properties, in conjunction with mechanical structures and loads, to educate the user on results that could occur post-print such as part stress, deflection, and heat transfers. After a mesh is generated from the patient image data, material properties are assigned to the area being modeled. Then, loads and boundary conditions, which are specific to the patient and procedure being performed (implant, reconstruction, graft, etc.), are added. The geometry of the implant/graft is then fed into a solver which is used for postprocessing and visualization.[6]

FEA provides an insight into the biomechanical properties of different tissue types that aid in the design of 3D printable implants, scaffolds, and surgical guides that are tailored directly to patient anatomy. Contrary to traditional implants, 3D printed parts can be made from a variety of biocompatible materials with varying porosity, flexibility, and dissolvability that better mimic natural function, reducing any mechanical stress on surrounding tissue.

The use of FEA has proven to be very impactful when designing implants and grafts for bone repair and replacement, especially in the field of prosthodontics. Traditional metallic implants can result in complications such as stress shielding and poor contact pressure at the bone interface.[7] Furthermore, misalignment of the implant can lead to poor vascularization, damage to surrounding tissue, damage to the implants such as cracking along the porcelain crown on a tooth surface,

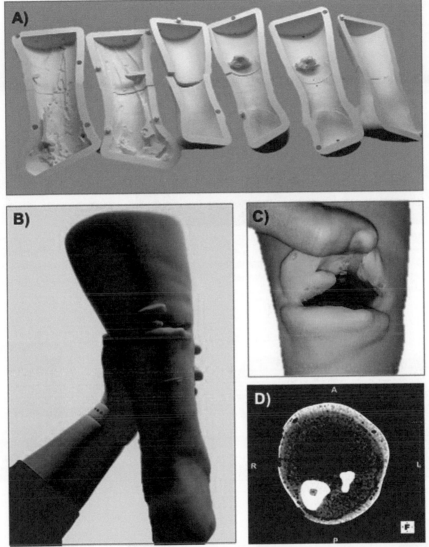

FIG. 4.7 **(A)** Multipart, multilayer molds for a lower leg model depicting a traumatic wound. From left to right: muscle mold, fat mold, skin mold. The molds are printed using binder jet technology (CJP460, 3D Systems, Rock Hill, SC). The powder surface produces a matte finish that closely resembles skin and is preferred at some facilities. 3D printed bones are placed inside the muscle mold, the mold is poured, cured, and removed and the part is placed in the fat mold. The process is repeated again for the fat and skin layers. **(B)** Completed multilayer mold of lower leg traumatic wound model showing internal layers with **(C)** zoomed in view. **(D)** CT scan of the lower leg molded model with 3D printed tibia and fibula, also printed with the CJP460 (3D Systems, Rock Hill, SC), embedded in the silicone.

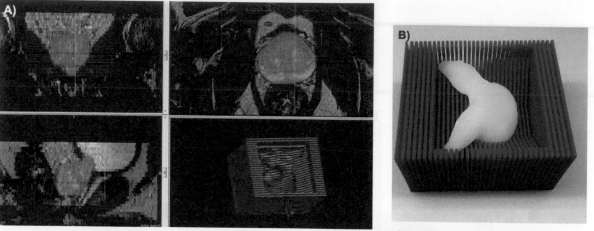

FIG. 4.8 **(A)** Image segmentation of the prostate (green) showing the coronal (top left), axial (top right), and sagittal views (bottom left) with the box shown surrounding the gland with gaps designed to represent the width of the knife with some clearance at the same angles and spacing as the edges of each MRI slice (bottom right). **(B)** The pink box was printed with material jetting (Objet 260 Connex 3, Stratasys, Eden Prairie, MN) and was filled with 30 shore silicone.

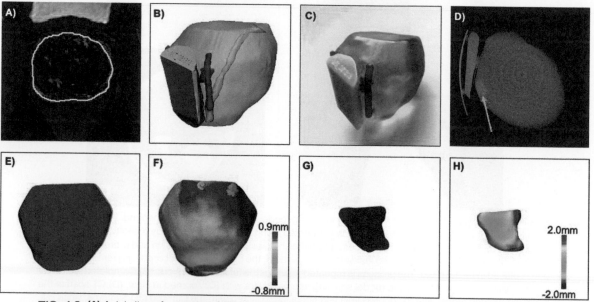

FIG. 4.9 **(A)** Axial slice of a prostate MRI showing prostate (yellow) and lesion (blue) segmentation. **(B)** CAD model of the prostate with the prostate (clear), lesion (blue), rectal wall (white), neurovascular bundles (pink), and urethra (yellow) with **(C)** corresponding 3D printed model printed with material jetting (J750, Stratasys, Eden Prairie, MN). **(D)** Micro-CT image of the 3D printed prostate model highlighting the lesion (yellow arrow). **(E)** and **(G)** Original CAD prostate and lesion models with CT scan model overlaid with **(F)** and **(H)** color map showing accuracy of model.

root fractures, or damage to the mandibular bones.[7–9] Proper contact between the implant and bone is critical for revascularization of surrounding tissue which, in turn, supports healthy function of the bones and/or joint.[9] Due to varying patient anatomy and bone porosity, FEA modeling can be used to derive patient-specific bone models to better predict the stress effects and contact between traditional implants to 3D printed implants that, subsequently, can be modified during post-processing to better mimic the biomechanical properties of the bone unique to the patient. Given that bone is an anisotropic material, calculating the deformation due to forces in various directions is key in determining areas with greater mechanical stress.[10] For instance, in one example, selective laser melting (SLM) of nickel–titanium (NiTi or Nitinol) was used to create a fixation plate with similar porosity to the patient's mandible. With the elastic response of NiTi, the resulting implant demonstrated a more normalized stress distribution and greater contact at the graft interface.[7]

The use of FEA goes beyond analysis for the customization of implants. This method is also used to analyze the progression of bone deterioration and cracking resulting from musculoskeletal diseases, such as arthritis or corrosion, and wear of contact surfaces of modular orthopedic implants. Given the stiffness of metal implants, mechanical mismatch could result in failures and need for surgical revision. In the United States, there are approximately 1 million hip replacements a year with 100,000 partial hip replacement procedures resulting from hip fractures and a growing need for surgical revisions.[11] Most of the loading in metal hip replacements is displaced to the more compliant, surrounding bone that is sensitive to mechanotransduction and reabsorption due to bone remodeling.[12] This is known as stress shielding. Attempts to reduce stress shielding have been made by altering the geometry and flexibility of metallic implants; however, this does not address the differences in porosity between the implant and bone. To combat this difference, FEA has been used in conjunction with 3D printing (SLM) to create a fully customized, porous implant for minimally invasive total hip arthroplasty that reduced stress shielding by 75%.[12] The steps of this design can be seen in Fig. 4.10.

In addition to hard tissue modeling, FEA can be utilized on soft tissue and, with advances in 3D bioprinting technologies, can be printed with similar biomechanical properties or used to generate treatment models. Natural and synthetic polymers can be used to create scaffolds for tissue engineering to aid in regeneration of tissue on vascular channels.[13] Use of other 3D printable materials, such as liquid crystal elastomers, shows promise in mimicking cartilage and other tissues with the softness to cushion with wear and compression-resistant properties.[14] Cartilage benefits from FEA in that it can be characterized into four structural zones with different characteristics: superficial, middle, deep, and calcified.[10] Similar to bone, cartilage is anisotropic. Recently, 3D printing has been used as a substitute for conventional ear transplant or reconstructive surgery. Jung et al. used CT images to create a 3D modeled scaffold, on which cartilage cells would be placed, of the unaffected ear and then mirrored to create the ear for transplant. The scaffold was made using the fused deposition 3D printing method with the biocompatible material polycaprolactone, which was printed with varying widths to accommodate different thicknesses of cartilage growth to mimic the structure and mechanics of an ear.[15] With a biocompatible 3D printed structure, the scaffold will hydrolyze as cells proliferate; however, the structure will still maintain its sturdiness as the ear takes shape (Fig. 4.11).[15]

Other soft tissues that benefit from FEA are ligaments, which have varying, time-dependent, and strain-dependent elastic properties and are also sensitive to varying temperatures. In one example, Serra et al. created a 3D printed lumbar cage for intervertebral disc degeneration treatment. Herein, FEA was used to evaluate different polymer cage architectures and filling densities that would provide similar stability to the traditional titanium cages, which improved osseointegration due to anatomical matching and higher load transfer.[16]

While FEA is a highly useful computational tool that provides information on how devices interact with human anatomy, computational fluid dynamics (discussed below) provides a greater insight into the varying performance of tissues under diseased states as well as how flow patterns are influenced by and impact the design of artificial components such as valve replacements, stent grafts, and flow diverters.

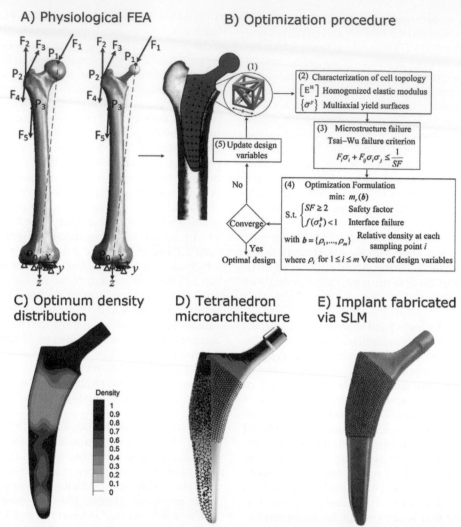

A) Physiological FEA

B) Optimization procedure

(1)

(2) Characterization of cell topology

$[E^H]$ Homogenized elastic modulus

$\{\sigma^y\}$ Multiaxial yield surfaces

(3) Microstructure failure
Tsai–Wu failure criterion
$$F_i\sigma_i + F_{ij}\sigma_i\sigma_j \leq \frac{1}{SF}$$

(5) Update design variables

No

(4) Optimization Formulation
min: $m_r(b)$
S.t. $\begin{cases} SF \geq 2 & \text{Safety factor} \\ f(\sigma_k^b) < 1 & \text{Interface failure} \end{cases}$
with $b = \{\rho_1,...,\rho_m\}$ Relative density at each sampling point i
where ρ_i for $1 \leq i \leq m$ Vector of design variables

Converge

Yes

Optimal design

C) Optimum density distribution

D) Tetrahedron microarchitecture

E) Implant fabricated via SLM

Density
1
0.9
0.8
0.7
0.6
0.5
0.4
0.3
0.2
0.1
0

FIG. 4.10 (A) Physiological FEA of the implanted femur. Forces F1–5, acting forces points P0–3, and boundary conditions applied to the intact and implanted femur during the gait cycle. **(B)** Computational scheme for multiscale mechanics and material property optimization of a minimally invasive 3D hip implant with minimum bone resorption. **(C)** Optimum relative density distribution of the fully porous implant. **(D)** Generation of lattice microarchitecture from optimal relative density distribution using a high strength tetrahedron topology. **(E)** Implant manufacturing via Selective Laser Melting. (Reproduced with permission from Arabnejad S, Johnston B, Tanzer M, Pasini D. Fully porous 3D printed titanium femoral stem to reduce stress-shielding following total hip arthroplasty. *J Orthop Res.* 2017;35(8):1774–1783.)

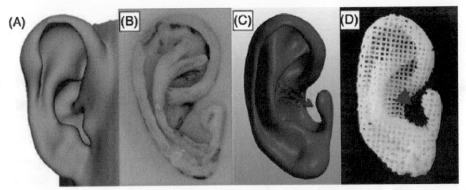

FIG. 4.11 **(A)** Final reconstruction of the 3D model, **(B)** real cartilage framework used in clinical ear reconstruction surgery with **(C)** and **(D)** modified design of the 3D scaffold (*red arrows*) to be suitable for the ear reconstruction surgery. (Reproduced with permission from Jung BK, Kim JY, Kim YS, et al. Ideal scaffold design for total ear reconstruction using a three-dimensional printing technique. *J Biomed Mater Res B Appl Biomater.* 2019;107(4):1295–1303.)

Computational Fluid Dynamics

Computational fluid dynamics (CFD) uses numerical analysis to analyze and solve problems that involve fluid flows. Computer algorithms are used to perform the calculations required to simulate the freestream flow of the fluid and the interaction of the fluid with the surface, as defined by boundary conditions. Flow patterns of a specific area such as the aorta, vessels in the brain, aneurysm, or plaque-filled artery may be simulated. Similar to FEA models, once the geometry is specified, a computational mesh is built, and appropriate variables are computed and stored within the model.

Long before current computer simulations, Leonardo da Vinci experimented with and analyzed blood flow through the aortic valve.[17] To accomplish this, he created a glass model and used seeds suspended in water to mimic circulation. He also proposed a model to cast a wax mold of a bull heart to use in the study of valve dynamics.[18] Da Vinci provided theories about turbulent flow through valves and the functioning of the heart. This experimentation and curiosity in fluid dynamics has been further enhanced by patient-specific 3D printing and CFD.

With advancements in computer technology, CFD modeling of arterial blood flow has recently become more common in surgical planning.[19-27] Flow diverter device implementation including coiling and deployment has been a subject of CFD modeling using patient-specific 3D models. A comparison of hemodynamic conditions with and without the flow diverter device can be performed to predict the likelihood of a successful aneurysm embolization.[19] In some cases, increased pressure due to the flow diverter device has shown to cause an increase in aneurysm rupture, further demonstrating the need of CFD prior to surgery to determine the best length and positioning of the device.[19,20] Prediction of aneurysm growth and rupture prior to surgery has proven to be more challenging. CFD takes into consideration hemodynamic factors, but does not include data such as age, smoking habits, family history, or other significant risk factors; however, recent combinations of CFD and deep learning algorithms have had an 86% success rate in discriminating between ruptured and unruptured aneurysms which could help with decisions when faced with the risk of hemorrhage versus surgery or endovascular treatment.[21] In other cases, hemodynamic flow pattern changes postsurgery can influence day-to-day activities. This is the case in patients with hypoplastic left or right heart syndrome. After a series of surgical interventions to reconstruct the ventricle, these patients have a Fontan circulation, which is where the venous blood bypasses the right ventricle and goes directly to the lungs through the pulmonary arteries.[22,23] CFD modeling of this complex flow pattern sheds light into physical limitations and outcomes of these surgeries. The viscous dissipation gathered from 4D MRI flow data and subsequent CFD results can be seen in Fig. 4.12.[23] In this case, CFD

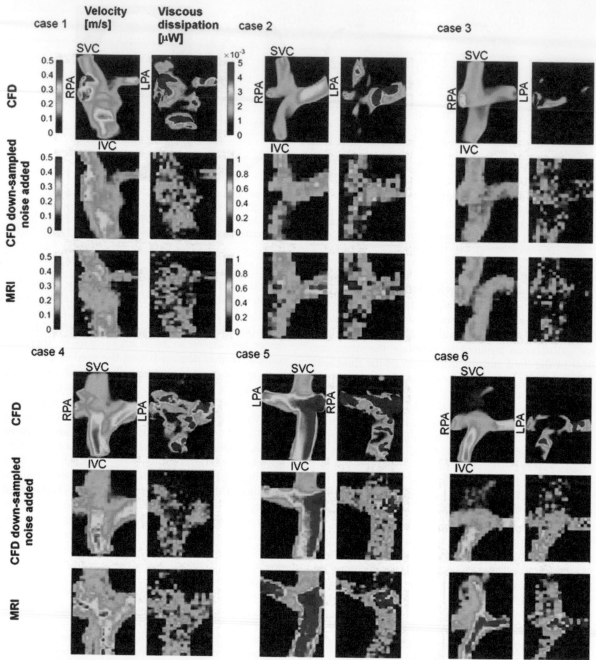

FIG. 4.12 Maximum intensity projection of velocity (left) and viscous dissipation (right) fields obtained by CFD, down-sampled CFD with added noise and 4D flow MRI shown for six subjects. The color maps given for case 1 are valid for all subjects. Note that the color-map scale of CFD-based viscous dissipation was 200 times smaller than others wince the volume of the voxels in CFD was ~1000 times smaller than those in MRI. Hence, viscous dissipation per voxel was also smaller. (Reproduced with permission from Cibis M, Jarvis K, Markl M, et al. The effect of resolution on viscous dissipation measured with 4D flow MRI in patients with Fontan circulation: Evaluation using computational fluid dynamics. *J Biomech*. 2015;48(12):2984—2989.)

was able to analyze viscous dissipation between patient regardless of MR image resolution and noise.[23]

When artificial materials are introduced into the cardiovascular system, such as a left ventricular assist device (LVAD) or an artificial valve, there runs a risk of hemolysis, or damage to the red blood cells. To mitigate this risk, simulation of flow dynamics can be performed to determine velocity, shear stress, and pressure along the cardiovascular system. In cases with higher shear forces, platelets can rupture, triggering a thrombogenic response. Models for hemolysis and platelet activation can be determined through CFD modeling.

Several studies using CFD to evaluate LVAD function have shown increased flow pressure in the ascending aorta, especially for lower anastamoses.[24,25] While most CFD studies of LVAD are not patient-specific, there is potential for better surgical placement and device selection based on anatomical differences. Patients with conditions such as ventricular or atrial septal defects or damaged chambers due to myocardial infarctions could benefit from flow analysis when determining the best course of treatment, whether it be an LVAD or valve replacement.

Arterial blood flow dynamics have been important in tracking the onset and progression of atherosclerosis. Build-up of activated platelets causes stenosis of the artery that, in turn, changes the dynamics of blood flow as the arterial wall thickens. Even with lesser degrees of stenosis, plaques can break loose, leading to myocardial infarction.[26] Ischemic stroke can also occur if there is stenosis of the carotid artery. For this reason, it is important to have CFD models to aid in identification of more vulnerable plaques. This has been accomplished by CFD to both plan surgery and predict the outcome. In carotid artery stenosis studies, use of CFD has accomplished 98.5% and 98.7% accuracy in blood flow reconstruction compared to ultrasound Doppler data gathered before and after surgery.[27]

INTEGRATING 3D PRINTING WITH SIMULATION MODELS

To validate computational models, the same mesh models that are used in simulations can be 3D printed and used for in vitro flow simulations. CAD measurements may be validated by reconstructing 3D printed phantom models and comparing the reconstructed geometries with the reference CAD geometries.[28] Similarly, quantitative measurements obtained in flow simulations can be compared to in vitro, 3D printed flow models. A few examples of studies that have shown good correlation between flow measurements, obtained in each method, are described below.[29–31] In one example, Clark et al. performed LVAD simulations with six different test configurations and compared CFD flow rates to in vitro flow rates using a 3D printed aortic arch model. Good correlation was found between CFD simulations and in vitro flow models, demonstrating that either computational or in vitro methods may be used to determine which VAD-OG (outflow graft) configuration without left coronary artery (LCA) bypass would lead to an optimal surgical implant configuration.[29] In another study, Vardhan et al. demonstrated the importance of side branches in modeling 3D hemodynamics.[30] Herein, coronary models were created from 2D biplane angiograms, which were then used to create a 3D phantom for in vitro validation.[30] CFD simulations were performed on both the complete coronary model generated from a reconstruction algorithm and the matched coronary model reconstruction from the angiogram. These flow dynamics were compared to the 3D printed model in which discernible features such as stenosis and bifurcation could be seen, mimicking that of both the original angiogram data and model.[30] Patient-specific 3D printed cardiovascular phantoms have also been used for clinical validation of CT-derived fractional flow reserve diagnostic software.[31]

CONCLUSIONS

CAD is a powerful tool that plays a key role in all aspects of medical 3D printing and modeling. From simple anatomic models, to facilitating computer-assisted surgery, to custom-made implants, as well as computational and in vitro simulation models, CAD can truly enhance patient care. Furthermore, with increasing capabilities in 3D CAD design allowing for enhanced simulations of patient-specific tissues and fluid dynamics, along with the continued development of printable tissues, it is expected that the transplant industry will be revolutionized in the future.

REFERENCES

1. Christensen A, Rybicki FJ. Maintaining safety and efficacy for 3D printing in medicine. *3D Print Med.* 2017;3(1):1.
2. Braid IG A, Lang C. *The 2008 Pierre Bezier Award Recipients.* Bezier Award. Solid Modeling Association; 2008. http://solidmodeling.org/awards/bezier-award/i-braid-a-grayer-and-c-lang/. Accessed August 17, 2020.
3. Lorensen WCH. Marching cubes: a high resolution 3D surface reconstruction algorithm. *ACM SIGGRAPH Comput Graph.* 1987;21(4).
4. Costa DN, Chatzinoff Y, Passoni NM, et al. Improved magnetic resonance imaging-pathology correlation with imaging-derived, 3D-printed, patient-specific whole-mount molds of the prostate. *Invest Radiol.* 2017;52(9): 507–513.
5. Priester A, Natarajan S, Khoshnoodi P, et al. Magnetic resonance imaging underestimation of prostate cancer geometry: use of patient specific molds to correlate images with whole mount pathology. *J Urol.* 2017;197(2):320–326.
6. Poelert S, Valstar E, Weinans H, Zadpoor AA. Patient-specific finite element modeling of bones. *Proc Inst Mech Eng H.* 2013;227(4):464–478.
7. Jahadakbar A, Shayesteh Moghaddam N, Amerinatanzi A, Dean D, Karaca HE, Elahinia M. Finite element simulation and additive manufacturing of stiffness-matched NiTi fixation hardware for mandibular reconstruction surgery. *Bioengineering (Basel).* 2016;3(4).
8. Oladapo BIAZS, Vahidnia F, Ikumapayi OM, Farooq MU. Three-dimensional finite element analysis of a porcelain crowned tooth. *Beni-Suef Univ J Basic Appl Sci.* 2018;7(4): 461–464.
9. Goh BT, Lee S, Tideman H, Stoelinga PJ. Mandibular reconstruction in adults: a review. *Int J Oral Maxillofac Surg.* 2008;37(7):597–605.
10. Yang Z. *Finite Element Analysis for Biomedical Engineering Applications.* CRC Press Taylor & Francis Group; 2019.
11. Maradit Kremers H, Larson DR, Crowson CS, et al. Prevalence of total hip and knee replacement in the United States. *J Bone Joint Surg Am.* 2015;97(17):1386–1397.
12. Arabnejad S, Johnston B, Tanzer M, Pasini D. Fully porous 3D printed titanium femoral stem to reduce stress-shielding following total hip arthroplasty. *J Orthop Res.* 2017;35(8):1774–1783.
13. Mondschein RJ, Kanitkar A, Williams CB, Verbridge SS, Long TE. Polymer structure-property requirements for stereolithographic 3D printing of soft tissue engineering scaffolds. *Biomaterials.* 2017;140:170–188.
14. Saed MO, Volpe RH, Traugutt NA, Visvanathan R, Clark NA, Yakacki CM. High strain actuation liquid crystal elastomers via modulation of mesophase structure. *Soft Matter.* 2017;13(41):7537–7547.
15. Jung BK, Kim JY, Kim YS, et al. Ideal scaffold design for total ear reconstruction using a three-dimensional printing technique. *J Biomed Mater Res B Appl Biomater.* 2019; 107(4):1295–1303.
16. Serra T, Capelli C, Toumpaniari R, et al. Design and fabrication of 3D-printed anatomically shaped lumbar cage for intervertebral disc (IVD) degeneration treatment. *Biofabrication.* 2016;8(3):035001.
17. Kemp M. Leonardo da Vinci's laboratory: studies in flow. *Nature.* 2019;571(7765):322–323.
18. Cambiaghi M, Hausse H. Leonardo da Vinci and his study of the heart. *Eur Heart J.* 2019;40(23):1823–1826.
19. Rayz VL, Cohen-Gadol AA. Hemodynamics of cerebral aneurysms: connecting medical imaging and biomechanical analysis. *Annu Rev Biomed Eng.* 2020;22:231–256.
20. Cebral JR, Mut F, Raschi M, et al. Aneurysm rupture following treatment with flow-diverting stents: computational hemodynamics analysis of treatment. *AJNR Am J Neuroradiol.* 2011;32(1):27–33.
21. Detmer FJ, Chung BJ, Mut F, et al. Development and internal validation of an aneurysm rupture probability model based on patient characteristics and aneurysm location, morphology, and hemodynamics. *Int J Comput Assist Radiol Surg.* 2018;13(11):1767–1779.
22. Khairy P, Poirier N, Mercier LA. Univentricular heart. *Circulation.* 2007;115(6):800–812.
23. Cibis M, Jarvis K, Markl M, et al. The effect of resolution on viscous dissipation measured with 4D flow MRI in patients with Fontan circulation: evaluation using computational fluid dynamics. *J Biomech.* 2015;48(12):2984–2989.
24. Karmonik C, Partovi S, Loebe M, et al. Computational fluid dynamics in patients with continuous-flow left ventricular assist device support show hemodynamic alterations in the ascending aorta. *J Thorac Cardiovasc Surg.* 2014;147(4), 1326-1333 e1321.
25. Callington A, Long Q, Mohite P, Simon A, Mittal TK. Computational fluid dynamic study of hemodynamic effects on aortic root blood flow of systematically varied left ventricular assist device graft anastomosis design. *J Thorac Cardiovasc Surg.* 2015;150(3):696–704.
26. Brunette J, Mongrain R, Laurier J, Galaz R, Tardif JC. 3D flow study in a mildly stenotic coronary artery phantom using a whole volume PIV method. *Med Eng Phys.* 2008; 30(9):1193–1200.
27. Polanczyk A, Podgorski M, Wozniak T, Stefancyk L, Strzelecki M. Computational fluid dynamics as an engineering tool for the reconstruction of hemodynamics after carotid artery stenosis operation. *Medicina (Kaunas).* 2018; 54(3).
28. Colombo M, Bologna M, Garbey M, et al. Computing patient-specific hemodynamics in stented femoral artery

models obtained from computed tomography using a validated 3D reconstruction method. *Med Eng Phys*. 2020;75:23–35.

29. Clark WD, Eslahpazir BA, Argueta-Morales IR, Kassab AJ, Divo EA, DeCampli WM. Comparison between benchtop and computational modelling of cerebral thromboembolism in ventricular assist device circulation. *Cardiovasc Eng Technol*. 2015;6(3):242–255.

30. Vardhan M, Gounley J, Chen SJ, Kahn AM, Leopold JA, Randles A. The importance of side branches in modeling 3D hemodynamics from angiograms for patients with coronary artery disease. *Sci Rep*. 2019;9(1):8854.

31. Sommer KN, Shepard L, Karkhanis NV, et al. 3D printed cardiovascular patient specific phantoms used for clinical validation of a CT derived FFR diagnostic software. *Proc SPIE-Int Soc Opt Eng*. 2018:10578.

CHAPTER 5

3D Printing Principles and Technologies

PETER LIACOURAS, PHD • NICOLE WAKE, PHD

INTRODUCTION

Three-dimensional (3D) printing, also known as additive manufacturing or rapid prototyping, originated in the 1980s and encompasses various processes that create physical 3D objects by fabricating them layer by layer from a digital file.[1,2] Whether the 3D printed part begins with radiological images or is designed from the ground up, specialized software is necessary to help generate the appropriate digital computer-aided design (CAD) file for each case. The stereolithography file format, sometimes known as the standard tessellation language or standard triangle language (STL), is the most widely utilized file format for printing. However, newer formats, such as the 3D Manufacturing Format (3MF), open the door to fine control over color, textures, and material properties, thus increase the power and options to the 3D printing community.

Once a part is ready to be printed, the CAD file is processed by a piece of software called a "slicer" or "build processor," which converts the 3D model into a series of thin layers and creates a build file containing instructions tailored to a specific printer. Within the slicing or build processing program, the user may be able to define and alter settings of the 3D printing build parameters such as color, layer height, print speed, support material location and attachment sites, infill, heat/intensity, and part orientation. Slicer programs are often proprietary to each brand of 3D printer, but there are some universal support generation and slicing programs available on the market.

The International Organization for Standardization (ISO) and American Standards for Testing and Materials (ASTM) have categorized 3D printing into seven groups of specific process categories or technologies: Vat Photopolymerization, Material Jetting, Binder Jetting, Material Extrusion, Powder Bed Fusion, Sheet Lamination, and Directed Energy Deposition.[3-5]

In this chapter, the five printing technologies generally utilized for medical applications will be discussed. Sheet lamination and directed energy deposition will not be discussed due to their limited popularity and adoption within the medical community. Having a basic understanding of 3D printing technologies will help radiologists to understand appropriate uses for each and determine which would be applicable in their practices.

VAT PHOTOPOLYMERIZATION

Vat photopolymerization is a process in which a liquid photopolymer is selectively cured by a high-intensity light, usually in the form of a laser or projection. The models or devices are constructed by each layer fusing together with each pass of the light source (usually less than an eighth of a millimeter of resin is cured at a time). After a new layer is solidified, the platform drops the object into the vat to expose a new layer of resin to be cured. This process continues until the entire model is completed (Fig. 5.1).

The most common forms of vat photopolymerization are stereolithography (SLA) and digital light processing (DLP). SLA has three basic components: (1) a high-intensity light source typically ultraviolet UV-A or UV-B, (2) a vat or tray that holds a photocurable liquid resin, and (3) a controlling system that directs the light source to selectively illuminate and solidify the resin. Mirrors, known as galvanometers or galvos, are located on the X- and Y-axes and these mirrors rapidly aim the laser beam across the vat curing and solidifying the resin as it goes along.

SLA machines can produce parts in two different orientations, bottom-up or top-down. Bottom-up printers have a light source positioned below a resin vat with a transparent bottom. Once a layer of the object is cured and becomes structurally stable, the object is raised by one layer, so that the next layer can be cured with the laser. For bottom-up printers, each layer may adhere to the build platform, therefore the printer performs a separation step which separates the layer from the base of the vat, before the build platform moves up

3D Printing for the Radiologist. https://doi.org/10.1016/B978-0-323-77573-1.00016-6

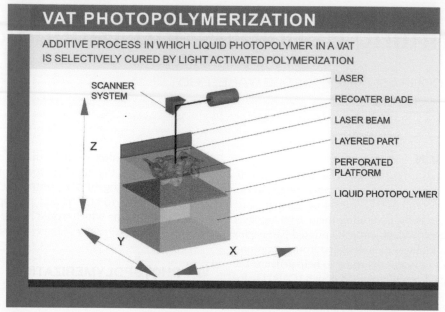

FIG. 5.1 Diagram of the top-down Vat Photopolymerization process. In this depiction, a laser is used to cure the photopolymer. Partial completed part resides within the resin tank and is only revealed upon completion. This is in contrast to bottom-up machines, where the part is suspended on the build platform. (Courtesy of Brandon Campbell, Walter Reed National Military Medical Center.)

one-layer thickness. Depending on the machine, this separation step may involve sliding, peeling, rotating, or shaking the vat. Bottom-up printers often have a nonstick coating (e.g., polydimethylsiloxane (PDMS) or fluorinated ethylene propylene (FEP)) applied to the base of the vat to assist with layer separation. In addition, a wiper may assist in oxygenating the PDMS/FEP coating, thus may help to improve the nonstick performance, while also ensuring that a fresh layer of resin is ready for the next layer. For bottom-up printers, another mechanism for reducing the bond forces exerted on parts during the active build layer, called Low Force Stereolithography, was recently introduced.[6] This method uses a flexible membrane which moves in coordination with the laser location, allowing for finer detail and greater clarity. As compared to bottom-up printers, top-down printers position the light source above the build platform. The build begins at the top of the resin vat and the build platform moves down layer by layer as the object prints. A blade assembly helps to apply a fresh even coat of resin before the laser cures the next layer. For top-down printers, once the build is complete, the part is raised out of the resin, allowed to drain, and removed from the build platform.

Both top-down and bottom-up printing technologies typically require supporting structures in the form

of lattices (Fig. 5.2). The necessity of structural support provides stabilization of the 3D printed part within the material during the build phase. For top-down printers, the support requirements are generally used to hold up overhanging areas, whereas for bottom-up machines, the supports are more complicated as they need to be able to hold the entire weight of the build to the platform.

Instead of using a laser and mirrors to dictate the area of the resin being cured, DLP, which was originally developed in 1987 by Larry Hornbeck of Texas Instruments, uses a digital projector to instantly illuminate the entire cross section of the layer being printed.[7] The projector is a digital screen, so the image of each layer is composed of square pixels, resulting in a layer formed from voxels. For parts which have complicated contours, DLP may be able to achieve faster print times than traditional SLA, as each layer is exposed at the same time, rather than being drawn out with a laser.

In 2017, a new method of bottom-up DLP called Continuous Liquid Interface Production (CLIP) was patented.[8] CLIP is a photochemical process that works by projecting light through an oxygen-permeable window into a reservoir of UV-curable resin. As a sequence of UV images are projected, the part solidifies and the build platform rises. The oxygen creates a dead-zone

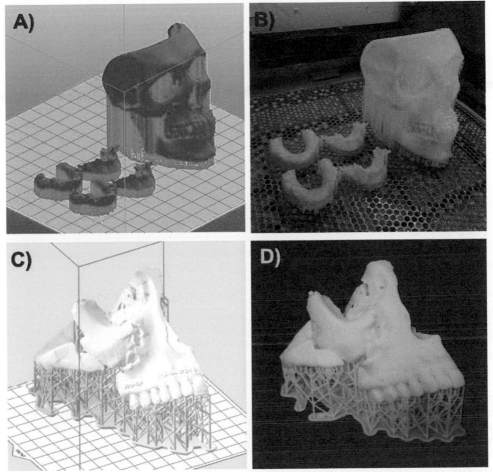

FIG. 5.2 **(A)** Anatomic models of the face and teeth (blue) are suspended with lattice-type supports (green). Once generated, the supports and models are sliced and saved as a build file for the Projet 7000HD (SD Systems, Rock Hill, SC). **(B)** The completed printed parts are shown in the postprocessing area with the supports still attached. **(C)** Anatomic model of the face with support structures on a bottom-up machine (Formlabs, Form 3, Cambridge, MA). **(D)** Printed model with supports still attached.

of uncured resin at the bottom of the vat, so the bottom of the print does not adhere to the resin tank, thus the separation step is eliminated allowing for significantly faster build times. This gives the illusion that the part is building in real time with no separation between layers. Since its introduction in 2017, other companies have adopted similar techniques to speed up the manufacturing process utilizing this oxygen-permeable membrane or window principle.[9,10]

After a model is printed with vat photopolymerization, the build platform is removed from the machine. The platform either with parts attached or the parts alone, after removal, are cleaned with a solvent, most commonly isopropyl alcohol, in a bath or parts washer.

Following the cleaning process, supports generated during fabrication are removed, and the model is placed into a chamber with special lights and possibly a heat source to harden any residual resin on the surface of the model. Some resins may specify that the part should be cured before support removal to limit any warping that may occur. In addition, some materials require a postbuild heat treatment, potentially several hours, to complete the polymerization process and obtain the proper material characteristics and properties.

Materials

Vat photopolymerization technologies use thermoset photopolymers which come in a liquid resin form.

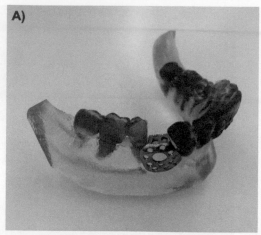
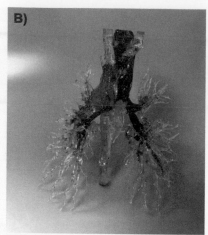

FIG. 5.3 Vat photopolymerization models printed with a Projet 7000HD (3D Systems, Rock Hill, SC) showing **(A)** teeth (amber) which have been overcured to show roots within the body of the mandible. This is being used to verify fixation screws for an implant so it will not penetrate a root. **(B)** lung vasculature (clear) and the airway (amber).

Some of the many resin choices include characteristics such as transparency, casting ability, durability, high temperature resistance, surgical/dental usability, and flexibility. As compared to larger industrial machines, some small- to medium-sized, bottom-up desktop machines have interchangeable resin vats, thus providing an easier option to change materials, adding to the systems versatility. Specific resins and printers can allow for extra exposure of energy to specific sections of the medical models, thereby darkening or changing the color of the resin and enabling multiple structures to be depicted within a single model (Fig. 5.3). Materials in this category were initially limited and were predominantly brittle; however, now there seems to be a resin for almost every application with the major advances coming in durability and flexibility.

Medical Applications

Most frequently, vat photopolymerization is used to create solid, plastic, 3D objects from medical scans or 3D designs in a matter of minutes, hours, or days to provide doctors with true-to-scale physical presurgical and planning models that they can handle and manipulate prior to procedures. As described above, dual-colored models may also be created by overcuring certain regions. Empty cavities within a model may also be created to be colored with paint or dye, thus allowing for pathology such as tumors or nerves, to be incorporated into designs. Many of the smaller bottom-up machines have become extremely popular in the dentistry industry for dental implant guides, night guards, aligners, and dentures.

MATERIAL EXTRUSION

Material extrusion is a process where a material is selectively dispensed through a nozzle. In most cases, heat is used to melt/soften material for the extrusion process. Melted material passes through the nozzle in a continuous stream under constant pressure and is selectively deposited onto the build tray or previous section of the printed part layer by layer (Fig. 5.4). Material extrusion is commonly referred to as fused filament fabrication (FFF), and it is also widely known under a trademarked term fused deposition modeling (FDM).[11]

The resolution of the printed part is defined by the nozzle diameter, filament diameter, and layer height. Parameters such as motor speed, part infill, extrusion speed, and nozzle temperature can be adjusted on most material extrusion machines to achieve the desired print. To save on the amount of material utilized, material extrusion parts can be printed with an internal, low-density structure known as infill. Infill percentage and shape can vary based on the application of a part as well as the type of printer being used. Common infill geometries include triangular, rectangular, and honeycomb. While the material extrusion process has many factors that may influence the quality of the final model, when these factors are controlled successfully, extremely strong and versatile parts can be produced.

Similar to parts that are printed using vat photopolymerization, material extrusion parts require support material to print successfully, where the support material prevents the model from falling down. The support material may be printed with the same nozzle as the main model material or with a separate nozzle using a different

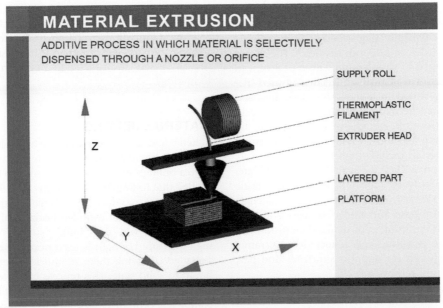

MATERIAL EXTRUSION

ADDITIVE PROCESS IN WHICH MATERIAL IS SELECTIVELY
DISPENSED THROUGH A NOZZLE OR ORIFICE

SUPPLY ROLL

THERMOPLASTIC
FILAMENT

EXTRUDER HEAD

LAYERED PART

PLATFORM

Z

Y

X

FIG. 5.4 Diagram of the Material Extrusion process showing a spool of filament which is heated and laid onto the platform or the previous layer of the build. Some machines use multiple filaments, thus allowing models to feature multiple colors or use a dissolvable support material to allow for more complex or overhanging geometry. Depending on the machine, either the platform lowers or extruder head raises before printing the next layer. (Courtesy of Brandon Campbell, Walter Reed National Military Medical Center.)

material, some material which can be dissolved in a hot water bath or solvent (e.g., alkaline solution). If a non-dissolvable or identical material is used for the supports, then these support structures are broken away from the part manually. If an alkaline bath is used, the part is rinsed in a water bath afterward and allowed to dry. Depending on the material, support structures may only have the option to be breakaway even if they are a different material. In some cases, a part may also be oriented on the build platform so that no supports are needed. Fig. 5.5 shows a tibia model printed using material extrusion with its support structures and infill geometry.

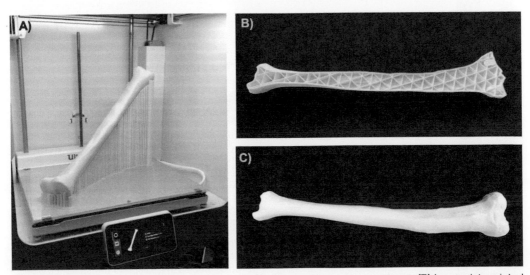

FIG. 5.5 (A) Tibia model printed on the Ultimaker S5 shown with support structures. **(B)** Incomplete printed part with a 30% triangular infill geometry. **(C)** Final 3D printed tibia model. ((A) Photograph courtesy of Matthew Griffin, Ultimaker.)

Materials

Material extrusion printers have a wide selection of materials which are typically 1 kg spools of thermoplastic filament with a 1.75 or 3.00 mm diameter. The spools are usually shipped in shrink wrap with a desiccant to reduce humidity. It is recommended that unused filament spools be stored in a cool, dry, dark area and only opened when needed for printing. Polylactic acid (PLA) and acrylonitrile butadiene styrene (ABS) are the most common and most widely utilized materials. Some other materials include high-impact polystyrene, nylon, polycarbonate (PC), polyethylene terephthalate, polyetherimide, polyvinyl alcohol, and thermoplastic polyurethane (TPU). In addition, creative materials with infiltrates of glass and fibers are also available. Finally, metal 3D printing with material extrusion has recently become possible, and it includes a ceramic release layer between the support structures and part to enhance support removal.[12]

Medical Applications

Most frequently, material extrusion technology is used to create monochrome plastic parts with larger anatomical features such as bones. 3D designs for assistive technology and orthotics are also commonly manufactured with material extrusion technologies. Multifilament machines have allowed medical models that include two or more materials or colors in the same build. Due to the resolution limitations and limited multicolor and multimaterial capabilities, superfine features such as smaller branch vessels are difficult to manufacture using this technology.

MATERIAL JETTING

Material jetting is a process in which droplets of material, typically a liquid photopolymer, are selectively deposited onto a build platform and are cured with UV light or solidified due to ambient conditions (Fig. 5.6). Similar to conventional two-dimensional ink-jet printers, material is jetted, sprayed, or extruded horizontally along the X- and Y-axes on the build surface. Most often, high-intensity UV light is used next to cure the layer of polymers allowing them to quickly transition from a liquid to solid state. This process is repeated, with each new layer bonding to the previous, until the object is complete. Some machines may use a wax and ambient temperatures in lieu of the photopolymer and light. These wax models may be used to make a cast using a burn out procedure, commonly called "lost wax." After the build is complete, the object is removed from the platform and temporary supports are eliminated using

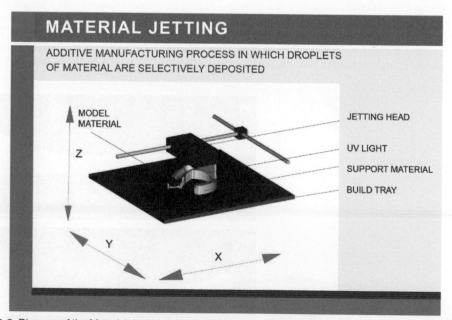

FIG. 5.6 Diagram of the Material Jetting process. Multiple print heads are used to jet material onto a platform and this material is usually solidified with UV light. After each layer, the platform lowers or the printhead rises. Some machines can mix materials together allowing for full-color models in addition to transparent models showing colored internal anatomical features. (Courtesy of Brandon Campbell, Walter Reed National Military Medical Center.)

a pressure washer, heat, or bath of basic solution. 3D printed models printed with material jetting can then be polished or coated, to achieve optimal visualization properties.

Materials

Many material jetting machines have the capability to utilize multiple materials with different colors, transparencies, shore values, and/or mechanical properties. Some can even mix different materials together to obtain new substances/materials in different colors, opacities, or even durometers. Various materials in this technology category can also mimic some of the vat photopolymerization material characteristics such as transparency, casting ability, durability, high temperature resistance, surgical/dental usability, and flexibility.

Medical Applications

Since material jetting technologies can print with transparent or semitransparent materials, one of the most utilized features of material jetting in medical modeling is depicting distinct external and internal anatomy, items such as metal hardware, teeth roots, and tumors (Fig. 5.7). These machines usually print at finer layer thicknesses than the other technologies, allowing for fine-detailed structures to be well depicted. Many of these models aid medical personnel in surgical planning and prefitting equipment for both routine and highly complex surgical procedures.

Due to the ability to print with multiple types of materials including both flexible and rigid materials simultaneously, material jetting is well suited to create simulation/training models. Figure 5.8 shows an

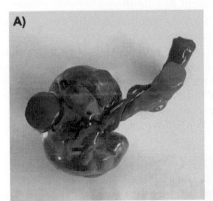
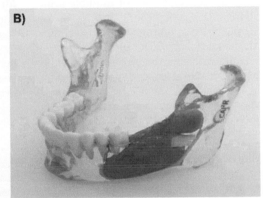

FIG. 5.7 **(A)** A kidney model with the kidney parenchyma (clear), tumor (pink), arteries (red), veins (blue), and collecting system (green). **(B)** A mandible model with the bone (clear), teeth (white), tumor (blue), and nerve (green). Both of these models were printed on the Stratasys J750 (Stratasys, Rehovot, Israel).

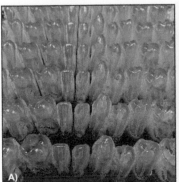
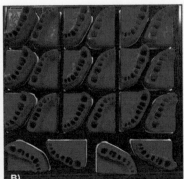
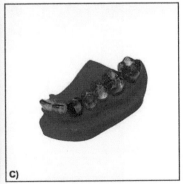

FIG. 5.8 **(A)** Teeth printed with material jetting on a Connex500 (Stratasys, Rehovot, Israel) still attached to the build platform with the body of the teeth (clear), and root canals highlighted with a very thin (faint) layer of blue and allowed to fill with support material. **(B)** Base model of the mandible with gums printed on a Fortus250mc (Stratasys, Rehovot, Israel) to hold the teeth during the simulation. **(C)** Final assembled model including the mandible/gums and teeth.

example of 3D printed root canal models printed on a material jetting machine (Connex500, Stratasys, Rehovot, Israel) with the teeth clear, the root canals highlighted in a light blue resin, and support material filling the inner canal. These teeth are used in combination with a base so dental residents and providers can practice root canal procedures.

BINDER JETTING

Binder jetting is a 3D printing process where a liquid bonding agent (binder/glue) is selectively added to join powder materials layer by layer (Fig. 5.9). In this process, the liquid substance is used to create an initial bond between the powder particles; however, usually the bond is weak and needs to be reinforced using infiltrates, a heat process, or both. The process begins with a layer of powder on a platform. One or multiple print heads move horizontally along the X- and Y-axes of the platform, applying a bonding agent(s) and, if equipped, color to the powder. As the material hardens, a new powder layer is drawn across the bed after the build platform lowers. The object is self-supported within the unbound powder bed, and once the part is completed, the remaining unbound material from around the part can be eliminated with a vacuum and

recycled. Upon removing the fragile model, all residual powder on the part is then blown away with air in an enclosed chamber. Finally, the brittle surface is hardened by infiltrating with cyanoacrylate, wax, resin, or another compound depending on the desired mechanical properties of the printed part.

Materials

Binder jetting materials can be divided into two main categories: sandstone such as gypsum printing and metal printing using metal powders. Full-colored parts can be printed with gypsum (using colored binders/inks and/or clear binders), but these models tend to be fragile with limited mechanical properties. Different types of metal powders are available including stainless steel, titanium, copper, and tungsten.

Medical Applications

For medical purposes, binder jetting systems are well suited to build colored anatomical training and presurgical planning models but can also serve as molds for the fabrication of facial prostheses, medical simulators, and specialty devices. Models created using this category may include veins, arteries, and other pathology where color can emphasize a distinct anatomical feature (Fig. 5.10).

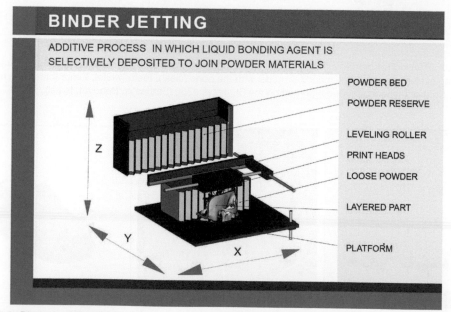

BINDER JETTING

ADDITIVE PROCESS IN WHICH LIQUID BONDING AGENT IS SELECTIVELY DEPOSITED TO JOIN POWDER MATERIALS

POWDER BED
POWDER RESERVE
LEVELING ROLLER
PRINT HEADS
LOOSE POWDER
LAYERED PART
PLATFORM

FIG. 5.9 Diagram of the Binder Jetting process. In this process, a binder is jetted on top of a powder layer. These machines have the ability to use color binders or print color onto a bound layer of the part. After these parts are built, an extraction and infusion process is needed to acquire a finished part. For metal parts, debinding and heat treatment steps are required. (Courtesy of Brandon Campbell, Walter Reed National Military Medical Center.)

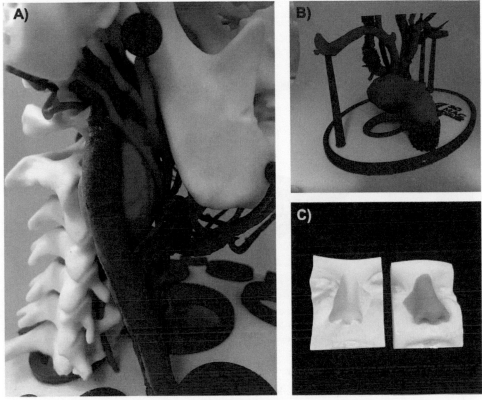

FIG. 5.10 Examples of models printed with binder jetting using a Zprinter 650, now known as Projet 660 Pro (3D Systems, Rock Hill, SC). **(A)** A paraganglioma (orange), in relation to the bony (white) and vascular anatomy of the neck with the veins (blue) and arteries (red). **(B)** An aortic arch aneurysm with surrounding and branching vessels along with a previously placed stent. **(C)** Mold (left) used to create a custom facial nasal prosthesis. The prosthesis (silicone nose) was molded using a flesh pigment within the silicone mixture.

POWDER BED FUSION

Powder bed fusion is a 3D printing process that uses thermal energy to selectively fuse precise regions of a powder bed's surface. The fusion is usually accomplished with an electron beam or laser. There are several common techniques which all fall under the powder bed fusion method including selective laser sintering (SLS), selective laser melting (SLM), electron beam melting (EBM), direct metal laser sintering (DMLS), direct metal laser melting (DMLM), and multi jet fusion. For each, the thermal energy used is the primary difference. Generally, powder bed fusion machines are capable of building some of the strongest 3D objects by sintering or melting polymers, pure metals, or metal alloys.

Materials

All powder bed fusion technologies use metals, except for SLS and multi jet fusion which use polymers. The most common polymers for SLS are nylons, which are lightweight and strong. Some other polymers include polyetherketones, polyaryletherketones, PC, polystyrenes, and thermoplastic elastomers (e.g., TPU). Metal powders used for SLM, DMLM, DMLS, or EBM include aluminum, gold, platinum, palladium, and pure titanium. Metal alloys such as cobalt chromium, titanium alloys, and stainless steel can also be used. The most common metals for medical applications are commercial pure titanium, titanium grade 23 (Ti6Al4V ELI), and cobalt chrome.

Polymer Printing (SLS and Multi Jet Fusion)

The SLS process begins with a blade or roller spreading thin layers of powder, over a platform from a reservoir of fresh material. As the platform lowers, a laser beam then selectively sinters the powder to solidify it. Once the layer is complete, a new layer of powdered material is deposited on top of the recently sintered layer, and this process proceeds layer by layer until the build is

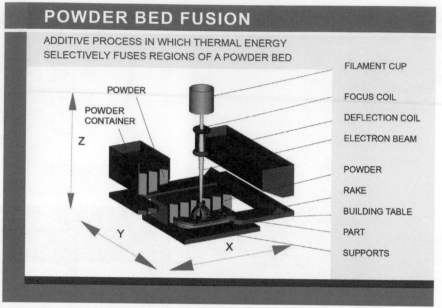

FIG. 5.11 Diagram of the Powder Bed Fusion process (Electron Beam Melting). Electron beam melting is used for melting metal powder together layer by layer using a high-energy beam (rather than a laser) to induce fusion between the metal powder. (Courtesy of Brandon Campbell, Walter Reed National Military Medical Center.)

complete. Support material is not necessary for building SLS parts, since the material which was not sintered/melted remains in place to support the model.

Multi jet fusion technology combines the thermal energy used for the fusion of materials, such as nylon or TPU, with the precise jetting of fusing and detailing agents onto the surface of the powder bed. These fusing and detailing agents along with fine temperature control allow for the manufacturing of highly accurate geometries. In addition, coloring agents can be added to the nylon material to achieve full color parts and models.

After printing, for both SLS and multi jet fusion, the parts remain hot and need to be allowed to cool before removal. After the cooling period, the manufactured parts, which are encapsulated in a block of lightly sintered powder, are blasted with air and other materials to remove the unfused powder. A part that is free of clumps and major debris with some remaining material can be brushed off manually or can be placed in a bead blaster to remove excess powder.

Metal Printing (DMLS, SLM, EBM, DMLM)

Metal powder bed fusion machines produce parts similar to SLS, with the main difference being that these machine types refer to melting metal media. SLM and DMLS both use a laser to melt metal powder forming

a physical 3D model. These laser builds require support structures in order to limit distortions and warping from occurring during the printing process by holding the part securely to the build platform. After printing, these parts require a heat treatment in order to relieve any residual stresses and then the models need to be physically cut from the build platform. Once the models are recovered, the fabricated supports are eliminated during post-processing by breaking them away from the part. Depending on the intended use, each piece is manually or mechanically finished, polished, cleaned with bead blasting, and possibly ultrasonically washed. Similarly, DMLM is a 3D printing process that builds parts by using a laser to selectively sinter (heat and fuse) a powdered material layer by layer.

EBM is a technology that uses a high-energy electron beam to melt, or essentially weld, raw metal materials, layer by layer in a vacuum (Fig. 5.11). Since this is a hot process with a heated bed and since the machine maintains elevated temperatures throughout the powder bed, these machines require longer cool-down phases. A postheat treatment to relieve residual stresses is not mandatory. However, this hot process causes the melted parts to be encapsulated in a block of lightly sintered powder, so the excess powder needs to be blasted away with identical powder to expose the part.

Medical Applications

The polymer powder bed fusion machines are usually used for medical models, surgical guides, orthotics, and prosthetic components which are generally manufactured from nylon. The metal-based machines allow numerous medical devices to be manufactured including implants, guides, and fixations for craniofacial injuries, dental and surgical devices, and orthopedic reconstructions, as well as specialty components or devices for prosthetics. Some examples of 3D printed metal parts printed with EBM are shown in Fig. 5.12.

DISCUSSION

As demonstrated above, a wide range of technologies can be utilized to create different types of 3D printed medical models. The type of technology will ultimately depend on what the model is being used for and what structures need to be visualized within the model.

In regard to materials, it should be noted that models used in the sterile field must be printed with biocompatible, sterilizable materials. For companies manufacturing and selling medical devices that come in direct or indirect contact with the human body, appropriate biological evaluation is carried out in accordance with FDA-2013-D-0350 or ISO 10993-1.[13] Currently, there is no formal guidance document for sterilization of medical devices which are printed in hospitals that come in direct or indirect contact with patients. However, several companies manufacture biocompatible materials and have recommended sterilization protocols which should be followed by anybody printing models in-house that will be utilized in the sterile field.

Different sterilization methods including steam sterilization (autoclave), ethylene oxide gas, and gamma ray ionizing radiation may be utilized[14,15]; and the appropriate method will depend on the printed material

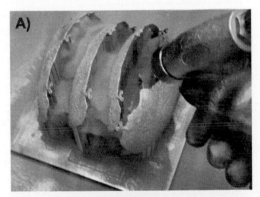
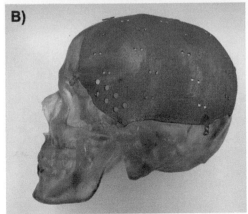
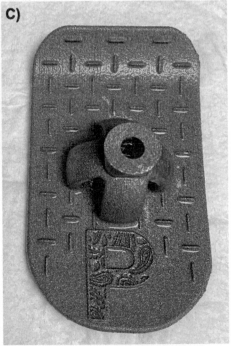

FIG. 5.12 Powder Bed Fusion parts printed with Arcam A1 (GE Additive, Cincinnati, OH). **(A)** Custom cranial implant plates being revealed, by blasting with additional titanium alloy powder, from a lightly sintered powder block after printing. **(B)** The finished 3D printed plate with fit verification on a skull printed with stereolithography. **(C)** This device, called a shorty foot, can be worn by bilateral above the knee amputees giving them the ability to ambulate like they are walking on their knees.

type. To validate proper sterilization, a combination of mechanical, chemical, biological, and cytotoxicity tests should be performed. Hospitals should establish internal validation methods and may partner with an external company to execute performance testing and validation on finished products printed and sterilized at the point of care. Upon model delivery, an instruction for use document should be included to ensure proper cleaning, sterilization, and storage prior to use.[14]

There have been many advancements of 3D printing over the past several years. Two of the major landscape changes have included the following: (1) large corporations have entered the field and have introduced new machines, materials, or acquired established companies within the 3D printing industry; and (2) major material companies have started to produce consumables for the 3D printing industry. These major trends across most technologies allow for increased speed of deliverables and provide a larger variety of materials.

Smaller, cheaper machines within vat photopolymerization and material extrusion (approximately a 5th to 10th the cost of previous machines) are changing the landscape with regard to the availability of onsite hospital manufacturing. This cost reduction has allowed many hospitals economic freedom to purchase this technology and print smaller cases in house. In addition, material extrusion has seen the introduction of machines with larger build platforms (1 m × 1 m or larger). These larger machines may not be widely utilized in anatomical modeling; however, medium to large machines may be useful in prosthetics and assistive technology applications. Material extrusion was the first technology type to have open platform capabilities and less restrictions on the materials, most likely stemming from the maker movement. This has allowed a whole host of different materials infiltrated with anything from carbon fiber to metals. Many of these machines can now print layer thicknesses near or below 100 microns. Material extrusion has also seen the implementation of labeling and coloring the filament with inks during the printing process enabling the creation of full-colored material extrusion parts.[16] There are also machines that increase bond strength of the layers within a part by nanocoating filaments and using electrical current.[17]

Similar to vat photopolymerization, material jetting has also seen many changes over the past several years. The major enhancement has been the introduction of machines which can have up to seven different materials loaded at a time. This enables the operator the ability to print in the full color spectrum, or different durometers by mixing the loaded materials. These printers, which have full color capability, are still priced on the upper end of the spectrum for both the technology and materials; however, the translucent capability in combination with multicolor internal geometry is currently unique to this printer technology. Other advancements include one manufacturer meeting the Pantone Validated standards of color quality and realism and the use of materials and structures to mimic biological tissues.[18] Smaller, cheaper, full-color machines have been launched, however, by price, would still be viewed as commercial systems.[19] There have been no major trends seen by the authors in regard to the creations of open systems for material jetting.

Binder jetting has stayed pretty similar to its roots in regard to medical 3D printing. The main printers used for medical purposes still use gypsum-based compounds as their base element and then binders/colorants are used to bond the parts together. Infiltration after printing is still done using primarily cyanoacrylate and/or wax. Recently, a renewed rise in metals has been seen, but this has yet to thoroughly impact the medical field, especially within a hospital. In addition, metal binder jetting usually involves additional postprocessing procedures which may include debinding soak and a heat treatment.

Metal powder bed fusion has seen advancements in build monitoring, surface finishing, and speed. The overall aspects of the process using a laser or electron beam remain unchanged. EBM has replaced the filament with a single crystalline cathode. Multibeam technology or multiple lasers have been incorporated to speed up build times. Many manufactures now have some simultaneous or "real-time" part quality verification systems.[20] In addition, a new method of printing nylon and TPU material has entered this category where activating and detailing agents are jetted on the surface of the powder and used in conjunction with a heat source to fuse layers together.

Currently, the overarching layering principle dictates the technology category; however, hybrid manufacturing methods are being developed to include multiple of the currently available technologies or by combining 3D printing technologies with subtractive processes. It is definitely certain that in the case of color and releasing agents, without these additives the machine would not be capable of providing these added benefits. Other new trends involving the digital "cloud," especially when relating to performance analysis, have been introduced. Cloud-based analyses allow manufacturing companies to monitor their system from abroad and, in some instances, predict when problems will arise.

In addition, "Open Platforms" have allowed major chemical companies to produce new materials changing the mechanical properties and economics of 3D printing materials, thus altering 3D printing as a whole. Open systems or modes allow users the freedom to choose from a multitude of material vendors, thus potentially leading to more choices, competition, and cost reductions. There has also been a focused reintroduction of flexible materials that can be used for a variety of applications ranging from vascular modeling to orthotics and simulators.

CONCLUSIONS

Each printing technology has its own advantages, and the optimal printer for medical applications will depend on the final use of the printed part. In addition, all printers have a specific cleaning method depending on the material and the use of the printed part. This post-processing generally requires additional auxiliary equipment requiring added floor or countertop space.

The information in this chapter has provided a general overview of 3D printing technologies, materials, and medical applications. When deciding which technology to purchase, a facility must consider initial hardware cost, size, speed, environment, materials, accessory equipment, and maintenance cost. In addition to all equipment considerations, labor needs to be a main priority. Dedicated or partially dedicated personnel to perform all digital operations and operate the equipment is essential to successfully running and maintaining a 3D printing lab. In the end, each facility needs to make decisions to meet their needs. In many cases, hospital-based 3D printing labs expand over the years as the applications increase, technology advances, costs decrease, and utilization becomes widespread. Further considerations for starting a 3D printing lab are discussed in Chapter 15.

REFERENCES

1. Hull C. *Apparatus for Production of Three-Dimensional Objects by Stereolithography*. United States patent US 4,575,330A; 1986. Available at: https://patents.google.com/patent/US4575330A/en.
2. Crump SS. *Apparatus and Method for Creating Three-Dimensional Objects*. United States patent US 5121329A; 1989. Available at: https:patents.google.com/patent/US5121329.
3. ISO. *Additive Manufacturing - General Principles - Part 1: Terminology*; 2015 [Cited 2020 June 27, 2020]. Available from: https://www.iso.org/obp/ui/#iso:std:iso:17296:-1:dis:ed-1:v1:en.
4. ISO. *Additive Manufacturing — General Principles — Part 2: Overview of Process Categories and Feedstock*; 2015 [Cited June 27, 2020]. Available from: https://www.iso.org/standard/61626.html.
5. ISO/ASTM. *ISO/ASTM 52900(en) Additive manufacturing — General principles — Terminology*; 2018 [Cited June 27, 2020]; Available from: https://www.iso.org/obp/ui/#iso:std:iso-astm:52900:dis:ed-2:v1:en.
6. Formlabs. *Form 3*; 2019 [Cited 2020 June 27, 2020]. Available from: https://formlabs.com/3d-printers/form-3/.
7. Hornbeck LJ. *Multi-level Digital Micromirror Device*. United States patent US5583688A; 1993. Available at: https://patents.google.com/patent/US5583688A/en.
8. Panzer M, Tumbleston J. *Continuous Liquid Interface Production with Upconversion Photopolymerization*. United States patent US20180126630A1; 2017. Available at: https://patents.google.com/patent/US20180126630A1/en?q=continuous+liquid+interface+production&oq=continuous | liquid | interface+production.
9. NewPro3D. *ILI(TM) Technology*; 2020 [Cited August 3, 2020]. Available from: https://newpro3d.com/ili-technology/.
10. 3DSystems. *Figure 4*; 2020 [August 3, 2020]. Available from: https://www.3dsystems.com/3d-printers/figure-4-standalone?smtNoRedir=1&_ga=2.83862038.1088134540.1596462088-2046461963.1596462088.
11. Stratasys. *FDM Trademark Information*; 1991 [June 27, 2020]. Available from: https://trademark.trademarkia.com/fdm-74133656.html.
12. DesktopMetal. *Studio System(TM)*; 2020 [August 5, 2020]. Available from: https://www.desktopmetal.com/products/studio.
13. FDA Center for Devices, Radiological Health. Use of International Standard ISO 10993-1, "Biological evaluation of medical devices — part 1: evaluation and testing within a risk management process". In: *Guidance for Industry and Food and Drug Administration Staff*; 2016 [August 3, 2020]. Available from: https://www.fda.gov/regulatory-information/search-fda-guidance-documents/use-international-standard-iso-10993-1-biological-evaluation-medical-devices-part-1-evaluation-and.
14. Association of Surgical Technologists. *Standards of Practice for the Decontamination of Surgical Instruments*. 2009.
15. Rutala WA, Weber DJ, The HICPAC. *Guideline for Disinfection and Sterilization in Healthcare Facilities*. 2008. Update: May 2019.
16. XRIZE. *The World's First Industrial 3D Printing Solution for Creating Vibrant, Full Color Functional Parts with Minimal Post-Processing*. [Cited August 3, 2020]. Available from:: https://rize3d.com/printers.
17. Essentium. *Flashfuse*. [Cited August 3, 2020]. Available from:: https://www.essentium.com/flashfuse/.
18. Stratasys. *3D Printing with PANTONE® Colors*; 2020 [Cited August 3, 2020]. Available from: https://www.stratasys.com/fr/~/media/Files/Best%20Practices/BP_PJ_3DPrintingWithPantone_0419a.
19. Stratasys. *Stratasys J55™ 3D Printer*; 2020 [Cited August 3, 2020]. Available from: https://www.stratasys.com/3d-printers/j55.
20. SLM Solutions. *Additive Quality*. [Cited August 3, 2020]. Available from:: https://www.slm-solutions.com/en/products/software/additivequality/.

CHAPTER 6

3D Printed Anatomic Models and Guides

AMY E. ALEXANDER, BME, MS • NICOLE WAKE, PHD

INTRODUCTION

Three-dimensional (3D) printed anatomic models and guides designed from volumetric medical imaging data are used clinically to provide increased comprehension of anatomy, more exact pathology evaluation, and more precise surgical intervention. Historically, obtaining a 3D printed patient-specific anatomic model was typically made possible through independent companies, several of which began building anatomic models for surgeons in the early to mid-1990s.[1–3] Today, a variety of third party companies provide services in which they accept medical imaging data and produce high quality 3D printed anatomic models. However, in order to bring 3D printing closer to the patient, decrease costs, and expedite the time required to get patient-specific 3D printed models and guides, many hospitals in the United States (US) and world are building 3D printing labs to provide this service in-house, in real time, and in response to trauma and other time-sensitive procedures.[4,5] From 2010 to 2016, the number of hospitals in the US with a centralized 3D printing laboratory grew from 3 to 99.[4,5] As of July 2019, at least 268 hospitals worldwide have adopted this innovative approach to patient care.[4,5] Given the consistent growth in production of 3D printed anatomic models and guides at the point of care over the last decade, continued growth is expected.[4–6] Through the use of illustrative case examples, this chapter provides readers with a detailed understanding of this advanced application of 3D printing technology in today's medical practice.

ANATOMIC MODELS

3D printed anatomic models offer a tangible extension of medical imaging that can be understood by a diverse audience quickly and easily. An anatomic model can help physicians communicate with their patients with a high level of clarity and understanding; two-dimensional (2D) imaging on a flat screen cannot compete. Trying to explain imaging findings with 2D imaging to patients who may not have in-depth knowledge of cross-sectional anatomy may prove challenging. By isolating individual anatomies, implanted devices, and pathologies, radiologists are able to relay spatial relationships of internal anatomical components that are otherwise difficult to view.

Anatomic models are built from 3D meshes of anatomy generated through the segmentation of medical imaging data and subsequent computer-aided design (CAD) modeling.[6,7] First, Digital Imaging and Communication in Medicine (DICOM) images are acquired from any imaging modality with volumetric imaging capability.[6] Commonly used modalities include computed tomography (CT), magnetic resonance imaging (MRI), or ultrasound.[6] High spatial resolution images with low signal-to-noise ratio and thin slice thicknesses are preferred.[6] Once imaging is selected, segmentation is performed via placement of regions of interest (ROIs) around the desired tissues.[6] Various dedicated software packages are available for the segmentation of 3D medical images, and the segmentation of appropriate ROIs can be obtained automatically using algorithms such as thresholding, edge detection, and region growing, or manually (see Chapter 3). Segmentation times range substantially and will depend on the imaging quality, use of automated techniques, and user's experience level. Segmented ROIs are then converted to a CAD file format such as the commonly used stereolithography (STL) format for editing and exportation to facilitate recognition by 3D printing software.[8] The STL format is currently the most common file type and it is used in all cases in this chapter.

Before printing, STL files are verified to ensure anatomical accuracy through a defined quality assurance plan, and then imported to the designated 3D printing software.[7,9] The model is oriented to minimize

3D Printing for the Radiologist. https://doi.org/10.1016/B978-0-323-77573-1.00017-8

printing time and optimize final part material properties, and printing materials are selected based on provider needs, printer specifications, and anatomic tissue type. Next, STL files are sent to the printer, and the 3D model is printed. Printing times vary depending on printer type, printing layer height and resolution, number of materials, and size of the object. Finally, post-processing is performed to remove support material and to enhance the appearance of the printed item. As this process of converting DICOM data to STL format is unfamiliar to many radiologists, a typical workflow is demonstrated in Table 6.1.[6,7,9]

Fig. 6.1 illustrates the creation of a life-sized model of a thoracic cavity tumor surrounded by important

TABLE 6.1
Overview of General 3D Printing Workflow Used to Create Anatomic Models and Guides From Radiological Imaging Data.[7,8]

1. Image Acquisition	2. Image Segmentation	3. CAD Modeling	4. 3D Printing
- High-resolution volumetric dataset - CT, MRI, or ultrasound are most common - Other volumetric modalities or surface scanning may be used	- Select anatomical structures by delineating different ROIs - Confirm contours of segmented anatomy pre-CAD	- Create digital models - Perform minor or major modifications to anatomic model - Confirm contours of anatomic models post-CAD	- Select printer and materials - Print model - Perform model postprocessing - Perform QA

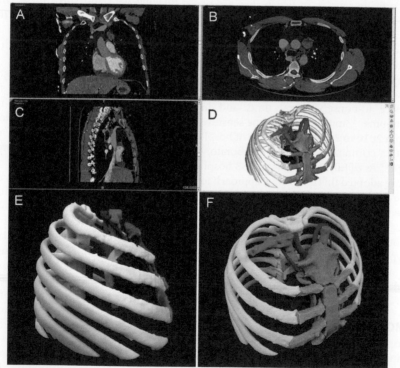

FIG. 6.1 Segmentation, CAD, and 3D printed anatomic model of adult malignant thymoma tumor. Included: thymoma tumor (dark purple), adjacent thrombus (teal), aorta (magenta), superior vena cava (dark blue), spine and ribs (white), sternum (light purple), and cartilage (pink). **(A)**: Coronal view of segmentation. **(B)**: Axial view of segmentation. **(C)**: Sagittal view of segmentation. **(D)**: Isometric view CAD model generated from segmented anatomies. **(E)**: Sagittal view of 3D printed anatomic model. **(F)**: Isometric view of 3D printed anatomic model. Mayo Clinic, Rochester, MN, USA.

structures including the ribs and sternum, cartilage, lungs, cardiac structures, aorta, and superior and inferior vena cava. This type of model can help to quickly bring a surgical team up to speed on how the tumor is entangled in otherwise healthy tissue and can help to form a communication bridge between radiologist, surgeon, operating room (OR) team, and patient.[9–11] When printed in tissue mimicking materials, anatomic models such as this can also facilitate the rehearsal and practice of complex procedures on a patient's specific anatomy prior to entering the OR.[11]

Simple Anatomic Models

Anatomic models are all derived from some variety of medical imaging, and radiology plays in integral role in model generation. Whether they are simple single-part or complex multimodality models, 3D printed anatomic models can be used as powerful communication tools between surgeon and patient, surgeon and care team, and surgeon and pathologist. Two use cases are shown to illustrate the clinical need behind the creation of a simple anatomic model. To generalize, a simple model is created from one data series from one imaging study and does not require advanced manipulation of data, e.g., coregistration of multiple imaging modalities or use of advanced CAD tools. Development and design of a simple model may require less time, but time required is still affected by quality of imaging and complexity of ROI. Simple models are held to the same high standard of quality assurance as complex models.[7,9]

Case 1

An orthopedic surgeon prepared to treat a 67-year-old male with a massive rotator cuff tear and osteoarthritis of the right shoulder with a reverse total shoulder arthroplasty, a procedure in which implants are used to turn the proximal humerus into the socket and the scapular glenoid into the ball of the joint.[12] Day one of patient care included CT imaging and surgical consultation; surgery was planned for day four, so segmentation, CAD, printing, cleaning, and post-processing all took place within a 48 h period. The orthopedic surgeon requested 3D printed models of the humerus and scapula to rehearse the procedure and reference during the operation. Since bone is best depicted on CT and no vasculature was requested, the imaging series selected was a soft-tissue reconstruction kernel with 2.0 mm slice thickness and no intravenous contrast. Choosing the soft-tissue kernel as opposed to the sharp for bone segmentation may seem counterintuitive, but the soft-tissue series is superior for medical imaging segmentation due to the noise that can occur in a sharp-kernel reconstruction, which translates to the mesh surfaces. The humerus and scapula were segmented and initial ROI contours were reviewed by a radiologist. In the CAD environment, the 3D meshes of the bones were run through a smoothing algorithm with appropriate parameters so as to not alter the overall surface contours of the parts. The humerus and scapula were stamped with an accession number from the original modeling order for traceability, and contours of the final STLs were reviewed over the imaging to confirm anatomical accuracy. The 3D printing technology was selected in accordance with the surgeon's needs. In this case, a ProJet CJP 660Pro (3D Systems, Rock Hill, SC) binder jetting printer was selected. Since this technology allows input files with color, both parts were assigned Pantone's "Bone" RGB values and exported as ZPR files for input to the ProJet CJP 660Pro. The files were printed and the final parts were infiltrated in paraffin wax to best simulate the feel of bone in accordance with the surgeon's preference (Fig. 6.2).

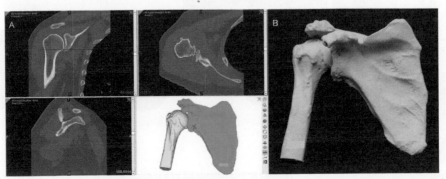

FIG. 6.2 Segmentation, CAD, and 3D printed anatomic model of the proximal right humerus and full right scapula for use in planning and rehearsal for a reverse TSA. **(A)**: Image segmentation with virtual model shown in lower right quadrant. **(B)**: 3D printed scapula and humerus printed in Pantone Bone White© and infiltrated with paraffin wax. Mayo Clinic, Rochester, MN, USA.

Case 2

A vascular surgeon prepared to treat a 41-year-old female with a Type A aortic dissection in the arch and right subclavian arteries and engulfing the ascending aorta. Treatment options, including the endovascular placement of a commercial stent, were being evaluated and a model of the true and false lumens was requested. In order to properly segment the blood pool and capture the false lumen wall, a high quality contrast-enhanced CT was selected, and a series with 2.0 mm slice thickness and a soft-tissue reconstruction kernel was selected. The true and false lumens were segmented as separate parts and calculated into 3D meshes, smoothed, and the descending aorta was trimmed just inferior to the heart. To best visualize the dissection, the model was printed with material jetting on an Objet500 Connex3 printer (Stratasys, Eden Prairie, MN). When loading the STLs into the printing software as an assembly, the true lumen was assigned a semiclear material and the false lumen was assigned an opaque magenta. To maximize the transparency of the true lumen, the model was clear-coated after support material was removal via water jetting. The final model worked to illustrate the extent of the false lumen within the true lumen (Fig. 6.3).

Complex Anatomic Models

Complex anatomic models can include more than one bone or anatomic part, and are often derived from a number of data series. In many cases, coregistration of either imaging data from multiple series or even modalities is required. Coregistration is also commonly performed on 3D parts from a variety of series data, where bone is often the fixed entity and all other

elements align. Complex models may also include anatomy that has been significantly altered or manipulated from the "as-scanned" state to further facilitate surgical planning or other intervention. Examples include mirroring anatomy, resecting or reconstructing anatomy, or designing grafts.[9,13] Developing a complex anatomic model with multiple parts follows a similar workflow as described for a simple anatomic model. The imaging series is selected, segmentation takes place, CAD modeling follows, contour review is performed, and the model is 3D printed. Several use cases for complex anatomic models are described below.

Case 1

An orthopedic surgeon prepared to treat a 26-year-old female with a right posterior pelvic osteosarcoma tumor and a complex venous malformation. In this case, the surgeon requested a pelvic tumor model which included bone, veins, arteries, ureters, bladder, and tumor to assist with surgical planning of tumor resection amidst the dangerous vascular malformation. Therefore, imaging that allowed for reasonable segmentation of each requested anatomic element was required. A triphase contrast-enhanced CT study was selected as it was the optimal choice with arterial, venous, and urogram phases. All three reconstructions were done with a soft-tissue kernel and had slice thicknesses of 2.0 mm. Each of the three phase series was segmented accordingly: the arterial phase was used to segment bone and arteries, the venous phase was used to segment veins, and the urogram phase was used to segment the ureters and bladder. Since a triphase study is collected sequentially as the contrast moves through the circulatory system, either the imaging series

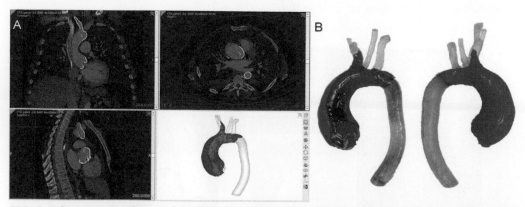

FIG. 6.3 Segmentation, CAD, and 3D printed anatomic model of the ascending aorta with Type A dissection for use in planning surgical intervention. **(A)**: Image segmentation with virtual model shown in lower right quadrant with the true lumen (clear) and the false lumen (magenta). **(B)**: Anterior and posterior views of the 3D printed model. Mayo Clinic, Rochester, MN, USA.

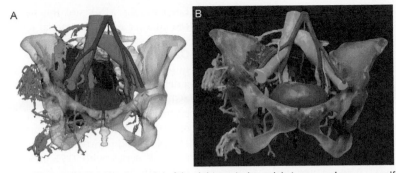

FIG. 6.4 CAD and 3D printed anatomic model of the right posterior pelvic tumor and venous malformation. **(A)**: Snapshot of the CAD model. **(B)**: 3D printed model; bones (clear) connecting cylinders (clear), arteries (magenta), veins and venous malformation (blue), bladder and ureters (clear/pink). Mayo Clinic, Rochester, MN, USA.

themselves or the corresponding segmented parts needed to be coregistered to one primary series to account for differences in timing and motion. In this case, the primary series selected was the arterial phase as it was used to segment bone, and the parts segmented from the venous and urogram phases were coregistered using N-point registration of the pelvic bone and accompanying anatomic elements. Additional CAD modeling was necessary to ensure that each part remained in its proper anatomical position after 3D printing. Thin cylinders were added as struts to strengthen the model at specific weak points, e.g., the venous malformation on the patient's right side was connected to the bone. This case was built on a material jetting printer (Objet500 Connex3, Stratasys, Eden Prairie, MN) with the bone in a clear material to allow for visualization of the intrusion of the tumor (dark purple) along with the other pertinent anatomical structures (Fig. 6.4).

Case 2

An ear, nose, and throat surgeon prepared to treat a 19-year-old male with a left lymphovascular tumor and vascular malformation. The model was requested to aid in surgical planning and discussion of options with the care team, and the extent of the tumor and vascular malformation were of high importance. To properly segment both the tumor and the vascular malformation in addition to the bone and detail of the orthodontia hardware, a noncontrast soft-tissue reconstruction kernel CT image series with a slice thickness of 0.6 mm was selected. Maxilla, mandible, hardware, vascular malformation, and tumor were segmented from this series. An important element of the model was to visualize bone interacting with tumor, which could require a multimaterial printer with clear material loaded, as shown in Complex Case 1. Alternatively, in this case, the surfaces of the vascular malformation and tumor meshes were converted to lattices as illustrated in Fig. 6.5. This is a

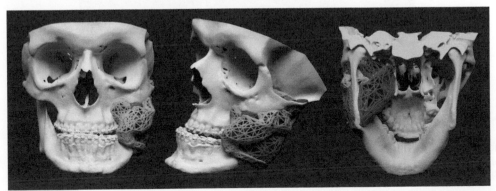

FIG. 6.5 3D printed model of mandible and maxilla including orthodontia hardware and both vascular malformation (blue) and tumor (red). Mayo Clinic, Rochester, MN, USA.

highly technical CAD operation, and works well to provide transparency on a single-material printer. This model was printed on a powder bed fusion printer (HP Jet Fusion 580 Color, HP, Palo Alto, CA).

Case 3

An orthopedic surgeon prepared to treat a 28-year-old female with rapidly progressive thoracolumbar spinal deformity and dural ectasia (DE). Medical history included a spinal fusion at age 5, which is the source of the hardware shown in the models. In order to best visualize the remaining native spine and hardware, the bone, the DE, and hardware were segmented from a noncontrast soft-tissue reconstruction kernel CT series with 0.75 mm slices. Two models with different goals were 3D printed. In the first model, bone, including a short distance of ribs and sacrum, was printed in white with hardware in blue. A second model was developed specifically to show the extent of the DE in the thoracic and lumbar spine, so bone was printed in a clear material, the DE in a clear/blue, and the hardware in blue. The bone in the second model was trimmed to decrease print time. Both models were printed with material jetting on an Objet500 Connex3 printer (Stratasys,

Eden Prairie, MN) and the second model was clear-coated after support material removal (Fig. 6.6).

Case 4

In some cases, mirroring healthy anatomy to the side of a defect can help in symmetrical reconstruction.[9] Here, a plastic surgeon specializing in facial reconstruction prepared to treat a 20-year-old male with a trauma-related right orbital floor fracture with a MEDPOR TITAN implant (Stryker, Kalamazoo, MI). A noncontrast CT series with 0.75 mm slice thickness and a soft-tissue reconstruction kernel was selected for segmentation. The skull, including maxilla and orbits, was segmented into one part and brought into the CAD environment. A sagittal midline plane through the center of the nasal and clivus bones was placed by the surgeon and radiologist. The skull was then mirrored about that plane in order to generate a carbon copy of the healthy left orbit on the patient's right side. The surgeon fine-tuned the location of the mirrored orbital floor using translate and rotate tools, and the mirrored part was fused with the patient's native fractured bone. A trimmed version of this fusion was printed in a biocompatible material that could be

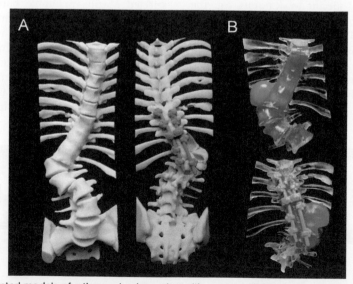

FIG. 6.6 3D printed models of a thoracolumbar spine with osseous deformity and dural ectasia (DE). **(A)**: Anterior (left) and posterior (right) views of the full spine model with bone (white) and hardware (blue). **(B)**: Anterior (top) and posterior (bottom) views of the trimmed spine model with bone (clear), DE (clear/blue), and hardware (blue). Mayo Clinic, Rochester, MN, USA.

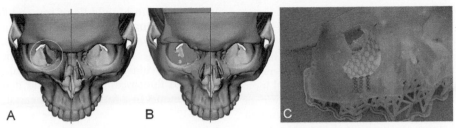

FIG. 6.7 3D printed anatomic model for orbital floor implant preparation. **(A)**: Illustration of right orbital floor fracture and midline plane. **(B)**: Healthy left orbital floor mirrored about the midline plane to the patient's right side. **(C)**: 3D print of the mirrored left fused with fractured right orbit to allow for implant contouring in the OR. Mayo Clinic, Rochester, MN, USA.

sterilized via steam sterilization and used in the OR to contour the implant (Fig. 6.7).

Another way to enhance the visibility of inner structures is to make planar cuts within the model, print in multiple pieces, and attach anatomic elements with magnets. When including a magnetic component, generating properly sized holes in the planes prior to printing is required, with magnets glued in after model postprocessing. The hole can be generated by subtracting a cylinder that is slightly larger the magnet in the magnet's location; offsetting the magnet dimensions by 0.15 mm in both diameter and depth to allow for glue is typically sufficient. Hollowing out the segmented anatomy can also serve to generate a fabricated wall of an arbitrary thickness chosen to ensure structural integrity of the model.

Case 5

A cardiac and endovascular surgery team prepared to treat a 67-year-old male with an aortic pseudoaneurysm with endovascular placement stent-graft.[13] A contrast-enhanced cardiac CT scan captured during diastole with 0.75 mm slices and a soft-tissue reconstruction kernel was selected for segmentation. The blood pool, pseudoaneurysm, and existing prosthesis were segmented as separate parts. This cardiac model, printed with binder jetting on a ProJet 660Pro (3D Systems, Rock Hill, SC), shows the hollowing technique to create an artificial but semirealistic rigid wall around the segmented blood pool, as well as the coronal planar cut and magnet additions (Fig. 6.8).

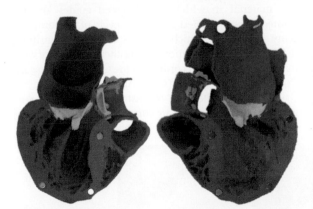

FIG. 6.8 Rigid 3D printed anatomic model of the left ventricle (red), pseudoaneurysm (beige), and prosthesis (gray). Model split at the long axis with embedded magnets to facilitate internal anatomical visibility. Mayo Clinic, Rochester, MN, USA.

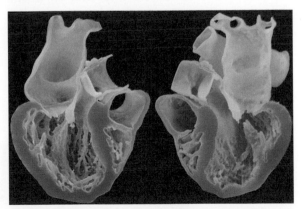

FIG. 6.9 Flexible 3D printed anatomic model of the left ventricle (pink), pseudoaneurysm (clear/white), and prosthesis (white). Model split at the long axis to facilitate internal anatomical visibility, and printed in flexible materials to aid in surgical rehearsal. Mayo Clinic, Rochester, MN, USA.

Anatomic Models for Simulation and Rehearsal

Printing models in materials that are tissue-mimicking that can be used for surgical simulation and rehearsal takes anatomic modeling a step further. By leveraging 3D printing technologies with multiple material input options, anatomic models with structures of varying flexibilities and hardness qualities can be created. Soft-tissue structures can be printed in soft materials or mixtures of materials that print in different durometers. One common application of this technique is printing cardiac models with structures in varying levels of stiffness for hands-on training of congenital and structural heart surgery techniques.[14-16]

Case 1

The same model as shown in Fig. 6.8 was printed with the Objet500 Connex3 material jetting printer (Stratasys, Eden Prairie, MN) in a flexible material without magnet holes for use as a simulation model (Fig. 6.9). Printing with different 3D printing technologies to expand the model's usability is a clever and efficient way to increase the value of the segmentation and CAD work.

Case 2

Hollowed patient-specific vascular models for procedural rehearsal with fluoroscopy are another example of how 3D printing can be used for surgical simulation.[17-20] Herein, an endovascular surgeon prepared to treat a 78-year-old male with an 85 mm abdominal aortic aneurysm using a fenestrated endograft. A contrast-enhanced CT with a 0.75 mm slice thickness and a soft-tissue reconstruction kernel was used to segment the blood pool. The 3D mesh was smoothed, hollowed, and specially designed connectors were added to facilitate connection to a pulsatile pump.[18] The model was printed with material jetting (Objet500 Connex3, Stratasys, Eden Prairie, MN),

using a mixture of rigid VeroClear and flexible Agilus (Fig. 6.10). Once connected to the 3D printed model, a pump ran water at physiological pressure, temperature, flow rate, and rhythm through the model, and the endovascular team catheterized, injected contrast, and used fluoroscopy to place and deploy the stent on the model in a full surgical rehearsal.

ANATOMIC GUIDES

3D printed anatomic guides are patient-specific tools built from medical imaging data that offer assistance with procedures and tasks requiring a high level of precision.[21-44] The use of patient-specific anatomic guides in surgical procedures has been shown to decrease surgical time and improve both accuracy and patient outcomes.[21-44] Patient-specific anatomic guides are built from the digital surface meshes of anatomic models. Therefore, the same foundational image acquisition, segmentation, and CAD principles are involved and required to develop an accurate, patient-specific anatomic guide. In the surgical practice, anatomic guides are often referred to as surgical guides. When designing surgical guides, biomedical engineers receive input from a surgical team on how the procedure will be carried out. Next, this multidisciplinary team discusses the possibilities and anatomic access during the procedure, and chooses a feasible and surgically assistive anatomic guide plan. Patient-specific and procedure-specific surgical anatomic guides are then designed to help carry out the surgical plan in the OR. The material in which the designed guides are 3D printed must be tested to certain levels of biocompatibility and sterility, which can be done through sensitization, toxicity, and irritation testing after compliance with instructions for use according to the Centers for Disease Control and Prevention (CDC, Atlanta, GA, USA).

In craniomaxillofacial reconstructive and facial surgery, free flap procedures are common; digitally planning

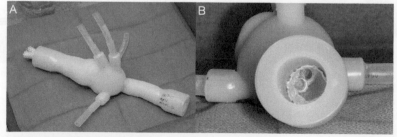

FIG. 6.10 Semiflexible 3D printed anatomic model of an abdominal aortic aneurysm. **(A)**: Hollowed abdominal aortic aneurysm model designed to connect to a pulsatile water pump which simulates vascular flow during practice catheterization and stent deployment under fluoroscopy. **(B)**: Axial view of fenestrated endograft deployed within the 3D printed model. Mayo Clinic, Rochester, MN, USA.

the resections and reconstructions serves as a precursor to the design and 3D print of patient-specific anatomic cutting and templating guides.[22–27,29,33,38,40–43] In a free flap procedure, either autologous or donor bone is used to reconstruct an area where bone was lacking, and one of the most common free flaps selected is the fibula.[45,46] The precision of the lengths and angles at which the fibula is cut are paramount to successful craniomaxillofacial reconstruction for both function and aesthetics. Therefore, using guides that effectively carry out the surgeon's digital plan is growing in popularity worldwide.[22–27,29,33,38,40–43] In orthopedic surgery, an osteotomy plane, or set of planes, may be digitally placed, and an anatomic guide can be designed and printed to fit to bone and guide the surgical saw to complete the osteotomy.[28,30–32,34,39,44] In the pathology practice, anatomic guides, referred to as cutting guides, can be used to cut through specimens at exact thicknesses.[21] Cutting through specimen tissue at the same axial slice thickness as preoperative medical imaging is one example of this application. Cutting guides may be designed for a particular specimen, 3D printed, and used to slice the specimen with a high degree of precision. For example, a prostate specimen with cancerous lesions sliced using a cutting guide allows for analysis at a level more consistent with pathological standards (See Fig. 4.8). In addition, specimens sliced at the same interval as preoperative radiological data allow for slice-by-slice comparisons for educational purposes.

Common types of anatomic guides created in the hospital setting include osteotomy cutting guides and drilling trajectory guides. In the following clinical illustrative examples, segmentation and CAD of the anatomic structures are completed before the surgical team is called in to digitally place osteotomies.

Case 1

An otorhinolaryngology surgeon prepared to treat a 55-year-old female with anterior mandible secondary malignant neoplasm and osteonecrosis due to substance abuse with a three-segment vascularized left fibular free flap mandibular reconstruction.[45,46] A noncontrast-enhanced CT with a 0.75 mm slice thickness and a soft-tissue reconstruction kernel was selected to segment remaining native bone. The mandibular bone was segmented and the surgical team was called upon to place the osteotomy planes and perform the digital reconstruction with the fibula. Fig. 6.11 shows the placement of osteotomy planes, utilization of the anatomic guide to execute the osteotomies, resection of the defect

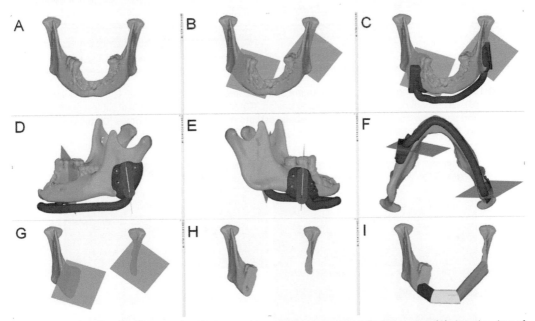

FIG. 6.11 Mandibular cutting guide for reconstruction with three-segment fibula free flap. **(A)**: Anterior view of native mandible bone with osteonecrosis. **(B)**: Osteotomy planes placed by surgeon. **(C)**: Mandibular cutting guide designed by biomedical engineer. **(D)**: Left view of mandibular cutting guide. **(E)**: Right view of mandibular cutting guide. **(F)**: Inferior view of mandibular cutting guide. **(G)**: Native remaining mandible bones with osteotomy planes. **(H)**: Native remaining mandible bones. **(I)**: Final reconstructed mandible with three-segment fibular free flap. Mayo Clinic, Rochester, MN, USA.

and resulting remaining native mandibular bones, and proposed mandibular reconstruction with a three-segment fibular free flap. Fig. 6.12 shows an additional guide created to aid in the osteotomies for the three-segment fibular flap. Fig. 6.13 shows a final quality assurance step of reviewing contours of the designed cutting guide on the original radiological imaging data to ensure the osteotomy planes designed in the guide would indeed carry out the cuts planned by the surgeon. All guides for this case were printed in Dental SG resin on a Form 2 (Formlabs, Cambridge, MA), a vat photopolymerization printer, post-processed, including ultraviolet (UV) curing, and sterilized via steam sterilization, also known as autoclave, prior to use in the OR.

Case 2

An orthopedic surgeon prepared to treat a 15-year-old male with periosteal osteosarcoma tumor of the left femur measuring 6.0 × 6.0 × 14.0 cm. The preferred treatment was a femoral resection and reconstruction with a left femoral allograft donated from a cadaver. To prepare for digital reconstruction, both the patient and the allograft were scanned. First, to segment the native bone and osteosarcoma, a noncontrast-enhanced CT with a 1.0 mm slice thickness and a soft-tissue reconstruction kernel was utilized. In addition, to best identify the true extent of the tumor and its margins, and because soft tissue is generally better visualized and segmented from MRI data, a T2-weighted

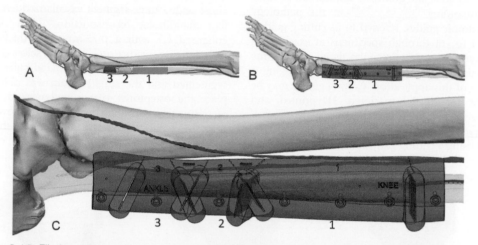

FIG. 6.12 Fibular cutting guide for three-segment fibular free flap. **(A)**: Segments 1, 2, and 3 selected by surgeon. **(B)**: Gross view of fibular cutting guide design. **(C)**: Magnified view of fibular cutting guide with segment and anatomic and segment number labels, osteotomy slots, and screw holes for guide attachment. Mayo Clinic, Rochester, MN, USA.

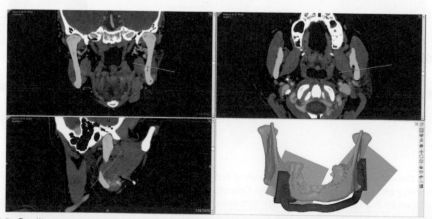

FIG. 6.13 Quality assurance of contours for the mandibular cutting guide design. Mask, 3D mesh, and contours of the mandible (blue), 3D mesh and contours of the osteotomy planes (green), and 3D mesh and contours of the mandibular anatomic guide (orange). Mayo Clinic, Rochester, MN, USA.

coronal MRI with a 0.66 mm × 0.66 mm pixel resolution and a 5.0 mm slice thickness was used to segment the tumor and a rough estimate of bone, focusing on landmarks that would facilitate boney alignment to the CT scan. The MR-segmented tumor and bone were then coregistered to the patient's CT scan to build the most accurate tumor segmentation prior to surgical planning. The surgeon met with the radiologist and engineer to place digital osteotomy planes on the patient's left femur, which resulted in a 19.0 cm resection. Surgical anatomic guides were designed and 3D printed to facilitate the exact osteotomies on the patient's bone (Fig. 6.14).

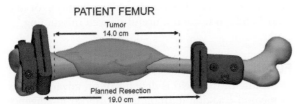

FIG. 6.14 Patient's left femur in blue, segmented osteosarcoma in green, and proximal and distal surgical anatomic guides shown in orange. Mayo Clinic, Rochester, MN, USA.

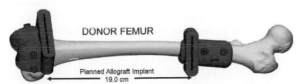

FIG. 6.15 Cadaver donor left femur allograft in yellow and proximal and distal surgical anatomic guides shown in orange. Mayo Clinic, Rochester, MN, USA.

A CT of the donor allograft femur was also performed and a series with a 0.75 mm slice thickness and soft-tissue reconstruction kernel was selected for segmentation. Next, the surgeon selected the segment of the allograft femur to be used in the reconstruction based on bone widths and shape, and separate surgical anatomic guides were designed specifically for the donor femur (Fig. 6.15).

All guides for this case were printed with vat photopolymerization using Dental SG resin on a Form 2 (Formlabs, Cambridge, MA). Postprocessing, including UV curing and sterilization via steam sterilization were performed prior to use in the OR.

3D Printed Patient-Specific Implant Considerations

Patient-specific 3D printed implants may be created for complex reconstructions, typically in cases for which currently available commercial products are not suited or available. Once the anatomic structures have been appropriately delineated, these anatomic models can be sent to 3D printing service bureaus with FDA clearance to, with express surgical input, design and manufacture biocompatible patient-specific implants. At the time of writing, most patient-specific 3D printed implants are built by third-party companies with teams who work closely with the radiology, surgery, and engineering teams to design an optimized implant. However, a small number of hospitals are 3D printing implants for their own patients. Similar to hospitals printing their own anatomic models and guides, those point of care implant manufacturing operations require in-house engineering and a host of additional resources to segment, perform CAD, run and maintain 3D printers, and post-process the implants.

An advantage of performing a digital reconstruction prior to surgery is the option to utilize the reconstructed 3D meshes to design and 3D print a patient-specific implant. When such an implant is ordered for manufacturing prior to surgery, there are additional considerations for segmentation and CAD. Figure 6.16 shows a two-segment fibular free flap reconstruction of the mandible with a patient-specific titanium alloy mandibular plate.

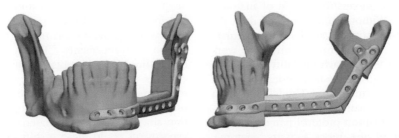

FIG. 6.16 Patient-specific 3D printed mandible plate in a titanium alloy, KLS Martin Group Individualized Patient Solutions, Tuttlingen, Germany. Mayo Clinic, Rochester, MN, USA.

In this example, the mandible plate contours to native bone; in order to avoid tooth root and nerve, those anatomies should be segmented separately in the initial segmentation and provided to the plate designer. Choosing a CT scan with a soft-tissue reconstruction kernel is of particular importance in this case because the designer will use the existing bone mesh to build the plate and a sharp-kernel series will yield a noisy bone surface. If there are any irregularities in the 3D mesh due to noise or artifact, the patient-specific plate may not fit properly in the OR.

DISCUSSION
Clinical Appropriateness

The Radiological Society of North America (RSNA) 3D Printing Special Interest Group (SIG) developed and published initial guidelines for medical 3D printing and clinical appropriateness criteria in 2018.[6] In this publication, a subset of clinical applications including congenital heart disease, vascular, craniomaxillofacial, musculoskeletal, genitourinary, and breast pathologies were reviewed, and consensus methodology recommendations were made for each application. Recommendations for abdominal, hepatobiliary, and gastrointestinal conditions have also recently been published by the RSNA SIG.[47] The criteria set forth by the RSNA 3D SIG provide a framework for physicians to decide when anatomic modeling is appropriate in their practice. The technical and professional work that goes into image acquisition, segmentation, CAD, and 3D printing of an anatomic model may not be appropriate for a routine procedure in a case with normal anatomy. For routine simple cases 3D printed models and guides may not be necessary, but for complex cases they can help to improve patient outcomes and add value to clinical care.

At this time, the corresponding clinical scenarios and appropriate guidance document for other clinical scenarios and anatomic guides are being developed. Modality-specific medical imaging acquisition protocols are paramount to successful creation of anatomic models and guides. Without sufficient input data, the resulting mesh may not be suitable for accurate anatomic modeling. Medical imaging physicists work to develop protocols within each modality that, when combined with existing diagnostic protocols, provide high quality data for segmentation. Guidelines within the first RSNA 3D SIG document include some recommended imaging acquisition protocol parameters that allow for creation of the most accurate anatomic mesh.[6] Commonly used modalities for segmentation include CT and MRI, and properly acquired ultrasound and 3D surface scanning data are also viable options. The mesh resulting from segmentation of the anatomy must accurately represent the patient's anatomy, or it is counterproductive to the mission of adding insight to the case based on the scan(s). The ultimate goal of anatomic models and guides is to extend the utility of medical imaging data. Therefore, any alteration or manipulation of anatomic 3D meshes should be done so with forethought and care. Using the original imaging to confirm contours of any parts prior to printing is an important quality assurance step.[7] Furthermore, validating 3D printer performance is equally important; what is input should match what is output to a tightly defined tolerance depending on application, or the model and guide are not useful or even misguiding.[7]

FUTURE INSIGHT

The future of this field is dependent on advancements in medical imaging technologies, artificial intelligence algorithms for automatic segmentation, automated scripting in anatomic modeling and guide generation, 3D printed material science, and 3D printing processes. Segmentation is recognized as a bottleneck to anatomic modeling and guide generation because it still requires a significant amount of manual intervention by a trained user in order to create physiologically accurate anatomic 3D meshes. Advances in automatic segmentation would alleviate some of that process strain.[48] The software used for digital surgical reconstruction is not typically user friendly and requires an operator with advanced knowledge and experience to confer with the surgeon. Advances in surgical planning software, perhaps utilizing augmented reality and granting surgeons increased control, would alleviate some of the difficulties around on-screen digital planning.[49] Advances in augmented reality including coregistration to live patients would allow for a more comprehensive provider–patient consultation with regard to diagnosis and procedure planning. In addition, utilizing augmented reality in the OR suite to make use of medical imaging data while a patient is on the operating table would prove a concurrent benefits of live coregistration advancements. Finally, bioprinting and bioplotting advancements will affect the way surgeons consider their approach to surgical intervention and reconstructing the body.[50] The fibula free flap has been a gold standard for craniomaxillofacial reconstruction since 1989, but biomaterial and bioprinting advancements could mean a shift to a simple reprint of the patient's own mandibular shape.[46]

3D printed anatomic models and guides have truly paved the way for 3D printing at the point of care. As 3D printing in hospitals becomes more widely utilized, advanced technologies such as augmented reality and virtual reality are combined with 3D printing, artificial intelligence algorithms are developed to facilitate the 3D printing workflow, and bioprinting of patient-specific structures comes into fruition, new degrees of personalized treatment will be implemented and these will revolutionize patient care.

REFERENCES

1. Mankovich NK, Cheeseman AM, Stoker NG. The display of three-dimensional anatomy with stereolithographic models. *J Digit Imag.* 1990;3(3):200−203.
2. Stoker NG, Mankovich NJ, Valentino D. Stereolithographic models for surgical planning: a preliminary report. *J Oral Maxillofac Surg.* 1992;50:466−471.
3. Mottart X, Slagmolen P. *3D Lab in a Hospital Environment. Materialise White Paper;* 2018. https://www.materialise.com/system/files/resources/Medical_WhitePaper_Formlabs_v3.pdf. Accessed August 5, 2020.
4. Pietila T. *How Medical 3D Printing is Gaining Ground in Top Hospitals.* Materialise Medical Blog; 2018. https://www.materialise.com/en/blog/3D-printing-hospitals. Accessed August 5, 2020.
5. Wang K. Clinical 3D printing: status, challenges, and opportunities. *Radiol Soc N Am News;* 2019. https://www.rsna.org/en/news/2019/January/Clinical-3D-printing-Status-Challenges-and-Opportunities. Accessed August 5, 2020.
6. Chepelev L, Wake N, Ryan J, et al. Radiological Society of North America (RSNA) 3D printing Special Interest Group (SIG): guidelines for medical 3D printing and appropriateness for clinical scenarios. *3D Print Med.* 2018;4(11):1−38.
7. Leng S, McGee K, Morris J, et al. Anatomic modeling using 3D printing: quality assurance and optimization. *3D Print Med.* 2017;3(1):6.
8. Hull CW, Lewis CW, 3D Systems, Inc. *Methods and Apparatus for Production of Three-Dimensional Objects by Stereolithography;* 1991. United States Patent 4,999,143 http://patft.uspto.gov. Accessed August 5, 2020.
9. Christensen A, Rybicki FJ. Maintaining safety and efficacy for 3D printing in medicine. *3D Print Med.* 2017;3(1).
10. Gillaspie E, Matsumoto J, Morris NE, et al. From 3D printing to 5D printing: enhancing thoracic surgical planning and resection of complex tumors. *Ann Thorac Surg.* 2016;101(5):1958−1962.
11. von Rundstedt FC, Scovell JM, Agrawal S, Zaneveld J, Link RE. Utility of patient-specific silicone renal models for planning and rehearsal of complex tumour resections prior to robot-assisted laparoscopic partial nephrectomy. *BJU Int.* 2017;199(4).
12. Sanchez-Sotelo J. Reverse total shoulder arthroplasty. *Clin Anat.* 2009;22(2):172−182.
13. Erben Y, Oderich G, Duncan AA. Endovascular repair of aortic coarctation psuedoaneurysm using an off-label "hourglass" stent-graft configuration. *J Endovasc Ther.* 2015;22(3):460−465.
14. Yoo SJ, Spray T, Austin EH, Yun TJ, van Arsdell GS. Hands-on surgical training of congenital heart surgery using 3-dimensional print models. *J Thorac Cardiovasc Surg.* 2017;153(6):1530−1540.
15. Hussein N, Lim A, Honjo O, et al. Development and validation of a procedure-specific assessment tool for hands-on surgical training in congenital heart surgery. *J Thorac Cardiovasc Surg.* 2020;160(1), 229-240.e1.
16. Sabbagh AE, Eleid MF, Matsumoto JM, et al. Three-dimensional prototyping for procedural simulation of transcatheter mitral valve replacement in patients with mitral annular calcification. *Catheter Cardiovasc Interv.* 2018;92(7):E537−E549.
17. Bundy JJ, Weadock WJ, Forris Beecham Chick J, et al. Three-dimensional printing facilitates creation of a biliary endoscopy phantom for interventional radiology-operated endoscopy training. *Curr Probl Diagn Radiol.* 2019;48(5):456−461.
18. Karkkainen JM, Sandri G, Tenoria ER, et al. Simulation of endovascular aortic repair using 3D printed abdominal aortic aneurysm model and fluid pump. *Cardiovasc Intervent Radiol.* 2019;42(11):1627−1634.
19. Itagaki M. Using 3D printed models for planning and guidance during endovascular intervention: a technical advance. *Diagn Interv Radiol.* 2015;21(4):338−341.
20. Weiss MY, Melnyk R, Mix D, Ghazi A, Vates GE, Stone JJ. Design and validation of a cervical laminectomy simulator using 3D printing and hydrogel phantoms. *Oper Neurosurg.* 2020;18(2):202−208.
21. Rutkowski DR, Wells SA, Johnson B, et al. MRI-based cancer lesion analysis with 3D printed patient specific prostate cutting guides. *Am J Clin Exp Urol.* 2019;7(4):215−222.
22. Hirsch DL, Garfein ES, Christensen AM, Weimer KA, Saadeh PB, Levine JP. Use of computer-aided design and computer-aided manufacturing to produce orthognathically ideal surgical outcomes: a paradigm shift in head and neck reconstruction. *J Oral Maxillofac Surg.* 2009;67(10):2115−2122.
23. Roser SM, Ramachandra S, Blair H, et al. The accuracy of virtual surgical planning in free fibula mandibular reconstruction: comparison of planned and final results. *J Oral Maxillofac Surg.* 2010;68(11):2824−2832.
24. Tepper OM, Sorice S, Hershman GN, Saadeh P, Levine JP. Use of virtual 3-dimensional surgery in post-traumatic craniomaxillofacial reconstruction. *J Oral Maxillofac Surg.* 2011;69(3):733−741.
25. Anthony AK, Chen WF, Kolokythas A, Weimer KA, Cohen MN. Use of virtual surgery and stereolithography-guided osteotomy for mandibular reconstruction with the free fibula. *Plast Reconstr Surg.* 2011;128(5):1080−1084.
26. Foley BD, Thayer WP, Honeybrook A, McKenna S, Press S. Mandibular reconstruction using computer-aided design

and computer-aided manufacturing: an analysis of surgical results. *J Oral Maxillofac Surg.* 2012;71(2):e111—e119.

27. Mardini S, Alsubaie S, Cayci C, Chim H, Wetjen N. Three-dimensional preoperative virtual planning and template use for surgical correction of craniosynostosis. *J Plast Reconstr Aesthet Surg.* 2014;67(3):336—343.

28. Helguero CG, Kao I, Komatsu DE, et al. Improving the accuracy of wide resection of bone tumors and enhancing implant fit: a cadaveric study. *J Orthop.* 2015;12(2):S188—S194.

29. Luu K, Pakel A, Wang E, Prisman E. In house virtual surgery and 3D complex head and neck reconstruction. *J Otolaryngol Head Neck Surg.* 2018;47(1):75.

30. Park JW, Kang HG, Lim KM, Park DW, Kim JH, Kim HS. Bone tumor resection guide using three-dimensional printing for limb salvage surgery. *J Surg Oncol.* 2018;118(6):898—905.

31. Imhoff FB, Schnell J, Magana A, et al. Single cut distal femoral osteotomy for correction of femoral torsion and valgus malformity in patellofemoral malalignment — proof of application of new trigonometrical calculations and 3D-printed cutting guides. *BMC Musculoskelet Disord.* 2018;19(1):215.

32. Donnez M, Ollivier M, Munier M, et al. Are three-dimensional patient-specific cutting guides for open wedge high tibial osteotomy accurate? An in vitro study. *J Orthop Surg Res.* 2018;13(1):171.

33. McAllister P, Watson E, Burke E. A cost-effective, in-house, positioning and cutting guide system for orthognathic surgery. *J Maxillofac Oral Surg.* 2018;17(1):112—114.

34. Jacquet C, Chan-Yu-Kin J, Sharma A, Argenson JN, Parratte S, Ollivier M. More accurate correction using "patient-specific" cutting guides in opening wedge distal femur varization osteotomies. *Int Orthop.* 2019;43(10):2285—2291.

35. Kim J, Rajadurai J, Choy WJ, et al. Three-dimensional patient-specific guides for intraoperative navigation for cortical screw trajectory pedicle fixation. *World Neurosurg.* 2019;122:674—679.

36. Garg B, Gupta M, Singh M, Kalyanasundaram D. Outcome and safety analysis of 3D-printed patient-specific pedicle screw jigs for complex spinal deformities: a comparative study. *Spine J.* 2019;19(1):56—64.

37. Pijpker P, Kraeima J, Witjes MJH, et al. Accuracy assessment of pedicle and lateral mass screw insertion assisted by customized 3D-printed drill guides: a human cadaver study. *Oper Neurosurg.* 2019;16(1):94—102.

38. Bowen L, Benech R, Shafi A, et al. Custom-made three-dimensional models for craniosynostosis. *J Craniofac Surg.* 2020;31(1):292—293.

39. Dagneaux L, Canovas F. 3D printed patient-specific cutting guide for anterior midfoot tarsectomy. *Foot Ankle Int.* 2020;41(2):211—215.

40. Brouwer de Koning SG, ter Braak TP, Geldorf F, et al. Evaluating the accuracy of resection planes in mandibular surgery using a preoperative, intraoperative, and postoperative approach. *Int J Oral Maxillofac Surg.* 2020 (in press).

41. Batut C, Pare A, Kulker D, Listrat A, Laure B. How accurate is computer-assisted orbital hypertelorism surgery? Comparison of the three-dimensional surgical planning with postoperative outcomes. *Facial Plast Surg Aesthet Med.* 2020 (in press).

42. Haas Junior OL, Farina R, Hernandez-Alfaro F, de Oliveira RB. Minimally invasive intraoral proportional condylectomy with a three-dimensionally printed cutting guide. *Int J Oral Maxillofac Surg.* 2020 (in press).

43. Zavattero E, Fasolis M, Novaresio A, Gerbino G, Borbon C, Ramieri G. The shape of things to come: in-hospital three-dimensional printing for mandibular reconstruction using fibula free flap. *Laryngoscope.* 2020 (in press).

44. Park JW, Kang HG, Kim JH, Kim HS. The application of 3D-printing technology in pelvic tumor surgery. *J Ortho Sci.* 2020 (in press).

45. Wei FC, Mardini S. Fibula flap. In: *Flaps and Reconstructive Surgery.* Philadelphia: Saunders/Elsevier; 2009:597—612.

46. Steel BJ, Cope MR. A brief history of vascularized free flaps in the oral and maxillofacial region. *J Oral Maxillofac Surg.* 2015;73(4), 786.e1-11.

47. Ballard DH, Wake N, Witowski J, Rybicki FJ, Sheikh A, RSNA Voting Group. Radiological Society of North America (RSNA) 3D Printing Special Interest Group (SIG) clinical situations for which 3D printing is considered an appropriate representation or extension of data contained in a medical imaging examination: abdominal, hepatobiliary, and gastrointestinal conditions. *3D Print Med.* 2020;4, 11.

48. Wang G, Li W, Zuluaga MA, et al. Interactive medical image segmentation using deep learning with image-specific fine tuning. *IEEE Trans Med Imag.* 2018;37(7). https://doi.org/10.1109/TMI.2018.2791721.

49. Pietruski P, Majak M, Swiatek-Najwer E, et al. Supporting mandibular reconstruction with intraoperative navigation utilizing augmented reality technology — a proof of concept study. *J Cranio-Maxillofacial Surg.* 2019;47(6). https://doi.org/10.1016/j.jcms.2019.03.004.

50. Essig H, Lindhorst D, Gander T, et al. Patient-specific biodegradable implant in pediatric craniofacial surgery. *J Cranio-Maxillofacial Surg.* 2017;45(2). https://doi.org/10.1016/j.jcms.2016.11.015.

CHAPTER 7

Quality Assurance of 3D Printed Anatomic Models

NICOLE WAKE, PHD • BENJAMIN JOHNSON, BS • SHUAI LENG, PHD, FAAPM

Quality Assurance (QA), defined as the maintenance of a desired level of quality in a service or a product, is a subset of the quality management system (QMS) and provides the framework that ensures quality requirements are met. A proper QA program has many components that objectively demonstrate confidence in product or service quality to the user. A QA program includes components such as document controls, purchasing controls, process controls, traceability, acceptance standards, and training. Ultimately, the QA program must be commensurate with the product and the potential risk of product failure.

QA IN RADIOLOGY

In radiology, a QA program ensures the correct operation of imaging systems for the delivery of optimal patient care. Facilities should have documented policies and procedures in place to monitor and evaluate the proper performance, management, and safety of imaging equipment. Ultimately, a radiologist's final report is the final product being evaluated and the images and imaging equipment are auxiliary.

Errors can occur at many stages and may include the following:

1. Improperly calibrated image acquisition devices
2. Inappropriate examination technique
3. Operator and transcriptional errors
4. Improperly calibrated display devices
5. Incorrect interpretation of images

There are many stakeholders within a radiology department who should be involved in a QA program (Table 7.1); and a QA committee including all these stakeholders should meet periodically to review QA issues.

A process map is a graphical representation of a process including the sequence of all steps that transform inputs to outputs. For a radiological imaging exam, the process is outlined in Fig. 7.1.

TABLE 7.1
Roles and Responsibilities for QA.

Personnel Type	Responsibilities
Radiologic technologist	1. Perform imaging exam and ensure images are delivered to physician 2. Process must be in place to verify arrival of images and a mechanism to detect and correct errors in delivery
Imaging informatics professional	3. Ensure appropriate imaging display, transfer, and archiving into PACS
Medical physicist	4. Acceptance testing of imaging equipment (verifies compliance with local regulatory requirements, compliance with special contractual terms, and compliance with manufacturer's specifications) 5. Ensure proper calibration and performance of imaging equipment 6. Implement Quality Control (QC) program
Radiologist	7. Support QA program by controlling resources and priorities in imaging departments 8. Demand accountability for image quality and availability
Radiology administrator	9. Allocate resources for QA program and coordinate QA efforts 10. Enforce QA policies and procedures

Derived from Samei, E, et al. Assessment of display performance for medical imaging systems: executive summary of AAPM TG18 report. *Med Phys.* 2005;32(4): 1205–1225 and Mawlawi OS, Kemp B, Jordan DW, et al. PET/CT Acceptance Testing and Quality Assurance: The Report of AAPM Task Group 126. AAPM; 2019.

3D Printing for the Radiologist. https://doi.org/10.1016/B978-0-323-77573-1.00003-8

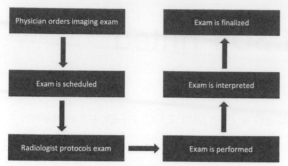

FIG. 7.1 Process map for diagnostic radiological imaging examinations.

Medical physicists are responsible for acceptance testing and verifying the appropriate setup and performance of imaging equipment. The American Association of Physicists in Medicine (AAPM) has established many Task Groups which focus on QA of medical imaging systems for each specific imaging modality.

In one example, Task Group 18 of the Diagnostic Committee of the AAPM has established a standard of performance for Quality Control (QC) of medical imaging displays.[1] As compared to QA, which is process oriented, QC is part of a quality system which is product oriented and focuses on defect identification. In another example, Task Group 126 is responsible for Positron Emission Tomography/Computed Tomography (PET/CT) acceptance testing and QA; and this group provides recommendations for testing preparations, PET spatial resolution, and PET/CT registration evaluation, PET sensitivity evaluation, PET count rate performance and accuracy of corrections evaluation, PET image contrast and scatter/attenuation correction evaluation, PET image uniformity assessment, and PET scanner QC.[2]

In the United States (US), medical imaging equipment used for diagnosis is considered a medical device and governed by the Food and Drug Administration (FDA). Medical imaging equipment such as CT and magnetic resonance imaging (MRI) scanners are accredited by an accreditation organization, such as the American College of Radiology (ACR) or joint commission. Measurable indicators of the quality of a diagnostic image can be described by contrast, resolution, and noise. Imaging phantoms, objects with specific dimensions and imaging properties, are used as standards to ensure that imaging systems are operating correctly. Tests are performed daily, monthly, and annually depending on the accreditation requirements. Geometric accuracy and spatial resolution are routinely assessed[3,4] (Fig. 7.2).

Proper interpretation of radiological exams can be assessed by peer review. In peer review, a peer radiologist is asked to re-read cases and determine if he or she agrees with initial report. Radiologists who are outliers among their peers for the number of radiology reports in disagreement can be identified and improvement plans can be implemented.[5] An alternative method for measuring professional outcomes is to score radiological examinations that have a reference standard proof such as knee MRI which can be compared to knee arthroscopy, coronary CT angiography compared to conventional coronary angiography, or CT colonography which is compared with colonoscopy.[5] These methods are preferred since they measure true outcomes for radiologic reports.

QA OF 3D PRINTED PARTS IN MEDICINE

To be useful to the clinician, 3D printed models must be a reliable representation of the patient's anatomy. To address this need, the 3D printing process and output should be covered by a QA program. Similar to QA in radiology, each step of the process must be analyzed from image acquisition to printed part to identify potential pitfalls and risks that could affect part performance. Key steps in the process include image acquisition, image data segmentation, model design, printing, and part post-processing. At minimum, finished parts should go through a QC process to ensure compliance to the device's quality requirements. The QC process could be a simple visual inspection ensuring that the model is free from manufacturing defects or could be more complex with verification of mechanical performance and measurement of critical model features for accuracy. The level of QC needed will be dependent on the QC plan established for the model as dictated by the QA program.

In the medical device industry, QA is a requirement of the quality system regulation law in many jurisdictions. For example, in the US, a manufacturer of medical devices is charged with establishing and maintaining a quality system that is appropriate for the scope of medical devices that are being produced. The QMS directs the entire scope of activities necessary to ensure confidence in the finished device inclusive of management responsibilities, QA, and QC. Within the QMS, a set of procedures and documents describe the product realization lifecycle from concept to

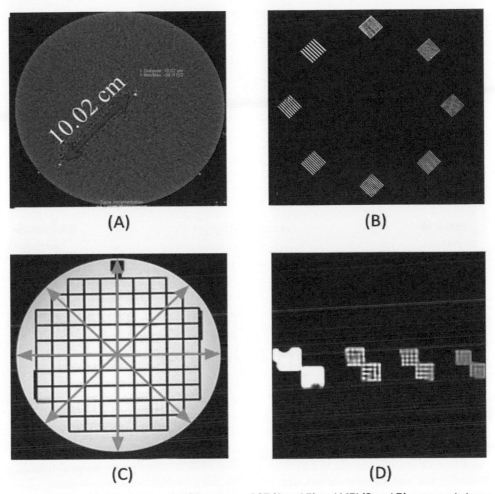

FIG. 7.2 Phantom images showing the QA process of CT **(A** and **B)** and MRI **(C** and **D)** scanners in terms of geometrical accuracy **(A** and **C)** and spatial resolution **(B** and **D)**.

development to production. An important input to product realization during the design control process is the concept of risk. Risk analysis is utilized to identify, assess, and mitigate all potential hazards associated with the medical device. Oftentimes, risk mitigation strategies will involve verification of product requirements through QC inspection.

The internationally recognized QMS standard for medical devices is ISO 13485:2016.[6] This standard specifies the QMS requirements needed by an organization to demonstrate its ability to provide medical devices and related services that consistently meet customer and regulatory obligations. Application of specific clauses in the standard is dependent on the organization's activities; some requirements can be excluded based on organizational scope.

At 3D Systems, a 3D printing company with medical device development and manufacturing operations, the requirements of ISO 13485:2016 and their relationships are depicted as shown in Fig. 7.3.

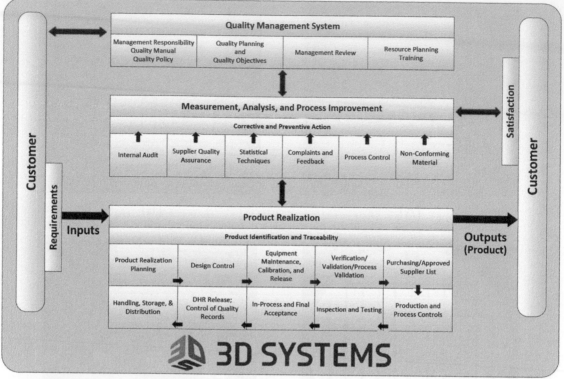

FIG. 7.3 Illustration of the 3D Systems Quality Management System components. (Image courtesy of 3D Systems.)

As Fig. 7.3 illustrates, quality is ingrained into all aspects of the organization, which is essential to the production of high quality safe and effective devices that are intended to diagnose, treat, cure, mitigate, or prevent disease. Inherent within the quality system is the application of risk management as described in ISO 14971:2019.[7] Importantly, considerations regarding QA and QC of a medical device need to be done with proper identification of the hazards, evaluation of the associated risks, and implementation of controls to mitigate risks to acceptable levels with monitoring of the effectiveness of the controls.

BRIDGING THE GAP BETWEEN RADIOLOGY AND MANUFACTURING

With the growing use of 3D printing in hospitals, ensuring the accuracy and reproducibility of the final 3D printed models with a comprehensive QA program is essential. Since 3D printing in hospitals is a relatively new area, there is currently no guidance for the application of relevant standards. Therefore, the onus of responsibility to ensure patient safety is placed on the clinical team. For example, the fabrication of an anatomic model from imaging data intended to aid the clinical team with surgical planning typically includes the following process steps:

1. Image Acquisition
2. Image Segmentation and Processing
3. Anatomic Model Design
4. 3D Printing Preparation
5. 3D Printing
6. Anatomic Model Post-processing
7. Packaging and Delivery to Clinical Team

Within each step, there is potential for failure that could propagate throughout the process and yield a model that does not meet device requirements for completeness and accuracy. Therefore, the 3D printing personnel at the hospital will need to evaluate each step and the potential for error to develop an acceptable control plan. Additionally, training of the hospital 3D printing staff on the QA procedures, control plan, and QC requirements is necessary to ensure compliance.

All hospital personnel involved in the 3D printing process (radiologic technologists, biomedical engineers, imaging informatics professionals, medical physicists, and radiologists) should be involved in developing the QA plan. Responsibilities for QA will vary across institutions, but should include at least the following:

1. Acceptance testing to verify appropriate setup of software, printing hardware, and postprocessing equipment
2. A process for verifying the accuracy of image acquisition, segmentation, and modeling
3. Methods to ensure that 3D printed parts are accurate and have the correct specifications
4. Methods to ensure appropriate biocompatibility and sterilization of models (for models that will be brought into the operating room (OR))
5. Methods to collect and analyze the QC data
6. A system for review, approval, and release of the model from the production team to the clinical team.

QA and Optimization of Image Acquisition and Segmentation for Anatomic Models

The first step in creating 3D printed patient-specific anatomic models is to acquire volumetric imaging of the patient. As described above, imaging systems such as CT and MRI machines are medical devices governed by FDA and accredited by an accreditation organization, such as the ACR, and QA of these systems is routinely performed by medical physicists.

Image acquisition and reconstruction parameters can affect image suitability for use in 3D printing, therefore protocols should be optimized. Major factors to consider include slice thickness, spatial resolution, signal-to-noise ratio and contrast-to-noise ratio, and image artifacts. More information regarding image acquisition and specific imaging artifacts can be found in Chapter 2 and will not be discussed here. However, in order to properly visualize and reconstruct the anatomy of interest and be suitable for 3D printing, the image dataset should be free of any major artifacts and visual inspection of the dataset should be performed prior to any modeling to ensure only acceptable artifacts are present. Image segmentation (discussed in detail in Chapter 3) involves separating the appropriate anatomic regions of interest from the surrounding anatomy and is an important step for converting medical images into 3D printed models. The accuracy of the image segmentation is critical to the process and requires a high attention to detail. After converting segmented regions of interest from medical images to 3D polygonal meshes, the mesh representation should be checked for accuracy. Accuracy of the image segmentation may be verified by overlying the final computer-aided design (CAD) file onto the original source images (Fig. 7.4).

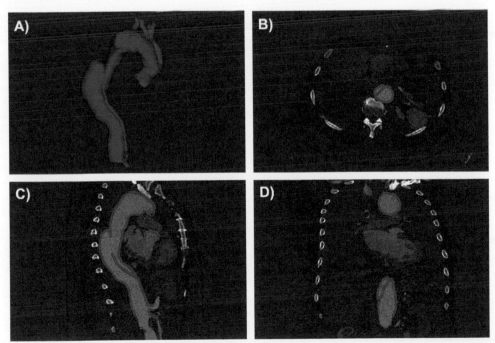

FIG. 7.4 **(A)** CAD file of an aortic aneurysm model with a dissection shown with overlying contours in the **(B)** axial, **(C)** sagittal, and **(D)** coronal orientations.

Model Design and Preparation for Printing

An important consideration in 3D printing is preparation of the CAD model before it is sent to the printer. Often, the clinical need, printing technology, and printing limitations will necessitate minor modifications of the segmented anatomy into a model design that is suitable.[8] This can include creating color differentiation in the model, splitting the segmented anatomy into multiple parts for enhancement of visualization, creating struts between anatomical structures to ensure a connected model, labeling of the model with information, and creating supports needed for a successful build. Each of these manipulations could affect the quality and accuracy of the model, and therefore should be done according to instructions or best practices. Typical failures during this step include accidental changes to important anatomy, lack of proper strutting that causes the model to fall apart, or improper supporting that causes the model to fail during the build. It is often best practice to have dedicated work instructions for model creation and labeling, as well as independent review from trained personnel on the model design and build file prior to sending the part to the printer.

3D Printing Hardware

Errors may occur during the printing process; therefore, it is important to ensure that the final 3D printed parts are accurate. Assessing the accuracy of 3D printed parts is not new and can be dated back to the early 1990s.[9] The type of error will depend on the printing technology but could include dimensional inaccuracies due to poor calibration or under–over printing of material, shrinking or wrapping, or lack of support in required areas. Table 7.2 describes printing considerations for the five major technologies currently used in hospitals to make 3D printed anatomic models and surgical guides. Other factors that can have an effect on the produced parts include the type of material, print settings, and design of the printed part.

In hospitals, when 3D printers are being used to create medical devices, it is imperative to ensure that the hardware is functioning properly and printing

TABLE 7.2
Summary of Dimensional Accuracy for Major 3D Printing Technologies Used in Hospitals.

Printing Technology	Dimensional Tolerance	Shrinkage or Warping	Support Requirements
Material extrusion	±0.5% (z-direction is typically more dimensionally accurate)	Thermoplastics with high print temperatures are most vulnerable. Shrinkage behavior is hard to predict and dependent on the design.	Essential for overhangs less than 45° and bridges longer than 20 mm.
Vat photopolymerization	±0.5% (lower limit ±0.15 mm)	Large flat surfaces and long unsupported parts are most likely to shrink or warp.	Essential. Orienting large, flat surfaces to an incline of 10−20° increases success rate of printing since the surface area is reduced, therefore the print is subject to less force when the build platform raises with each layer.
Material jetting	±0.1 mm	Large flat areas may warp or shrink.	Essential, but supports are dissolvable resulting in a smooth part finish.
Binder jetting	±0.2−0.3 mm	Shrinkage of ~0.8%−2% may occur due to secondary infiltration or sintering processes.	Not required.
Powder bed fusion	±0.1 mm	High risk of shrinkage or warping mitigated by design file offsets.	Variable depending on material.

Modified from Redwood et al. The 3D printing Handbook: Technologies, design and applications. ISBN 978-90-827485-0-5. 3D Hubs B.V. 2017.

accurate, reproducible parts. Each 3D printer should be properly set up and tested according to the manufacturer's instructions. In addition, routine preventative maintenance of 3D printing equipment should be performed and documented.

As part of a quality system for 3D printing in hospitals, coupons/phantoms should routinely be printed to ensure that the hardware is functioning properly. Different types of coupons may be created to assess calibrations, layer quality, geometric accuracy, tensile strength, compressive strength, flexure properties, and image resolution. The size and specific geometries of the coupon are defined in CAD software and can serve as ground truth for quantitative comparisons of the 3D printed parts. Printable coupons may be available from some 3D printing manufacturers. Researchers have come up with their own designs and methods to test certain machine types and printing technologies (Fig. 7.5).[10,11] There are also some 3D objects with known sizes available online that people may use as a coupon.[12] However, there are no standard phantoms like those used in QC of medical imaging equipment (e.g., CT and MRI).

In the future, we suspect that most 3D printing manufacturers will provide specific test coupons and instructions to customers for verification of accuracy. In addition, 3D printable coupons for certain clinical applications may become publicly available for hospitals across the world to use.

Cleaning and Post-processing

Post-processing of 3D printed parts depends greatly on the specific 3D printing technology (Table 7.3). Post-processing can be challenging for 3D printed models with complex or small structures as residual raw material can get stuck in the printed model. In addition, controls to prevent cross-contamination of foreign materials should be established and validated.

TABLE 7.3
Summary of Support Removal Techniques for Major Printing Technologies Utilized in the Hospital Setting.

Printing Technology	Support Removal Technique
Vat photopolymerization	Solvent bath sequence followed by a required UV postcure
Material extrusion	Solvent bath or manual removal of supports
Material jetting	Water/solvent bath and water jet stream
Binder jetting	Compressed air
Powder bed fusion	Heat treatment, manual removal of supports, and loose powder removal

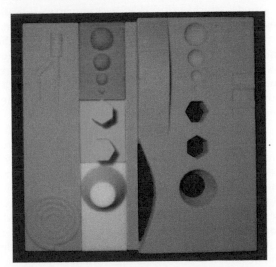

FIG. 7.5 A 3D printing QA phantom designed to test 3D printing accuracy and precision. The phantom contains various geometrical and anatomical objects with various size, shape, and surface curvature. Parts in the middle section are removable positive parts that can be used for fit tests to the corresponding negative counterparts.

Sterilization of 3D Printed Anatomic Models

Models that will be brought into the OR and used in the sterile field require an extra level of QA considerations. Sterility of a device cannot be verified without destructive testing; therefore, the sterilization process must be validated. Sterilization parameters must be established that ensure a sterility assurance level of 1×10^{-6}, or a 1 in 1,000,000 probability of a nonsterile product to be considered at an acceptable risk. Several ISO standards exist for common sterilization techniques available in hospitals including autoclave (also known as steam sterilization or moist heat),[13] ethylene oxide gas,[14] and gamma ray ionizing radiation.[15–17] Autoclave is used for materials that can withstand high temperatures, e.g., greater than 200°F.[17] Ethylene oxide gas and gamma ray ionizing radiation may be used in cases where lower temperatures are required to maintain structural integrity of the part.[17] Instructions for Use should accompany a 3D printed anatomic model or guide to the surgical core for proper cleaning, sterilization, and storage prior to surgery.[16]

VERIFICATION OF THE 3D PRINTED MODEL

After a model has been printed, visual inspection should be performed to ensure the model is free from obvious defects. A visual inspection can include a check that all structures printed properly, a check of the surface finish, an assessment of flatness or warping, and a check to ensure that no foreign objects or debris are in the model. Fig. 7.6 shows an example of a 3D printed model of a retroperitoneal mass in which part of the mass and duodenum did not print successfully and the error was easily identified with visual inspection.

After a 3D printed model has passed a visual inspection, additional measurement methods can be performed to ensure accuracy of the part including physical measurement with rulers or calipers or more sophisticated techniques such as surface scanning and/ or CT scanning.

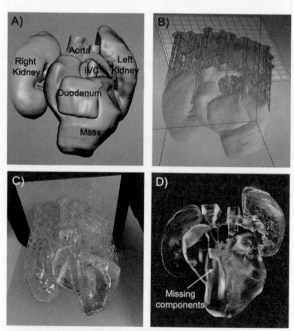

FIG. 7.6 3D printed model of a retroperitoneal mass showing **(A)** the digital design including the aorta, IVC, bilateral kidneys, duodenum adjacent to the mass, and the retroperitoneal mass, **(B)** setup of 3D printed model in Preform printing software (Formlabs, Cambridge, MA), **(C)** printed model with supports, and **(D)** final printed model with supports removed showing that part of the mass and duodenum failed to print.

CALIPER MEASUREMENTS

Calipers can be used to measure size of printed model and compare with the reference size obtained either from patient images or CAD designs (Fig. 7.7). Previous work of ours has demonstrated the accuracy of our methods to create 3D printed kidney tumor models, with tumor measurements obtained from the medical images and 3D printed models within 0.6% ± 1.9% of each other.[11] In addition to the overall sizes of the model, measurements of distances between predefined landmarks that are critical to the use of the model are also usually performed.[18] Measurement of nonstraight lines, e.g., perimeters of aortic valves, may be accomplished using flexible wires, following through the object and then straightened to compare against a ruler.[19] In addition, photography techniques have also been investigated by taking a photograph of the model and then performing a measurement of the images in a software program. Calibration is needed to take into consideration of the difference between physical size and size in the photograph.[19]

Surface Scanning and CT Scanning

Although caliper measurements are accurate and easy to perform, they are usually limited to external features and they only provide partial measurements of the model. To address these limitations, other techniques such as surface scanning and CT scanning have been investigated. Surface scanning can provide the external contour of the model, which can be loaded back into image processing software to perform various measurements and comparison with the reference model. In addition to the measurements that can be achieved with calipers, this technique might also allow more sophisticated measurements such as the curvature, area, and volume. With the volume data, it is also feasible to do a point-by-point comparison with the virtual model that was printed.[19]

Surface scanning is a great technique to use for models whose measurements of external structures and features are the main interest. It is challenging for measurement of any internal structures. Imaging methods that can provide information of the internal structures, such as CT and MRI, may accomplish these needs. These volumetric imaging techniques provide complete 3D information of the model, including internal structures. Comparison with the reference model can be achieved after registration, with analysis of conformality using various metrics, such as point-to-point distance or intersection over union.[10,20]

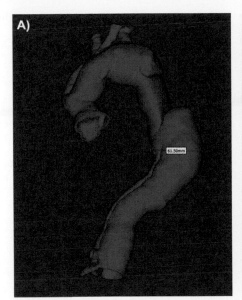
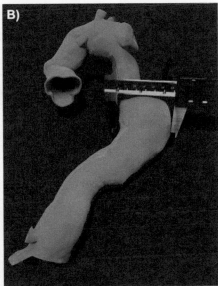

FIG. 7.7 Aortic aneurysm model from Fig. 7.4 shown **(A)** with a diameter measurement (61.50 mm) in the CAD software and **(B)** corresponding 3D printed model printed in powder bed fusion (HP Multi Jet 4200, HP, Palo Alto, CA) showing corresponding caliper measurement (61.44 mm).

CONCLUSION

QA programs for 3D printed medical models should be implemented within hospitals to ensure that patients have access to safe and effective 3D printed medical products. There are multiple factors that comprise a successful QA system, and there are several relevant standards that provide comprehensive guidance. Ultimately, the QA system deployed must be commensurate with the intended use and potential risk of the device. Additionally, the QC methods utilized to verify model characteristics will depend on various factors including the type of 3D printed models being created, equipment availability, software types, and available personnel. In this chapter, considerations for QA of 3D printing in medicine were discussed with a focus on 3D printed anatomic models. It should be noted that there are additional biocompatibility considerations for 3D printed surgical guides as well as patient-specific 3D printed implants.

REFERENCES

1. Samei E, et al. Assessment of display performance for medical imaging systems: executive summary of AAPM TG18 report. *Med Phys.* 2005;32(4):1205–1225.
2. Mawlawi OS, Kemp B, Jordan DW, et al. *PET/CT Acceptance Testing and Quality Assurance: The Report of AAPM Task Group 126.* AAPM; 2019.
3. Dillon C, Breeden W, Clements J, et al. *Computed Tomography Quality Control Manual.* ACR; 2017.
4. Price R, Allison J, Clarke G, et al. *Magnetic Resonance Imaging Quality Control Manual.* ACR; 2015.
5. Johnson CD, et al. Quality initiatives. developing a radiology quality and safety program: a primer. *Radiographics.* 2009;29(4):951–959.
6. ISO. *ISO 13485:2016 Medical Devices — Quality Management Systems — Requirements for Regulatory Purposes. 2020;* August 6, 2020. Available from: https://www.iso.org/standard/59752.html. Accessed August 6, 2020.
7. ISO. *ISO 14971:2019 Medical Devices — Application of Risk Management to Medical Devices. 2019;* August 6, 2020. Available from: https://www.iso.org/standard/59752.html. Accessed August 6, 2020.
8. Christensen A, Rybicki FJ. Maintaining safety and efficacy for 3D printing in medicine. *3D Print Med.* 2017;3(1).
9. Kruth JP. Material incress manufacturing by rapid prototyping techniques. *CIRP Annals.* 1991;40(2):603–614.
10. Leng S, et al. Anatomic modeling using 3D printing: quality assurance and optimization. *3D Print Med.* 2017;3(1):6.
11. Wake N, et al. 3D printed renal cancer models derived from MRI data: application in pre-surgical planning. *Abdom Radiol (NY).* 2017;42(5):1501–1509.
12. Creative Tools.se. *#3DBenchy - the Jolly 3D Printing Torture-Test,* 2015. https://www.thingiverse.com/thing:763622. Accessed August 14, 2020.
13. ISO. *ISO 17665-1:2006 Sterilization of Health Care Products - Moist Heat - Part 1: Requirements for the Development, Validation and Routine Control of a Sterilization Process for Medical Devices;* 2006. Last update 2016. Available from: https://

www.iso.org/standard/43187.html. Accessed August 14, 2020.

14. ISO. *ISO 11135:2014 Sterilization of health care products - Ethylene oxide -Requirements for the development, validation and routine control of a sterilization process for medical devices;* 2014. Available from: https://www.iso.org/standard/56137.html. Accessed August 14, 2020.

15. ISO. *ISO 11137-2:2013 Sterilization of Health Care Products - Radiation - Part 2: Establishing the Sterilization Dose;* 2013. Last update 2018. Available from: https://www.iso.org/standard/62442.html. Accessed August 14, 2020.

16. *Association of Surgical Technologists. Standards of Practice for the Decontamination of Surgical Instruments;* 2009. https://www.ast.org/uploadedFiles/Main_Site/Content/About_Us /Standard_Decontamination_%20Surgical_Instruments_.pdf. Accessed August 14, 2020.

17. Rutala WA, W D, The HICPAC. *Guideline for Disinfection and Sterilization in Healthcare Facilities, 2008 Update.* May 2019.

18. Galvez M, et al. Error measurement between anatomical porcine spine, CT images, and 3D printing. *Acad Radiol.* 2020;27(5):651−660.

19. Odeh M, et al. Methods for verification of 3D printed anatomic model accuracy using cardiac models as an example. *3D Print Med.* 2019;5(1):6.

20. George E, et al. Measuring and establishing the accuracy and reproducibility of 3D printed medical models. *Radiographics.* 2017;37(5):1424−1450.

CHAPTER 8

Documentation and Reimbursement for 3D Printed Anatomic Models and Guides

JANE M. MATSUMOTO, MD • KENNETH C. WANG, MD, PHD

INTRODUCTION

In the American healthcare system, standardized documentation is critical to ensure accurate medical billing and coding for appropriate reimbursement. An encounter for radiology services starts with a test order from a referring physician which includes the patient's signs/symptoms or a reason for performing the test. Once the imaging exam is performed, information about the exam and the diagnosis including the International Classification of Diseases-10 codes must be recorded. Next, providers or certified medical coders assign current procedural terminology (CPT) codes that denote procedures and services. Finally, payers will review these claims and render healthcare reimbursement. This chapter will discuss proper documentation for three-dimensional (3D) printed anatomic models and guides, CPT codes for 3D printing, and current efforts to demonstrate widespread use of 3D printing in medicine.

DOCUMENTATION

Medical record

The multiple steps of care including history, orders, vital signs, medications, lab, imaging and testing results, consultations, biopsies, procedures, clinical outcomes, and care plans are documented in the current comprehensive medical record which is largely in an electronic format. Most importantly, this record serves as the patient's clinical history for all care providers in order for them to give the patient optimal care. Information is also included in the medical record to describe the effort that goes into a patient's care such as which type of healthcare workers are involved, the amount of time spent, and the materials and techniques used.

Documentation of 3D printed anatomic models is largely reflective of documentation for other medical services. It starts with an electronic order which lists the important information to know for planning. This includes patient name, medical record number, ordering physician and contact number, indication or diagnosis, anatomic structures to include, date needed by, sidedness, and whether imaging has been performed yet. Additional questions on mirror imaging, need for guides, material, and color preferences are also helpful. For the best understanding of what is needed, it is important to talk directly to the ordering physician before starting.

Data storage organization

Secure backed up large capacity computer storage is needed to keep each patient's imaging data, segmentation, and computer-aided design (CAD) files, photos, and any videos which are created from the files. Other patient-specific information such as quality assurance measures can also be kept in these files. This information can be organized and listed by the patient's name and clinic number similar to filing in a classic medical record (Fig. 8.1).

Dictation

A formal dictation is placed in the medical record to document the creation of the model. The dictation can be organized in any number of ways depending on each institution's dictation guidelines and software. Completing the dictation can be easier if it is created with as many pick lists as possible to choose options from. Most dictation software has some type of pick list options. A dictation format similar to that used in interventional radiology procedures could be considered as it has a similar organization of history and

3D Printing for the Radiologist. https://doi.org/10.1016/B978-0-323-77573-1.00018-X

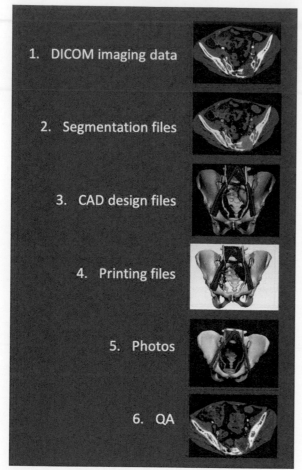

1. DICOM imaging data

2. Segmentation files

3. CAD design files

4. Printing files

5. Photos

6. QA

FIG. 8.1 Example of possible patient file organization for the various data files used during the creation of 3D printed anatomic models. The images are representative of the content of each file. These folders reflect the steps of the process. In addition, files can include information on the specific DICOM data used, type of segmentation and CAD software, number of structures segmented, printing technologies and materials used, post-processing techniques, and details regarding the QA process.

indication, findings, procedural technique, and final impression. The dictation report can begin with a short history and specific indication for the model. This would include the basic information from the request form including general anatomic structure, side, type and date of imaging used, contrast used, and laterality as needed.

The procedural technique would go through the multiple steps of model and guide creation which would make up the largest part of the dictation. This would include segmentation and CAD processing details including the design time with the level of staff that completed these and specific details including

how many and which anatomic structures are in the model. The dictation would also include the type of 3D printing technology, specific printer, and type of materials and colors used to create the model. Postprocessing procedures including cleaning and curing time would also be part of the technique. How and where guides are sterilized should be documented. Quality control measures done to check accuracy of the model and guides can also be noted.

The final impression would be a short synopsis of what type of model was created and for what use. Additional information could include date of model delivery, to whom it was delivered, and what department they are in. Color photos of the final model may be placed both with the dictation and in the imaging section of the medical record.

The extensive and detailed information in the dictation reflects the work, skill, and effort put into creating the models. These data are invaluable and are used for patient care, quality improvement, and to potentially include in research studies and registries. Importantly, components of the clinical and technical documentation are used to determine the appropriate level of reimbursement for services rendered by both government and private healthcare insurers.

REIMBURSEMENT
Current procedural terminology codes
In medicine, one of the major hurdles to development of 3D printed anatomic models and guides has been a lack of reimbursement. Obtaining reimbursement for a new service through governments and private insurance is a multiyear process which takes significant organization as well as institutional support and patience. It is about a 2- to 3-year process at best to go from CPT code application to inclusion in the Medicare Fee Schedule. Medical centers creating models for clinical care need to be able to absorb the cost of the models before they are able to create enough to demonstrate the models' efficacy. Development funding at many medical centers has been able to help bridge the gap between the cost of creating 3D printed models and insurance reimbursement.

In the United States (US), medical reimbursement is a complex process. It is overall based on the assumption that it is paying for physician or healthcare provider work and the resources used for medical services and procedures. Each of these services and procedures is itemized and has a specific code and reimbursement attached to them. The Healthcare Common Procedure Coding System (HCPCS), maintained by the Centers for Medicare and Medicaid Services (CMS), is ultimately in charge of developing, reviewing, and updating these codes. HCPCS is divided into two levels. HCPCS level I codes consist of the CPT codes which are set and published by the American Medical Association (AMA), whereas HCPCS level II codes use the HCPCS alphanumeric code and generally include nonphysician products, supplies, and services not included in CPT. CPT codes are currently accepted as the standard for healthcare providers throughout the US to report medical procedures and services.

CPT codes were first established by the AMA in 1966 and were used to help set standard terms and descriptors to document medical procedures. They were not initially associated with reimbursement. Over the next decades, the CPT codes were updated regularly and became more detailed. As the CPT system evolved, it became the national coding system for healthcare provider services and procedures in 2000. The CPT codes are regularly reviewed and updated by the CPT Editorial Panel which meets three times a year. The panel is made up of 17 members including healthcare and insurance providers, hospitals, and CMS. They are supported by the CPT Advisory Committee, a large group made up of multiple major medical societies and organizations representing healthcare providers, and act as a resource for the CPT Editorial Panel. There are high standards for requirements of confidentiality and disclosure of any conflict of interest for the panel.[1]

There are currently three CPT code categories: Category I, II, and III. Category I CPT codes are established medical services and have met the requirements of wide clinical use and documented efficacy. Category I CPT codes use the familiar five-digit codes for healthcare provider services. For example, the code 74177 is used for computed tomography (CT) of the abdomen and pelvis with contrast, and the code 74178 is used for CT of the abdomen and pelvis, with and without contrast. Category I codes are billable for reimbursement.

Category II codes are supplemental tracking codes for reporting quality performance measures that reflect good clinical care. The reporting of Category II codes is optional, and these codes are not used in place of Category I codes. Category II codes contain five characters—the first four are numerical, followed by an alphabetical fifth character, the letter "F." These codes are not associated with any relative value units (RVUs); therefore, they are billed with a $0 billable charge amount. Although not reimbursed, the use of Category II codes is expanding as the emphasis on quality care grows.

Category III CPT codes were established in 2001 and are used for data collection for emerging technologies that are not yet mature and do not yet meet Category I criteria. They need to show medical specialty support, peer-reviewed literature showing growth, and ongoing clinical studies to evaluate their efficacy. When approved, they are assigned a four-digit code followed by the letter "T" as an identifier. The Category III codes are used to demonstrate how widespread their use is and for data collection in investigational protocols. They are only voluntarily reimbursable and RVUs are not assigned to them. Under HIPAA, Category III codes, though, are accepted by all healthcare payers. Local payments may be sought from local insurance carriers or through local Medicare contractors. Category III codes are temporary and can only be used for 5 years. After that time, they sunset if not converted into Category I codes. A 5-year extension for Category III codes may be obtained if approved by the CPT Editorial panel.[2,3]

Establishment of CPT codes for 3D printed anatomic models and guides

In the spring of 2018, the American College of Radiology (ACR) CPT Advisory Team, after many months of work and with consultation with the Radiological Society of North America (RSNA) 3D Printing Special Interest Group, submitted a Category III CPT code application to the CPT Editorial Panel of the AMA for 3D printed anatomic models and guides. A Category III code was thought to be the most appropriate because 3D printing of anatomic models represents a relatively new technology with developing use in patient care. The Category III application outlined the extensive process of creating anatomic models using imaging data including physician effort and the multiple technical inputs of performing image segmentation, creating CAD files, 3D printing the files, and post-processing the printed models. The application also included multiple peer-review medical articles supporting the clinical value of the models and guides and documentation of use of the models for patient care in multiple medical centers in the US.

The codes requested were based on the number of anatomic components included in the model. This approach seemed to best reflect the complexity and work needed to create the model. It was recognized that 3D printing and associated technologies such as segmentation software are a dynamic changing landscape and that over time, things would evolve and the work effort and technical input may well change. The submitted codes were the best effort to gather information on the technology as it stood at that point of time. This situation was a good fit for the exploratory Category III code category and would not constrain using a different measure of work and cost for a subsequent Category I application.

The CPT Editorial Panel reviewed the application over the summer of 2018 and requested input from the CPT Advisory Committee which is a group made up of multiple medical societies. In September 2018, the application was reviewed by the full CPT Editorial Panel at an open AMA CPT meeting in Boston. The ACR CPT Advisory Team formally presented the application and answered questions from the panel. The panel voted in private and the results were announced in late October that the four Category III codes for 3D printing of anatomic models and guides were approved (Table 8.1). The codes became available for submission for billing use for services provided as of July 1, 2019.[4–6]

Once the codes became available, medical centers could integrate these codes into their charge master billing system and begin to submit charges for reimbursement. Although Category III codes are voluntarily reimbursable, they may be reimbursed both by CMS and private insurers. A CMS reimbursement was announced for 0559T (anatomic model with single anatomic structure) and 0561T (single anatomic guide).[7,8] Private insurers payments may reflect the CMS payment or can be negotiated or set separately. The amount a medical center charges for their services is determined independently at each medical center. Each medical center determines physician or qualified healthcare provider effort and technical input costs such as space, equipment, material, and allied health to come up with a charge.

The Category III codes approved for reporting creation of 3D printed anatomic models from an individual's imaging dataset for patient care are 0559T and +0560T. Code 0559T is used to report the only or dominant anatomic structure which is individually segmented and processed to create the 3D printed anatomic model. An anatomic structure is a well-defined recognized component of anatomy such as bone, heart, arteries, veins, muscles, or visceral organs. A 3D printed anatomic model can, though, be made up of more than one anatomic structure (Fig. 8.2).

TABLE 8.1
List of the four Category III CPT codes for 3D printed anatomic models and guides.

CPT Code	Code Description
0559T	Anatomic model 3D printed from image dataset(s); first individually prepared and processed component of an anatomic structure
0560T	Each additional individually prepared and processed component of an anatomic structure (list separately in addition to code for primary procedure) (use 0560T in conjunction with 0559T)
0561T	Anatomic guide 3D printed and designed from image dataset(s); first anatomic guide
0562T	Each additional anatomic guide (list separately in addition to code for primary procedure) (use 0562T in conjunction with 0561T)

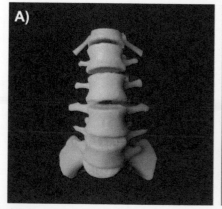 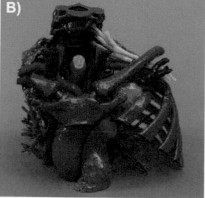

FIG. 8.2 **(A)** Anatomic model made up of a single anatomic structure (spine). **(B)** Anatomic model of Pancoast tumor of the chest made up of seven multiple anatomic structures with the bones—brown, aorta and arterial system—red, venous system—purple, trachea—orange, left brachial plexus—yellow, pulmonary veins—blue and tumor—green. Both models were printed with material jetting (Connex 500, Stratasys, Eden Prairie, MN).

The Category III code +0560T is an add-on code (as designated by the "+" symbol) and is used to report and list separately in conjunction with 0559T code if there is more than one anatomic structure included in the model.[9] This code is reported one time for each additional anatomic structure printed in addition to the base structure (which is reported with 0559T). An example of this would be a renal mass anatomic model (Fig. 8.3). The normal renal parenchyma (cortex) could be coded 0559T. The additional structures in the model would be coded using +0560T. This could include renal tumor (0560Tx1), renal arteries (0560Tx2), renal veins (0560Tx3), and collecting system (0560Tx4). The number of individual files used to print the anatomic model is generally a reflection of the number of anatomic structures to code for. 3D printed parts such as cylinders and connectors are not considered anatomic structures and would not be coded.

The Category III codes approved for reporting of 3D printed anatomic guides which are created using individualized imaging data for patient care are 0561T and +0562T. Guides are tools used for surgical and interventional procedures such as but not limited to cutting or drilling (Fig. 8.4). The code 0561T is used to report the first or main 3D printed anatomic guide. A second guide with a different design but using the same segmented image data may be created for the same procedure and would be coded with the add-on code of +0562T.[9] In addition, a 3D printed anatomic model

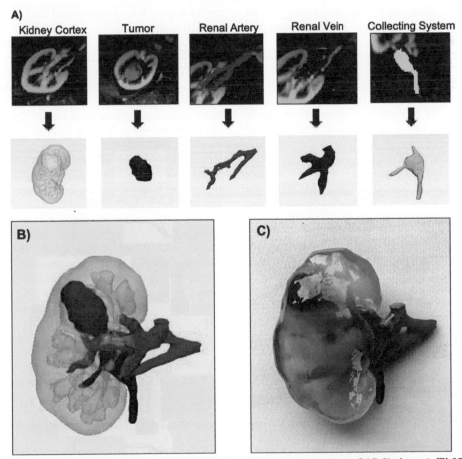

FIG. 8.3 **(A)** Image segmentation and conversion of each segmented region to CAD file format. **(B)** 3D CAD model showing all five structures, **(C)** 3D printed model showing all five structures. The model was printed on the Connex 500 (Stratasys, Rehovot, Israel) using Heart Print Flex material (Materialise, Leuven, Belgium) for the kidney and combinations of cyan and magenta materials (Stratasys, Eden Prairie, MN) to highlight the remaining four structures (Nicole Wake, PhD, NYU Langone Health, New York, NY).

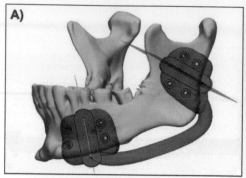
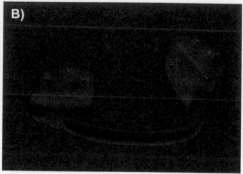

FIG. 8.4 Anatomic guide example showing a single mandibular guide **(A)** in the computer-aided design software (3-matic, Materialise, Leuven, Belgium), and **(B)** 3D printed anatomic guide printed using vat photopolymerization (Form2, Formlabs, Cambridge, MA) with a biocompatible surgical grade resin which was sterilized with autoclave prior to use. (Images courtesy of Amy Alexander, BME, MS, Mayo Clinic, Rochester, MN.)

may be created in conjunction with the guide(s) to assist as a surgical aid and this would be coded separately using 0559T and +0560T.

There is active discussion on what constitutes an anatomic guide and how it differs from an anatomic model. The difference between an anatomic model and anatomic guide could be distinguished based on its composition. A 3D printed anatomic model is composed of specific human anatomic structures, and is used in a number of ways as an aid for surgical planning. A 3D printed guide is a tool used to facilitate surgical procedures such as cutting and drilling and is not composed of specific anatomic structures. The data collected through the Category III CPT code and the registry will be helpful in evaluating the specific uses of guides and will be helpful to develop a clearer definition of what constitutes an "anatomic guide." This information can then be used in Category I code application.

Future application for Category I CPT code
Category III CPT codes are archived after 5 years from the initial publication or extension, unless a modification of the archival date is noted. Toward the end of the 5-year period of a Category III CPT code, application to the AMA for a Category I CPT code can be made. The bar for approval of a Category I code is much higher than a Category III code and the application must pass more rigorous criteria. Requirements include demonstration of clinical efficacy with abundant peer-reviewed literature. In addition, the service must be shown to be common practice at multiple US medical centers and there must be Food and Drug Administration clearance for all drugs and devices associated with the service. Category I applications are reviewed

by the same CPT Editorial Panel that reviews the Category III applications.

Once approved, the level of reimbursement of a Category I CPT code is complex and depends on several factors (Fig. 8.5). The approved code is reviewed by the Relative Value Scale Update Committee (RUC) of the AMA which is an advisory group to CMS. The RUC seeks input from an Advisory Council which is made up of representatives from all medical societies and is completely separate from the CPT Editorial Panel. Surveys are sought on the CPT code being reviewed from members of each specialty society that perform or have an interest in the procedure or service. The RUC analyzes the data on both physician effort and the technical inputs or practice expenses needed to provide the clinical service. They then make recommendations to CMS of an appropriate RVU for the CPT code. Budget neutrality is an important consideration for the RUC when considering valuation for new services. The total amount of money Medicare can spend is fixed by law and can only be changed by Congress. If the new level of spending exceeds this limit, a conversion factor (CF) is used to decrease compensation for all codes uniformly to ensure that the overall payments for Medicare remain within boundaries.

CMS utilizes the RUC recommendations in assigning RVUs for the CPT code associated with that service or procedure. The RVU, though, is not the final payment. Because of geographic cost differences, the RVU is adjusted by a geographic practice cost index for each Medicare location. The RVU is also multiplied by a CF of dollars per RVU for the final payment rate for the procedure. The submitted billing and payment are made through local Medicare carrier insurers who are contractors with the US government. CMS announces

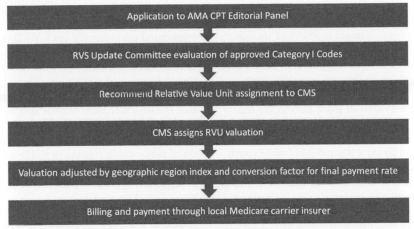

FIG. 8.5 Process for category I CPT approval and reimbursement.

the Medicare Fee Schedule for the next year through the Federal Register.[6,10] Private nongovernment health insurance payers use CPT codes and consider the RVU levels in setting their own reimbursement levels. Another option for reimbursement includes bundling the model and guide cost into broad surgical packages instead of pursuing a specific CPT.

RSNA-ACR 3D PRINTING REGISTRY

In July 2019, the RSNA and the ACR agreed to collaborate on a registry for 3D printing. The fundamental goal of this system is to collect information about clinical 3D printing across the US, conducted at the point of care (i.e., within hospitals or clinics, as opposed to services supplied by commercial vendors). Registry data will support two primary purposes: to enable institutional quality improvement and to provide evidence for potential future reimbursement. This section describes the RSNA—ACR 3D Printing Registry and discusses how it will be used to support these two purposes.

Registry design and implementation

The RSNA—ACR 3D Printing Registry was created with several factors in mind. First, with regard to scope, the registry is intended to mirror the existing Category III CPT codes for 3D printing which became active on July 1, 2019. Second, the registry is designed to capture case data to address quality improvement and reimbursement. Third, the registry is designed to promote ease of participation. By balancing these considerations, the registry intends to capture relevant information about clinical 3D printing at the point of care while limiting the burden on participating practices and institutions.

Registry scope: anatomic models and anatomic guides

As of this writing, the registry restricts data submission to two categories of 3D printing (i.e., anatomic models and anatomic guides) in order to mirror the data associated with the aforementioned CPT codes (0559T—0562T). While this addresses a large portion of the clinical 3D printing currently performed in hospitals and clinics, this restriction in scope does exclude some specific types of 3D printed objects, including external prostheses and implanted devices.

The registry classifies objects as either anatomic models or anatomic guides based on what is represented in the object, rather than by how the object is used. Anatomic models are defined as objects which consist primarily of anatomic structures, whereas anatomic guides have engineered features (such as flanges, slots, or latticework) as primary design elements. Note that anatomic models may still contain engineered elements, when these are used for some secondary function such as mechanical support. An object with multiple separate bony structures, using cylindrical connectors between bones to maintain alignment in the printed object, would be considered an anatomic model. The registry also defines several subtypes of anatomic models and anatomic guides, as detailed in the registry data dictionary.

Data dictionary

The registry data dictionary[11] defines the data fields collected by the registry for each submitted case. This document is divided into nine sections, addressing various portions of the clinical 3D printing workflow. The document also includes seven appendices, which define the terms used by the data fields. Such "controlled terminologies" serve to constrain possible responses and facilitate subsequent data analysis. Here, the use of anatomic terms in the data dictionary is described in detail.

The anatomic terms defined in Appendix A of the data dictionary are used both to describe imaging exams and to describe the parts of an anatomic model. These terms are organized into a system of three tiers: body region, subregion, and structure. This system enables users to describe many different anatomic structures in any part of the body while utilizing a limited number of words.

In order to describe imaging exams (see Section 2 of the data dictionary), it is typical to indicate a broad area of the body that is imaged, such as with "CT Chest" or "US abdomen" or "MRI pelvis." The nine body region terms described in Appendix A of the data dictionary (i.e., Head, Neck, Chest, Abdomen, Pelvis, Upper extremity, Lower extremity, Spine, Breast) provide these broad area descriptors. Often, body region alone suffices to characterize the anatomy of an imaging exam. Sometimes, imaging exam names may provide more anatomic specificity, such as when a particular imaging protocol is being described (e.g., "CT of the abdomen focusing on the liver" or "MRI of the head focusing on the orbits" or "MRI of the pelvis focusing on the prostate"). In such cases, the subregion and structure terms provide increasing levels of anatomic specificity.

It is important to note that the anatomic descriptors for an imaging exam are not expected to bear a direct one-to-one relationship with the segmented parts of a 3D printed object. Even if the printed object in a given case contains an arterial tree and nerve segments, as derived from imaging, it is not expected or necessarily desirable for the imaging description to explicitly reference such anatomic terms.

The same anatomic terms of Appendix A in the data dictionary are used again in Section 3 to describe the segmented parts created for the 3D printed object. The same system of tiers applies as above. Here, however, the most detailed terms (i.e., the terms in the "structure" tier of the system) will almost always be required to specifically identify the anatomy of a segmented part. Note that the structure term may be specific to a given region or subregion (e.g., the structure Pancreas is only present in the region Abdomen), may be specific to only a subset of the possible regions (e.g., the structure GI tract occurs only in the Chest, Abdomen, and Pelvis), or may occur in any region of the body (e.g., structure Artery). For selected anatomic regions, subregions, and structures, laterality must be specified. For example, laterality is always required for structures in the regions Upper extremity, Lower extremity, and Breast. Laterality is also relevant for selected other structures, such as Kidney. Table 8.2 shows several examples of anatomic parts described with the registry's system of anatomic terms.

Note an important difference in the use of anatomic terms for imaging exams versus segmented anatomic parts: while a structure term is often unnecessary when describing imaging exams, it is almost always required when describing segmented anatomic parts.

Registry participation

The registry has been implemented on the ACR National Radiology Data Registry (NRDR) platform.[12] NRDR was established in 2008 and now has thousands of facilities participating in a range of active registries. NRDR hosts well over 150 million cases and is widely recognized as a leading platform for imaging registries. The 3D printing registry benefits from the maturity, stability, security, maintenance, and support associated with the NRDR platform, and many institutions already have

TABLE 8.2
Examples of anatomic parts with appropriate anatomic terms selected as described in the registry data fields.

Part	Region	Subregion	Structure	Laterality
Pancreas	Abdomen	—	Pancreas	—
Prostate	Pelvis	—	Prostate	—
Vertebrobasilar arterial tree	Head	—	Artery	—
Right scapula	Upper extremity	Shoulder	Bone	Right
Left breast mass	Breast	—	Tumor	Left
Left ventricle	Chest	Heart	Left ventricle	—

experience submitting case data to other NRDR registries. Facilities may sign up to be a part of the registry through the NRDR site.[13] Facilities new to NRDR need to create a new corporate account and need to sign a Participation Agreement and Business Associate Agreement, establishing a formal relationship between the facility and the ACR. Once registered, the 3D printing registry will show up on the user's account and cases may be submitted.

There are potential barriers to registry participation. One class of concerns relates to the privacy and security of clinical data. In order to address these concerns, the registry by design collects no protected health information (PHI). For example, the registry does not collect any of the following: individual names, institution names, dates other than year, age other than years (and no specific age in years for patients 90 years of age or older), and patient identifiers (e.g., medical record number, social security number, accession number). In addition, the registry has been reviewed by an Independent Review Board (IRB) on behalf of the ACR and found to be exempt from IRB oversight. By avoiding PHI, the 3D printing registry limits the potential for breach of privacy. Another potential barrier to registry participation relates to the work required for data collection and case submission. Toward this end, the registry makes some data fields optional. For example, all of the user assessment questions (Section 8 of the data dictionary) are optional. While it is useful to know the opinions of clinical users regarding 3D printed anatomic models and anatomic guides, the realities of the clinical workflow may prohibit the collection of such responses. By making fields such as these optional, the registry recognizes these constraints and allows submission of cases without these data.

Registry data for institutional quality improvement and to support reimbursement

The use of registries for quality improvement is well established,[14,15] and this is a primary purpose of the ACR NRDR platform. Some of the ways in which registry data can contribute to quality improvement include the benchmarking of current practice, the assessment of appropriateness, and the identification of variation in clinical practice and outcomes. By establishing norms, and identifying variation, registries empower participants to evaluate their own practice in a broader context. For example, the ACR Dose Index Registry allows participating institutions to compare their own CT radiation doses with aggregated dose data from across the registry. Such comparison may highlight opportunities for dose reduction.

As a relatively new area of clinical practice, medical 3D printing in hospitals continues to evolve and mature. The RSNA–ACR 3D Printing Registry will enable the most detailed and broad-based characterizations to-date of clinical practice in this field. Such characterizations will include information about the distribution of case volumes, the scope of clinical indications, and the 3D printing technologies used. By informing the continued development of guidelines and best practices, this type of information will be useful for quality improvement efforts at the level of individual institutions, as well as for the clinical 3D printing community as a whole.

In addition to quality improvement, registry data will be useful in demonstrating the value of point of care 3D printing, quantifying the effort involved, and making a case for reimbursement.

CONCLUSIONS

Proper documentation is required in order to ensure suitable reimbursement for 3D printed anatomic and guides. Today, limited reimbursement may be obtained using the established Category III CPT codes for 3D printing. Hopefully, in the future, there will be Category I CPT codes for 3D printed anatomic models and guides that will offer more robust reimbursement. The RSNA–ACR 3D Printing Registry is collecting data on 3D printed anatomic models and anatomic guides, produced at the point of care, and the registry data will support future efforts relating to reimbursement for clinical 3D printing. Institutions interested in contributing to these efforts should consider using the relevant Category III CPT codes and participating in the registry.

REFERENCES

1. Thorwarth Jr WT. CPT: an open system that describes all that you do. *J Am Coll Radiol.* 2008;5:555–560.
2. Hirsch JA, Leslie-Mazwi TM, Nicola GN, et al. Current procedural terminology; a primer. *J NeuroIntervent Surg.* 2015; 7:309–312.   https://doi.org/10.1136/neurintsurg-2014-011156.
3. CPT Editorial Team. *The CPT Code Process*; September 25, 2019. Retrieved from: https://www.ama-assn.org/about/cpt-editorial-panel/cpt-code-process.
4. American Medical Association. *September 2018 CPT Editorial Summary of Panel Actions*; 2018. https://www.ama-assn.org/system/files/2018-10/september-2018-summary-panel-actions.pdf. Accessed August 11, 2020.
5. CPT Changes. *An Insider's View: Spiralbound*. America Medical Association; 2020:213–214. https://commerce.ama-assn.org/store/ui/catalog/productDetail?product_id=prod2950005&navAction=push. Accessed August 11, 2020.

6. American Medical Association. *CPT® 2020 Professional Edition*. Chicago: American Medical Association; 2020.

7. *July 2019 Update of the Hospital Outpatient Prospective Payment System (OPPS)*. CMS Manual System, Pub 100-04, Transmittal #R4313CP; May 24, 2019. Change request 11318 https://www.cms.gov/Regulations-and-Guidance/Guidance/Transmittals/2019-Transmittals-Items/R4313CP. Accessed August 11, 2020.

8. MLN Matters®. *July 2019 Update of the Hospital Outpatient Prospective Payment System (OPPS), MM 11318*; 2019. https://www.cms.gov/Outreach-and-Education/Medicare-Learning-Network-MLN/MLNMattersArticles/downloads/MM11318.pdf. Accessed August 10, 2020.

9. Clinical examples in radiology. *AMA/ACR*. Spring 2019; 15(Issue 2):6–8. https://commerce.ama-assn.org/store/ui/catalog/productDetail?product_id=prod1270029&navAction=push. Accessed August 10, 2020.

10. Thorwarth Jr WT. From concept to CPT code to compensation: how the payment system works. *J Am Coll Radiol*. 2004;1:48–53.

11. Radiologic Society of North America and American College of Radiology. *3D Printing Registry Data Dictionary*; 2020. August 11, 2020 https://nrdrsupport.acr.org/support/solutions/articles/11000073770-3d-printing-data-dictionary.

12. American College of Radiology. *Introducing the NRDR*; 2019. https://nrdrsupport.acr.org/support/solutions/articles/11000030671-introducing-the-nrdr.

13. American College of Radiology. *National Radiology Data Registry New Corporate Account Registration*; 2020. https://nrdr.acr.org/Portal/Nrdr/Main/NewCorporateAccountRegistration/page.aspx. Accessed August 10, 2020.

14. McNeil JJ, Evans SM, Johnson NP, Cameron PA. Clinical-quality registries: their role in quality improvement. *Med J Aust*. 2010;192:244–245.

15. Stey AM, Russell MM, Ko CY, Sacks GD, Dawes AJ, Gibbons MM. Clinical registries and quality measurement in surgery: a systematic review. *Surgery*. 2015;157:381–395.

CHAPTER 9

Regulatory Perspectives for 3D Printing in Hospitals

ANDY CHRISTENSEN, BS, FSME • NICOLE WAKE, PHD

INTRODUCTION

The United States (US) Food and Drug Administration (FDA) has overseen medical device marketing in the US since May 28, 1976, when the Medical Device Amendments to the Federal Food, Drug and Cosmetic Act were passed.[1] The system that was established has first and foremost the public safety in mind, focusing on regulations for the marketing of medical devices in the US. While safety is the first priority, the FDA also has purview to mandate evidence of efficacy for any devices it chooses, but certainly for devices that are either novel or high risk. A key point is that the FDA regulates the medical device industry which designs, manufactures, and sells medical devices to physicians and hospitals. The FDA does not typically regulate hospitals or individual physicians. Physicians operate with certifications from the state and their medical society along with privileges to practice medicine at a specific medical facility or hospital. This is the concept of the "practice of medicine."[2] Dating back to 1908, the "practice of medicine" derived its name from the custom of administering so-called "medicines."[3] Today, the "practice of medicine" is defined as diagnosing, treating, operating, or prescribing for any human disease, pain, injury, deformity, or physical condition.[2] Licensed physicians or healthcare professionals with appropriate state and hospital privileges can treat patients as they see fit under the "practice of medicine."

A medical device is defined by the FDA as follows:[4]

Per Section 201(h) of the Food, Drug, and Cosmetic Act, a medical device is: An instrument, apparatus, implement, machine, contrivance, implant, in vitro reagent, or other similar or related article, including a component part, or accessory which is:

1. recognized in the official National Formulary, or the US Pharmacopoeia, or any supplement to them,
2. intended for use in the diagnosis of disease or other conditions, or in the cure, mitigation, treatment, or prevention of disease, in man or other animals, or
3. intended to affect the structure or any function of the body of man or other animals, and which does not achieve its primary intended purposes through chemical action within or on the body of man or other animals and
4. which does not achieve its primary intended purposes through chemical action within or on the body of man or other animals and which is not dependent upon being metabolized for the achievement of its primary intended purposes. The term "device" does not include software functions excluded pursuant to section 520(o).

The key takeaways from the definition include that a medical device is meant for diagnosis or in the cure, mitigation, treatment, or prevention of disease. Medical device products range from simple gauze and surgical tape to very complex total joint implants and pacemakers. In the US, diagnostic imaging equipment such as ultrasound devices, computed tomography (CT) systems, and magnetic resonance imaging (MRI) machines are also included and regulated as medical devices.

Medical Device Classification

The FDA uses a classification system based on risk of the device and the regulatory controls necessary to provide a reasonable assurance of safety and effectiveness.[5] Medical devices are categorized into one of three classes—Class I, II, or III (Table 9.1). All device manufacturers, regardless of device class, must follow "general controls," i.e., have a quality system, maintain records, and perform duties such as adverse event reporting in addition to registering and listing the device with the FDA.

3D Printing for the Radiologist. https://doi.org/10.1016/B978-0-323-77573-1.00015-4

TABLE 9.1
Overview of FDA Medical Device Classes I–III.

	Class I	Class II	Class III
Risk level	Low	Moderate	High
Type of FDA submission	Typically none	510(k)	Premarket approval (PMA)
Clinical data required?	No	Mostly no	Yes

Low-risk devices fall into **Class I** and typically do not require premarket notification or approval from the FDA. If a manufacturer would like to sell a Class I product which does not require premarket notification or premarket approval (PMA), they must comply with general controls, register as a manufacturer with the FDA, and list the products with the FDA prior to selling. It is estimated that just under half of all medical devices fall into the Class I category.

Class II devices contain higher, but still moderate levels of patient risk and are typically subject to premarket notification. Premarket notification for Class II medical devices typically involves filing a 510(k) application which provides safety data and compares the product to a known, previously approved "predicate device." The predicate device must have the same indications for use and risk profile as the subject device. The use of predicate devices is key to the way the FDA has worked for over three decades. Again, just under half of all products fall into the Class II category, including most implants (e.g., total knee implants, facial fracture plating) and diagnostic imaging systems such as CT scanners or MRI machines.

Class III devices are considered high-risk devices and may be life-supporting, life-sustaining, or important in preventing impairment of human health. If the risk to the patient is high and/or there is little known about similar devices in the market, the FDA will require more data and assurance about the device. Class III devices represent less than 10% of all devices on the market and this category is reserved for either high-risk devices or devices without adequate historical market data. These devices typically require a PMA application to be filed and most times the FDA requires clinical data in support of these PMAs. When the PMA is cleared by the FDA, it is cleared for both safety and efficacy. Efficacy (or effectiveness) is something that the lower Class I and II categories cannot claim because

their submissions typically are not forced to contain these data. Only a product cleared through the PMA pathway can be claimed to be "FDA-Approved." All other clearances should be referred to as "marketing clearance" or "FDA-cleared" as it is inappropriate to use the term "approved" with devices which are not cleared through the PMA pathway.

Another key to the FDA's way of looking at the medical device market is that they clear or approve a specific medical device for a specific intended use. Here it is helpful to lookup specific FDA Product Codes (aka procodes) which list a specific medical device, its classification, and whether or not it typically requires a 510(k), a PMA, or is Exempt. Many of these product codes are agnostic to whether the product is personalized, this product code could refer to a patient-matched or a non–patient-matched product, depending on the applicant and product.

Let us take for example a cranioplasty device, product code GXN.[6] The title of the device is "Plate, Cranioplasty, Preformed, Non-Alterable." Looking at the listing, a more formal description in the Federal Register for product code GXN is found at 21 CFR Part 882.5330.[7] From the listing we can tell that this device is a Class II device that typically requires a 510(k) and is overseen by the Neurology review panel within the FDA. If Company A files a 510(k) and obtains clearance for a product in the GXN product category with the FDA, then this product will be a patient-matched cranioplasty product. They use an indication for use statement of "<Product Name> is designed individually for each patient and is intended to replace bony voids in the cranial skeleton." Indications statements are typically fairly short and to-the-point, although most are more than a single sentence. After getting the FDA's marketing clearance for their product, Company A can market the product freely within the US for this indication. If Company A were to market this product to fill voids in another areas of the skeletal structure (e.g., the pelvis), this would be outside of the cleared indications for the product. The FDA considers this practice misbranding and "off-label use" of the device. The FDA regulates companies and prohibits them from off-label promotion but the FDA does not regulate physicians who safely use devices off-label in order to provide a solution that will positively impact patient care. Many shades of gray are present with regard to off-label usage of medical devices, but this only applies when the device is a medical device and has some cleared indication for use. In this case, if a second company, Company B, wants to sell the exact same product for cranial reconstruction, they would also need to go through the 510(k) process with the FDA. They could use Company A's product as a predicate if they so desired. Preparing a 510(k) and choosing a predicate device is beyond scope for this chapter but there are many factors that would go into choosing a predicate, including access to the device and/or test data so as to use it for direct comparison to the new device.

Novel products called De Novo products are products which do not have an adequate predicate since they are new and follow an expanded pathway as compared to filing a traditional 510(k). Most times De Novo products end up in the Class II category. Future products after the first product is cleared through the De Novo pathway can be cleared using the De Novo product as a predicate with a traditional 510(k).

Another pathway for a Class III device targeting a small population is the Humanitarian Device Exemption pathway. These devices are cleared for limited numbers of patients per year and typically require submission of clinical data to which the FDA gives approval for safety and "probability of effectiveness."[8]

MEDICAL DEVICE REGULATIONS

FDA regulations, which only apply to the medical device industry, include commercially available, 3D printed medical devices consisting of instrumentation (e.g., surgical guides to assist with proper placement of a device), implants (e.g., cranial plates or joint arthroplasty components), and external prostheses (e.g., lower extremity prosthetics).[9] Between January 2010 and April 2016, more than 80 3D printed medical devices received 510(k) clearance, with the majority (83%) using powder bed fusion printing techniques.[10]

Anatomic models have historically been regarded by the medical device industry as very low–risk medical devices. Many questioned early on whether an anatomic model is actually a medical device at all. Starting around 2000 several companies providing services in this area submitted themselves to the FDA's scrutiny and listed products under a product code HWT— Template for Clinical Use, regulation number 888.4800.[11] HWT devices consist of a pattern or guide such as that intended to assist with selecting or positioning of orthopedic implants or guiding the marking of tissue before cutting.[12]

Although this was not a perfect fit for patient-specific 3D printed anatomic models, it seemed justifiable since these models are used for planning purposes. HWT is a Class I Exempt device, with the exemption allowing the product to bypass premarket notification or approval. The manufacturers of these devices are still required to abide by general controls, including company registration, device listing, maintaining a quality system, and adverse event reporting. Importantly, the fact that the manufacturer must register and list the device gives the FDA the authority to audit the manufacturer at any time it wishes. Companies that sold 3D printed anatomic models to physicians and hospitals used HWT as a "home" for anatomic models since approximately 2000. If the FDA disagreed with this classification, then they certainly did not make it known publicly, at least not until 2017.[13]

In August 2017, an important public meeting was held at the FDA's White Oak Campus (Silver Spring, MD) by and between the FDA and the Radiological Society of North America (RSNA) 3D Printing Special Interest Group (SIG). The meeting, which brought together different stakeholders (e.g., regulatory personnel, manufacturers, and healthcare professionals), was focused on 3D printed anatomic models and regulatory implications. The stated goals and objectives of the meeting were, as described on the FDA website,[13]

(1) To provide a forum for open discussion between experts in 3D printing anatomic models from the clinical, industry, hospital, and regulatory field.

(2) To map out priorities for developing scientific evidence, identifying critical quality attributes, and building best practices for the safe clinical use of 3D printed anatomic models derived from medical imaging data.

Both of these goals were met during the course of this meeting, and a few very interesting clarifications were made by the FDA. First, the FDA clearly explained that HWT was not the appropriate product code for a 3D printed anatomic model. They stated that a 3D printed anatomic model, if marketed for diagnostic use, was considered a Class II medical device and should be listed under product code LLZ, "System, Image Processing, Radiological."[14] LLZ is typically related to software for PACS and image processing, and several of the software historically used in image processing for 3D printing are cleared under product code LLZ. The FDA reiterated that the existing software cleared for image processing stopped short of the actual 3D printing and as such could not claim that the outputs of these software packages were "diagnostic use" anatomic models. In addition, the FDA clarified that they see the image processing software as the most important and critical portion of the workflow for creating a "diagnostic use" anatomic model.[12]

The term "diagnostic use" has been frequently misconstrued in the context of patient-specific 3D

What does the FDA's Division of Radiological Health (DRH) Consider to be Diagnostic Use for a 3D Printed Anatomic Model?
Use that <u>can</u> affect/change:
• Diagnosis
• Patient Management
• Patient Treatment
Examples:
• Models used to make diagnosis based on examination or a physical measurement of structural changes from the 3D model
• Using the model to size and/or select a device or surgical instrument based on a comparison, fitting, or measurements with the model
• Using the model to determine whether a specific surgical procedure may be viable

FIG. 9.1 Summary of "Diagnostic Use" anatomic models. (Reproduced from Kiarashi N. FDA current practices and regulations. *FDA/CDRH-RSNA SIG Joint Meeting on 3D Printed Patient-specific Anatomic Models*; 2017. https://www.fda.gov/media/107498/download. Accessed 1 June 2020.)

printed anatomic models. We will recall the word diagnosis appearing in the definition of a medical device. Many in the medical field have believed diagnosis was more of a literal word concerning the definitive prediction of the patient's medical condition. Radiologists diagnose from medical images on a daily basis. Indeed the FDA clarified that their interpretation of the term diagnostic use was broader by far than classification of illness. Diagnostic use of a 3D printed anatomic model was defined by the FDA as shown in Fig. 9.1.[12]

This expanded definition of what is considered "diagnostic use" links the use of almost any patient-specific anatomic model for visualization, surgical planning, and device sizing applications. From the FDA's perspective, if a 3D printed anatomic model is marketed for "diagnostic use," then it is considered a medical device. Because these are considered medical devices, and of a Class II nature, the FDA would require a company who wishes to market a diagnostic use 3D printed anatomic model to follow requirements, including submission of a 510(k) premarket notification for such a device.

At the August 2017 meeting, the FDA discussed a new methodology for industry to follow for 3D printing systems meant to produce diagnostic use anatomic models in a hospital environment. Using product code LLZ the image processing software would be the primary cleared device. Additionally, for production of a diagnostic use, 3D printed anatomic model, the 3D printer, 3D printing material, and anatomic location would be spelled out in the device's intended use. They clarified that the 3D printer and 3D printing materials would not technically be cleared, but these combinations of 3D printer and materials would be "validated" for the specific intended use. In order to receive 510(k) clearance, performance testing should be carried out and could include, but is not limited to, clinically relevant accuracy and precision measurements for a specific anatomy type, phantom-based testing to ensure detectable landmarks are accurately replicated in 3D printed anatomy, and 3D printer capability. At the time of writing, there are two companies which have LLZ-cleared software systems intended to produce diagnostic use 3D printed anatomic models,[15,16] and it is expected that more systems will be approved in the future.

3D Printed Guides

3D printed surgical guides, also known as anatomic guides, cutting guides, or drilling guides, first appeared on the market for dental implant applications in the early 2000s. Companies selling these guides focused on the software and FDA clearance but not on the guides, and they did not consider these guides medical devices on their own. By 2008, the applications were expanding, and the first 3D printed surgical guides for total knee arthroplasty began to be sold by the companies providing the implant systems. Companies including Biomet, Zimmer, and DePuy began to sell these guides; and they listed the guides under the HWT product code as Template for Clinical Use. However, the FDA later disagreed with this classification and sent warning letters to several companies asking them to justify their stance and explain why premarket notification via 510(k) was not required.[17] In the end, the FDA mandated that companies selling these surgical guides submit a 510(k) for the guides in the same product code and classification as the total joint implants, which were typically Class II.

Patient-Matched versus Custom Devices

Custom devices are often confused with patient-matched/patient-specific devices (Table 9.2). A truly custom device, defined under the FDA's Custom Device Exemption (CDE), is exempt from premarket review because it

TABLE 9.2
Comparison of Patient-Matched versus Custom Devices.

	Patient-Matched Devices	Custom Devices
FDA premarket notification/ approval needed	Yes	No
Limits to numbers available to sell	No	Limit of 5 per year per indication/ anatomic area
Can be freely marketed	Yes	No
Is based on medical imaging data	Yes	Not necessarily
Can be used even if there is another product on the market which could treat the intended use	Yes	No
Is exempt from general controls for medical devices	No	No
Requires yearly reporting to the FDA on numbers produced	No	Yes

the medical device industry, so much of this discussion is focused on medical device companies providing these products, not on hospitals making their own medical devices. More elaboration on this can be found below when talking about the future and the FDA's conceptual framework for hospital-based 3D printing.

Patient matched refers to a design where instead of a product being a discreet size (e.g., small, medium, large), the product will encompass a design envelope for a range of sizes. Patient-matched products are designed to fit a patient's anatomy many times using medical image data as a basis. That range allows one to determine what the worst-case product is from a testing standpoint to demonstrate the rest of the product within that range are going to perform as expected.[19] Patient-matched products may be cleared by the 510(k) pathway and widely marketed, unlike their custom device counterparts. Patient-matched and custom as terms have been used interchangeably in the past, but from an FDA standpoint the word "custom" has a specific meaning as described in the CDE and as such the word custom should not be used to describe a personalized, or patient-matched product which will have pre-market clearance.

Example of patient-matched device: cranioplasty

We have already explored the product code GXN for a cranioplasty product, used in neurosurgery to replace missing portions of the cranial bone. Several FDA-cleared products exist for a patient-matched cranioplasty plate, produced from a patient's CT scan data. The clearances for these devices would be material-specific (i.e. titanium or polyetheretherketone) and would have defined specifications, internal to the manufacturer, for thickness, minimum and/or maximum size, what type of fixation plating can be used with the device, and other characteristics. As long as the product produced follows these specifications it may be legally and freely marketed under the 510(k) clearance. This is not a custom product because it is the same product, being made for different individuals, sized based on their CT scan and produced under the auspices of a 510(k) clearance.

Example of custom device: femoral component of failed total knee replacement

In this theoretical example, the patient had a malignant lesion of the knee which required resection of some of the distal femur, the knee joint, and a portion of the proximal tibia. The reconstruction included a total knee replacement, and this procedure is typically referred to as a limb salvage procedure. This was originally carried out with off-the-shelf components which

is so unique that it does not make sense for that review.[19] The purpose of the regulation is to make clear which devices fall into this category and which do not. Most devices will not fall under this category, but it exists since the FDA wants medical device companies to be able to help physicians with very difficult, one-off surgical situations, and this is the intent of the CDE language.

If a procedure is performed frequently, then it is most likely not a candidate for this category. The confusion likely arises from the fact that the word "custom" is in some ways synonymous with personalized, and as such people assume that if something is personalized, then it must be a custom device. The FDA's most recent guidance document on the topic in 2014 limits what can be called a custom device to a very narrow scope.[18] Other parts of the world, Europe for instance, have historically taken a more liberal interpretation of devices that are exempt from premarket notification. Again, the FDA regulates were fit to the patient at the time of surgery. A decade later the femoral component has loosened and is failing, but the component in the proximal tibia is still functioning well. Surgeons decide they want to replace only the femoral component but the company which made the original component is no longer in business. A very special implant which is designed to fit this single patient and made to fit with existing, out of date, implant components is designed and produced. This is an example of a custom device, something that would fall under the FDA's CDE.

3D Printing in Hospitals

Hospitals that are creating 3D printed anatomic models and guides at the point of care need to look at the whole process and breakdown the most important steps of the workflow to ensure that models are being created safely. In order to ensure the best appropriate patient care, it is imperative that models are made with the highest possible quality and accuracy. Starting from the image acquisition going all the way to 3D printing and post-processing of the models, quality assurance (QA) measures should be taken to ensure that no errors occur during the process (see Chapter 7).

In regard to image postprocessing software, there are many choices (see Chapter 3), and these software range from freeware to fairly expensive proprietary software options. Typically, freeware is not FDA cleared, whereas proprietary software may have FDA clearance for visualization or even clearance for 3D printed, diagnostic use, anatomic model creation. When creating 3D printed models for clinical care (i.e., diagnostic use), the RSNA 3D printing SIG recommends that FDA-cleared software is utilized.[20]

As mentioned above, at this time, two companies offer FDA-cleared products for creating diagnostic use 3D printed anatomic models from medical imaging data.[15,16] The first received its clearance in 2018 and since this company does not manufacture its own printers approved several printers were validated in the workflow.[15] The other, received its clearance more recently in 2019; and this clearance involved proprietary software in conjunction with printers that were manufactured by the same company.[16] It is important to note that in both cases, only certain printers, materials, and use cases (anatomic areas) have been cleared. In the case that an anatomic model is desired which was not included with one of these clearances, hospitals are still able to make these models under the so-called "Practice of medicine"; however, it is imperative that hospitals ensure these models are accurate representations of the patient's anatomy or in the case of guides

that these models appropriately fit the patient's true anatomy. Proper selection of printing technologies and materials, especially for models that will be brought to the operating room and require sterilization, should also be considered. QA is discussed in detail in Chapter 7 so will not be discussed in detail here, but QA measures that are taken during each step of the 3D printing process will help to ensure high quality of the final product, and ultimately lead to improved satisfaction for use of models within the hospital environment and for outside regulatory bodies including the FDA.

FDA Conceptual Framework for 3D Printing in Hospitals

The ultimate goal of the FDA is to protect and promote human health; and the FDA is currently investigating what regulations should be implemented in a hospital which is performing 3D printing at the point of care. Ultimately, the FDA wants to ensure that the quality of a medical device being created in the hospital setting meets the same high standards as that which a company would sell and market to a hospital. The patient should have the same level of trust in a device made in a hospital as made by industry in regard to quality and safety. As hospitals are talking about producing devices such as implants, which are clearly more than minimal risk devices, this becomes even more important.

In May 2019, the FDA announced a "Conceptual Framework" for 3D printing at the point of care.[21] This was meant to be a starting point to the discussion between FDA and industry and physicians. These theoretical points are far from being something that is regarded as binding in this area. The FDA's ultimate goal is to ensure the safety and effectiveness of a medical device, regardless of where the device is manufactured. In this framework, six potential scenarios for 3D printing in hospitals were discussed (Fig. 9.2).

In Scenario A, 3D printed products would be considered to have minimal risk or harm to patients. These could be any range of low-risk medical devices which may include simple 3D printed anatomic models. Scenarios B and C both include devices or systems that are designed by a medical device manufacturer, cleared through existing FDA pathways, and sold for use to physicians and hospitals. In Scenario B, the system is fairly "closed" to changes whereby a user cannot make changes to the design process. For Scenario C, there may be additional requirements such as postprocessing that are not included in the validated process. This could include processing steps such as heat treatment or finish machining for additive metals products.

Potential 3D Printing Scenarios	
Scenario	**Description**
A	Minimal risk 3D printing by Healthcare Facility Personnel (HCFP)
B	Device designed by manufacturer using validated process • Turn-key system
C	Device designed by manufacturer using validated process • Additional HCFP capability requirements
D	Manufacturer co-located at the point of care
E	HCFP becomes a manufacturer
F	Others?

FIG. 9.2 Six potential scenarios for 3D printing in hospitals from the 2019 FDA Conceptual Framework. (Reproduced from FDA CDRH Additive Manufacturing Working Group. *3D Printing Medical Devices at the Point of Care*; 2019. https://cdn2.hubspot.net/hubfs/5268583/AMWG-FDA%20-%203DP%20at%20PoC%20V2.pdf?hsCtaTracking=8b212dad-9d50-4054-92a7-cdaeb1b27dec%7C1cbbfc11-6402-46e4-9a76-16a681e6d84a. Accessed 9 September 2020.)

Scenario D involves a situation where the manufacturer is co-located at the healthcare facility. In this case, the manufacturer operates under the traditional FDA guidelines using their own equipment and personnel, but it is expected that the close proximity to the point of care will enable improved workflows and patient care. To our knowledge, at this time there is one facility in the US that is planning to create a co-located manufacturing facility on the hospital campus.[22] In Scenario E, the healthcare facility produces a device with greater than minimal risk and becomes the medical device manufacturer and is thus responsible for all regulatory requirements. This would mean that these facilities would be registered as a medical device manufacturer with the FDA, list their products, and would need to have their 3D printed devices cleared via premarket submissions such as a 510(k) in the same manner as a traditional manufacturer. A final scenario, Scenario F, was left open for further discussion on the topic of 3D printed devices produced at the point of care.

The FDA has been closely monitoring 3D printing of medical devices for several years.[23,24] Dozens of product clearances and the monitoring of the companies providing these products have helped to inform the FDA's viewpoint of these technologies and their place in the manufacturing ecosystem. In order to ensure the safe and effective creation of 3D printed medical devices, it is expected that the FDA will continue to pay close attention to 3D printed medical devices that are created outside of the traditional manufacturing environment.

REFERENCES

1. U.S. Food and Drug Administration. *Medical Device Amendments of 1976*; 1976. https://www.govinfo.gov/content/pkg/STATUTE-90/pdf/STATUTE-90-Pg539.pdf.
2. NYSED.gov. *Article 131, Medicine*; 2010. http://www.op.nysed.gov/prof/med/article131.htm#. Accessed August 12, 2020.
3. What constitutes the practice of medicine? *J Am Med Assoc*. 1908;(5):368–369.
4. U.S. Food and Drug Administration. *Classification of Products as Drugs and Devices and Additional Product Classification Issues: Guidance for Industry and FDA Staff*; 2017. https://www.fda.gov/regulatory-information/search-fda-guidance-documents/classification-products-drugs-and-devices-and-additional-product-classification-issues#:~:text=For%20a%20medical%20product%20also,primary%20intended%20purposes%20through%20chemical. Accessed August 30, 2020.
5. U.S. Food and Drug Administration. *Overview of Medical Device Classification and Reclassification*; 2012. https://www.fda.gov/about-fda/cdrh-transparency/overview-medical-device-classification-and-reclassification. Accessed August 30, 2020.
6. U.S. Food and Drug Administration. *US Food & Drug Administration Product Classification, Device: Plate, Cranioplasty, Preformed, Non-Alterable, Product Code: GXN, Regulation Number: 882.5330*. https://www.accessdata.fda.gov/scripts/cdrh/cfdocs/cfPCD/classification.cfm?ID=3743. Accessed 30 August 2020.
7. U.S. Food and Drug Administration. *US Food & Drug Administration CFR- Code of Federal Regulations Title 21: CFR882.5330*. https://www.accessdata.fda.gov/scripts/cdrh/cfdocs/cfcfr/cfrsearch.cfm?fr=882.5330. Accessed 30 August 2020.

8. U.S. Food and Drug Administration. Humanitarian Device Exemption. https://www.fda.gov/medical-devices/premarket-submissions/humanitarian-device-exemption. Accessed November 16, 2020.

9. U.S. Food and Drug Administration. *Medical Applications of 3D Printing*; 2017. https://www.fda.gov/medical-devices/3d-printing-medical-devices/medical-applications-3d-printing.

10. Ricles LM, Coburn JC, Di Prima M, Oh SS. Regulating 3D-printed medical products. *Sci Transl Med.* 2018;10(461).

11. U.S. Food and Drug Administration. *Product Classification — Template.* https://www.accessdata.fda.gov/scripts/cdrh/cfdocs/cfpcd/classification.cfm?id=4595. Accessed 30 August 2020.

12. Kiarashi N. FDA Current practices and regulations. In: *FDA/CDRH-RSNA SIG Joint Meeting on 3D Printed Patient-specific Anatomic Models*; 2017. https://www.fda.gov/media/107498/download. Accessed June 1, 2020.

13. U.S. Food and Drug Administration. *FDA/CDRH — RSNA SIG Joint Meeting on 3D Printed Patient-specific Anatomic Models*; August 31, 2017. https://www.fda.gov/MedicalDevices/NewsEvents/WorkshopsConferences/ucm569452.htm. Accessed April 18, 2019.

14. U.S. Food and Drug Administration. *Product Classification — System, Image Processing, Radiological.* https://www.accessdata.fda.gov/scripts/cdrh/cfdocs/cfPCD/classification.cfm?ID=LLZ. Accessed 31 August 2020.

15. Materialise. *Materialise Mimics in Print: Regulatory Information*; 2018. https://www.materialise.com/en/medical/software/materialise-mimics-inprint/regulatory-information. Accessed April 18, 2019.

16. 3DSystems. *3D Systems Draws on Healthcare Expertise to Deliver FDA Cleared D2P™ — Industry's Only Company to Create Patient-specific, Diagnostic, Anatomic Models Using its Own Software and Printers*; 2019. https://www.3dsystems.com/press-releases/3d-systems-draws-healthcare-expertise-deliver-fda-cleared-d2p-industry-s-only. Accessed September 4, 2020.

17. Massdevice Staff. FDA warns Biomet on knee replacement planning system. *Mass Device*; 2010. https://www.massdevice.com/fda-warns-biomet-knee-replacement-planning-system/. Accessed August 30, 2020.

18. U.S. Food and Drug Administration. *Content of Premarket Submissions for Management of Cybersecurity in Medical Devices: Guidance for Industry and Food and Drug Administration Staff*; 2014. https://www.fda.gov/media/86174/download. Accessed August 30, 2020.

19. U.S. Food and Drug Administration. *Custom Device Exemption: Guidance for Industry and Food and Drug Administration Staff*; 2014. https://www.fda.gov/media/89897/download. Accessed August 30, 2020.

20. Chepelev L, Wake N, Ryan J, et al. Radiological Society of North America (RSNA) 3D printing Special Interest Group (SIG): guidelines for medical 3D printing and appropriateness for clinical scenarios. *3D Print Med.* 2018;4(1):11.

21. FDA CDRH Additive Manufacturing Working Group. *3D Printing Medical Devices at the Point of Care*; 2019. https://cdn2.hubspot.net/hubfs/5268583/AMWG-FDA%20-%203DP%20at%20PoC%20V2.pdf?hsCtaTracking=8b212dad-9d50-4054-92a7-cdaeb1b27dec%7C1cbbfc11-6402-46e4-9a76-16a681e6d84a. Accessed September 9, 2020.

22. Hospital for Special Surgery. *HSS and LimaCorporate 3D Printing Facility.* https://www.hss.edu/hss-lima-3d-printing.asp. Accessed 31 August 2020.

23. Di Prima M, Coburn J, Hwang D, Kelly J, Khairuzzaman A, Ricles L. Additively manufactured medical products — the FDA perspective. *3D Print Med.* 2016;2.

24. U.S. Food and Drug Administration. *Technical Considerations for Additive Manufactured Medical Devices: Guidance for Industry and Food and Drug Administration Staff*; 2017. https://www.fda.gov/regulatory-information/search-fda-guidance-documents/technical-considerations-additive-manufactured-medical-devices. Accessed August 30, 2020.

CHAPTER 10

3D Printing in Radiology Education

JUDAH BURNS, MD • MOHAMMAD MANSOURI, MD • NICOLE WAKE, PHD

INTRODUCTION

Diagnostic radiology programs currently encompass image-based diagnosis and image-guided therapeutic techniques using multiple available imaging modalities. Three-dimensional (3D) image post-processing of radiologic images routinely uses high-resolution computed tomography (CT) and magnetic resonance imaging (MRI) datasets for diagnostic evaluation and treatment planning. Dedicated training in 3D modeling may be incorporated into some radiology training programs, although it is not required, and formal training programs are limited. In radiology, a comprehensive medical 3D printing training program should prepare radiologists to be knowledgeable and proficient in creating 3D printed medical models from radiological imaging data. This chapter will give background on 3D modeling for medical education and will provide an overview of the fundamentals required for a radiological program that includes medical 3D printing.

HISTORICAL PERSPECTIVE ON 3D MODELING FOR MEDICAL EDUCATION

3D modeling in medical education has been used for generations. Together with two-dimensional (2D) drawings, scaled and realistic models have been used to record the discovery of anatomists, record unique and innovative patients and pathologies, and more recently, to widely disseminate both normal and abnormal teaching examples to students of anatomy, physiology, and medicine. 3D models are a staple of medical education; and the use of 3D models in medical schools is being expanded as the use of cadaveric dissection decreases. Surgical training has benefitted greatly from the availability of 3D models to plainly visualize pathology and simulate surgical approaches.[1] The addition of readily available, patient-specific 3D printed models is a further step in the progression toward more personalized medical and surgical care.

One of the earliest existing anatomical models is an Early Classic Mayan head, dated to 300—600 AD. Half of this sculpture shows the head in life and the other half shows the underlying bony skull. In 1027 in China, an imperial physician, Wang Wei-Yi had two life-size bronze statues made for teaching surface anatomy for locating the acupuncture points.[2] Sometime between 400—600 BC, an Indian sage named Sushruta was recorded to have used patient simulators for practice of surgical skills and suggested that such simulation-based education leads to competence and confidence. More recently, the 17th century father and son of the family Grégoire of Paris created obstetrical manikins for teaching midwives.[3] Also, in 17th century, Gaetano Giulio Zummo (1656—1701) a Sicilian abbot created 3D models from wax and recommended them for anatomy training.[4]

Over time, the materials used in creating realistic anatomic models have changed from wax to plaster and plastination.[5] Preparing plastination models is a time-consuming and expensive process, which requires expertise for model preparation. These models are realistic but degrade readily and are easily damaged.[6] More modern static models use plastic materials which rely on premade molds, limiting the flexibility of their application to individual patient care. As a tool for demonstration, however, virtual models and 3D printed models form the historical backbone and future for both hands-on learning and simulation.

3D PRINTING IN ANATOMY EDUCATION

Anatomy education, a traditional and key element of medical training, has evolved over the past few decades. The gold standard in anatomy education is cadaveric dissection, which is for many students their first encounter with a nonliving body. The process of dissection was traditionally viewed as a right-of-passage for students. Though this passage came with emotional and ethical conflict, dissection helped young physicians form a strong emotional connection to the form of the human body, which they sought to heal. Advances in technology have offered students even greater access to virtual dissection, which also closely mimics the way most nonsurgical physicians view clinical examples of pathology, that is, through imaging.[7]

Anatomical dissection promotes deep anatomical understanding, and because each cadaver represents a unique individual, the process of dissection underscores the breadth of possible anatomical variations.[8] As a 3D hands-on experience, cadaveric dissection offers tactile feedback and enhances manual skill sets.[9,10] Moreover, as students work in teams, cadaveric dissection promotes problem-based, team learning.[11]

The total number of hours spent in anatomy teaching labs has decreased over the past 20 years for several reasons:[12] the financial burden of having a fully equipped anatomy laboratory,[13] limited cadaver availability,[14] and the increased availability of e-learning platforms.[15] While e-learning platforms have not fully replaced cadaveric dissection, they have greatly changed the ways students traditionally accessed anatomical information. In addition, these computer-based models are popular with students; however, studies have shown that students who rely solely on computer-based models perform worse compared to students who use traditional resources in learning anatomy.[16]

3D printing as a novel method opens up opportunities to create anatomical models for medical training on an individual scale. Like all printed models, patient-specific 3D printed models allow students at all training levels to review both normal and abnormal anatomical structures outside the cadaveric laboratory. A wide variety of materials can be used to create 3D printed models, which can help accentuate anatomic details.[17–19] These models are reproducible, safe to handle, and can represent variety of normal and pathologic anatomy.[20]

When combined with cadaveric dissection (as many medical schools now perform CT scans on cadavers prior to dissection), 3D printing expands the possibilities for anatomy students. The creation of anatomical models by students which replicate the body's form promotes engagement with cadaveric specimens themselves. Pre-learning through 3D modeling stimulates anatomical review, forcing students to understand anatomical relationships on a more direct level and facilitates kinesthetic learning by engaging the tactile senses.[21]

Using 3D printing for anatomy training has its limitations. Compared to true anatomical dissection, fine details such as small nerve branches or microstructures,

which can be explored in the cadaveric subjects using expert techniques, can be difficult if not impossible to replicate with 3D printing techniques. Whole organ printing with detachable parts requires a tradeoff between precision-printing, and the form and function needed to facilitate active engagement with the printed model.

A further limitation of using 3D printed models as a cadaveric replacement is the model printing time, which may limit the routine use of 3D printing in an ongoing course of study. Industrial 3D printers are better suited to producing multicolored models suitable for visualizing finer structures; however, local efforts to print with such fine detail make routine and on-demand 3D printed models expensive for most training purposes.[22] Additionally, accurate size representation is an important element of student learning, which must be balanced by the time and material cost required for printing; the use of scaled 3D models is discouraged as it may potentially lead to an incomplete understanding of true organ size additional spatial relationships to nearby anatomical structures.[23] The utility of 3D printing for medical education is a growing field of study. One recent systematic review validated the utility of 3D printed models for teaching medical students; and it was postulated that these models positively impacted medical students, especially because of their limited knowledge of anatomy.[55]

3D PRINTED MODELS AS A TOOL IN CLINICAL RADIOLOGY TRAINING

Radiology practice, at its core, uses technology to visualize internal structures, assess anatomic relationships, and to infer pathology. These same tools are now used to quantify tissue structure and assess disease progression on a microstructural level. Key to success in radiology training programs is understanding anatomical relationships of increasingly greater complexity than those required of anatomy students, both in normal and in abnormal patients, as well as mastering anatomical description. 3D models can be used in education to visualize and conceptualize complex anatomical structures and are a useful tool for facilitating learning in a range of normal and abnormal patient-focused settings. Models can even include fine detailed structures such as ophthalmology anatomy and can be created based on cadaver prosections.[24] Furthermore, since a catalog of models may not be available in many clinical learning environments, 3D printing allows a resident or student to select a specific area of interest that may be difficult to evaluate, and facilitates using individually printed models to teach these relationships to others.

Normal and Complex Anatomical Relationships

Due to the inherent complexity of normal anatomic structures and the fact that the human body is not made up of straight lines, smooth edges, and 2D interfaces, normal anatomical relationships are often difficult to comprehend. 3D models can be used to visualize and conceptualize complex anatomical structures, and have been shown to be effective tools in medical training. Studies have shown the utility of 3D printed models for teaching complex surface anatomy[25] and as an alternative to traditional didactic instruction.[26]

Beyond identifying key structures on imaging, students often struggle to recognize the relationship between adjacent structures, for example, the ductal anatomy of the pancreas and common duct within the pancreas head. Surface anatomy and its relationship to underlying structures can be difficult to estimate using standard cross-sectional imaging. 3D models, in contrast, more easily demonstrate complex interfaces and allow students to better understand these spatial relationships. 3D printed models have similarly been used to teach complex segmental anatomy of organs such as lungs, liver, and prostate, or branching anatomy of the coronary arteries and circle of Willis.[27]

Another example of using 3D printing to visualize complex anatomical relationships relates to vascular structures in the setting of both common and less common anatomical variants. For example, the left renal vein typically crosses anterior to the aorta when communicating to the IVC. However, important vascular variants including retroaortic and circumaortic renal veins are critical to recognize. The relationship between the aorta, IVC, and renal veins is difficult to conceptualize and students who encounter this variant anatomy benefit from advanced 3D visualization. Similarly, the number and length of the renal veins and arteries is an important consideration that drives presurgical imaging prior to renal transplant surgery and can be difficult to accurately demonstrate to surgeons using 2D sectional anatomy alone (Fig. 10.1).

Abnormal Pathologies

There are many common injuries and pathologies which recur in a clinical setting for which trainees rely on representative examples to make diagnoses and highlight contrasts. This occurs most commonly on call, when residents practice with greater independence.

Understanding and referencing classification schemes for abnormal pathologies is a challenging task among radiology trainees for which they typically rely on external reference comparisons including anatomical models, textbooks, and case review examples when making a diagnosis. The opportunity to use patient-specific examples of complex anatomical structures can provide an added benefit in academic hospitals and training environments. Specialty reading rooms such as for musculoskeletal and neurological imaging are well suited to identify and to archive printed examples of these complex cases. Clinical conferences held together with surgeons serve to amplify the benefits to trainees in both diagnostic and procedural subspecialties when 3D models are available as a visual reference during case discussion.

For example, the classification of hip acetabulum fracture types or Le Fort midface fracture classifications can be aided by using printed models as a reference, given the complex anatomy and 3D geometry of these

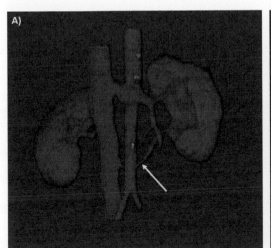
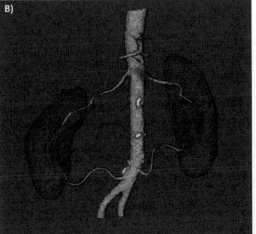

FIG. 10.1 **(A)** Patient with retroaortic left renal vein feeding the lower pole (*yellow arrow*) in addition to main left renal vein. **(B)** Patient with duplicate bilateral renal arteries feeding the upper and lower poles.

structures. A study on radiology residents showed that residents who received 3D printed models during a didactic lecture regarding acetabular fractures had better learning outcomes compared to control group which only received the didactic presentation.[28] Printed clinical examples move this teaching tool into the clinical learning environment.

Realistic Phantoms for Hardware and Software Evaluation

In radiology departments, phantoms with known material properties and geometries are utilized to properly calibrate imaging equipment and optimize image protocols. Commonly available phantoms are simple geometric phantoms or anthropomorphic phantoms which usually represent typical or average adult or pediatric patients. 3D printing allows for the creation of more realistic models based on patient-specific imaging data, thereby providing more accurate and reliable models for quality assurance (QA) and research investigation. In one example, patient-specific 3D printed phantoms of peripheral and central pulmonary embolism were used to optimize a CT pulmonary artery protocol. Researchers used varying kVp and pitch values and assessed their impact on radiation dose and image quality using 3D printed models of peripheral and central pulmonary embolism, achieving 80% dose reduction.[29,30] In addition to learning about radiation dosing including "image gently" and "as low as reasonably achievable," in a simulated environment without exposing a patient to radiation, using 3D printed phantoms gives an opportunity for trainees to experiment with the physics concepts in radiology. More details regarding 3D printed imaging phantoms can be found in Chapter 14.

3D PRINTED MODELS FOR RADIOLOGICAL PROCEDURAL PLANNING

3D printed models of patient-specific anatomy are being increasingly used for procedural planning and can facilitate understanding of a patient's complex or unique anatomy, thereby removing diagnostic uncertainty, decreasing procedure times, and potentially improving a patient's outcome. Surgeons-in-training can use 3D printing techniques, using anatomical or scaled models, to review surgical plans with senior surgeons and simulate their own approach, decreasing diagnostic uncertainty, procedure times, and potentially improving patient outcomes.

A complete description of the advantages and drawbacks of using 3D printed, patient-specific models is beyond the scope of this chapter. However, numerous individual case reports and small studies have highlighted the value of 3D printed models in making patient-specific surgical decisions.[31-37] 3D printed models have also been shown to help both radiology and surgical trainees better understand anatomical relationships and aid in enhancing surgical technique. Selected clinical case series describing the use of 3D printed models specifically for procedural training of residents in various academic training environments is summarized in Table 10.1.[24,38-43] In terms of training radiology residents, a recent review noted that available case reports and controlled studies were limited to simpler models and small sample sizes, and therefore could not show true learning benefit with high confidence.[55] This highlights the role for future cooperative research assessing the impact of 3D printing for resident education.

Procedure Planning and Simulation for Interventional Radiology Training and Radiological Procedures

Patient-specific 3D printed models present both a clinical benefit and a training aid to both students and junior faculty. Training in and the clinical performance of radiological procedures requires skill, preparation, and experience to develop proficiency and independence. Similar to planning for open surgical procedures, the availability of patient-specific models guides the clinical performance of image-guided procedures.

Use of these models has been shown to improve hand–eye coordination in trainees and optimize their image acquiring quality and positioning.[44] Moreover, as trainees learn to perform minimally invasive procedures, they need to practice using increasingly realistic and challenging simulator tools. Studies have shown benefit to training using realistic phantoms and models.[45] 3D printed models provide even more realistic opportunities to create models and phantoms at patient scale, which can be embedded within other materials such as ballistic gel and used in simulation training for both ultrasound and CT-guided procedures. Presurgical planning and procedure rehearsal can be especially more important in high risk and complicated procedures such as pediatric neurointerventional radiology and can even aid experienced interventional radiologists. For example, in one study, researchers showed that 3D models of pediatric arteriovenous malformations can be printed within 24 hours with a high degree of fidelity and use of these models resulted in a 12% reduction of procedure time.[47]

INTRODUCING TRAINING IN 3D PRINTING TO RESIDENT EDUCATION

3D printing in medicine is an evolving field, with a wide range of available tools, material, and challenging technical requirements. Moreover, as 3D printed models become further incorporated into clinical workflows

TABLE 10.1

Examples of Select Clinical Case Series Describing the Use of 3D Printed Models for Procedural Training of Residents in Various Academic Environments.

Specialty	Clinical Entities	Clinical Examples of Complex Anatomy, Delineated for Learners Using 3D Printing Tools
Ophthalmology	Orbital decompression training	• Using preoperative high-resolution orbital CT scan, trainees practiced orbital decompression techniques in the wet-lab setting, which can potentially improve the surgical outcome.[37]
Orthopedic surgery	Spinal surgery training	• 3D printed lumbar spine models were used for training the residents in free-hand pedicle screw instrumentation. The training on the 3D printed models decreased pedicle cortex perforations and length of time to completion. However, authors described that the "osseous feel" is different on printed models.[38] • Open source 3D printed spine models were created to facilitate resident training in lumbar spine pedicle screw placement during COVID-related elective surgical cancellation.[39]
Plastic surgery	Mandible reconstruction	• In a patient with progressive osteomyelitis, a complete mandible was 3D printed and successfully implanted. The model was constructed from titanium and customized with appropriate articulating condyles and muscle attachment cavities.[40]
Urology	Percutaneous nephrolithotripsy surgery	• A material extrusion method (fused deposition modeling) was used based on CT data of patients with unilateral complex renal stones. Urology residents demonstrated better understanding of renal calices anatomy, stone location, and optimal entry calix.[41]
	Locating prostate cancer	• 3D printed prostate models created from MRI improved medical students' accuracy of locating the prostate cancer.[42]
	Flexible ureteroscopic training	• 3D printed bladder, single-calyceal, and double-calyceal models were used to train junior residents, which resulted in improved mean post-course task completion times and overall performance scores compared to baseline and led to improved short-term technical skills.[43]

and patient-care scenarios, the requirements and degree of oversight needed to oversee and train others in appropriate use increase. Technical descriptions of the image acquisition and processing requirements and regulatory elements regarding 3D printing are covered elsewhere in this book. This section will focus on the advantages of incorporating didactic and hands-on teaching of 3D printing to radiology trainees.

Learning the Process of Obtaining 3D Models and 3D Lab Workflow

Creating anatomically precise models which accurately reflect clinical reality is an arduous process which requires training and expertise to effectively employ in patient care, where both precision and accuracy matter. There are pitfalls specific to each stage, from image acquisition, segmentation, computer-aided design, printing, and postprocessing. Errors at any stage have direct implications for patient care. Physicians who will interpret and report on 3D printed models must learn from case examples—both successful and unsuccessful examples—analogous to the process used in medical QA and morbidity and mortality conferences. In addition, akin to the didactic process used in classroom and patient-care settings, direct training in 3D processing is needed to both generate accurate models and interpret the implications of findings on these models for clinical use.

Clinical Infrastructure

3D printing is a time-intensive process that uses physical resources and currently carries limited clinical reimbursement. Although Category III Current Procedural Terminology (CPT) codes were introduced by the American Medical Association in July 2019[46], reimbursement is extremely limited and many 3D printing labs are funded externally. Rather than generating revenue, these 3D printing labs are typically internally funded and/or draw on donations, research, and educational funding sources. Successful labs employ dedicated managers, specialized technologists, and/or biomedical engineers to segment individual cases for clinical use and manage 3D printing resources. Trainees who receive hands-on experience in a training environment are exposed to the full range of processes and tools, engaging with requesting physicians, interpreting physicians, and technologists. Understanding the fundamental inputs used in running a 3D printing lab allows physicians-in-training to develop a business framework which effectively utilizes resources to balance between the clinical useful 3D printing, cost requirements, and leveraging the nonclinical advantages offered to departments which feature a 3D printing service.

While the reimbursement for medical 3D printing is limited, the opportunity for adding clinical benefit is great. Through engaging with specialty departments, forging effective collaborations, and demonstrating excellence in product and service, interdisciplinary programs are forged and led by those who manage the critical resources. Students in training develop communication and leadership skills by actively participating in these interdepartmental efforts.

In 2013, the Radiological Society of North America (RSNA) launched an educational program on 3D printing. At the time of writing, the RSNA features a dedicated category for scientific presentations and educational exhibits at their annual meeting highlighting advances using 3D Printing [49]. The RSNA 3D Printing Special Interest Group (SIG) has published consensus guidelines for the clinical implementation of 3D printing and offers a venue for scholarly collaboration.[47,48]

Developing a Research Infrastructure

3D printing has tested use cases not only in clinical practice but also is an evolving field. Using 3D printing tools as part of a research program offers diverse opportunities for residents to be recognized for their contributions to advancing scientific and technical knowledge in the field. New printing technologies, materials, segmentation techniques, and clinical applications require testing to be used effectively in the clinical environment. Both funded and industry-sponsored research opportunities are likely to grow, with opportunities available to programs that can demonstrate effective and efficient use of their available resources, as well as an ability to effectively scale to meet the needs of projects.

There are a range of research avenues using 3D printing which can engage trainees and be used to help build a platform for future academic growth. A major area for investigation includes demonstrating the value-added component of 3D printing in radiological and surgical practices. In addition, studies regarding techniques for improving image acquisition and segmentation protocols and assessing the true accuracy of created models through QA studies provide ample opportunities for radiologists engaged in testing new and evolving technologies.

SAMPLE CURRICULUM FOR A HANDS-ON RESIDENT MINICOURSE IN 3D PRINTING AND VISUALIZATION

What should a training course in 3D printing for trainees look like? Structure, didactic education, and hands-on experience are all needed. What follows is a sample curriculum that can be adapted to different training programs, depending on local resources and time availability. Elements of a structured curriculum for trainee education in 3D printing are included in Table 10.2. Specific elements of the curriculum are discussed in the following section.

Introduction to 3D Printing

One of the main objectives of the hands-on minicourse in 3D printing is to teach the principles of 3D printing. 3D printing describes all technologies in which 3D objects are built by adding sequential layers of material. Seven unique processes have been described by the International Organization for Standardization (ISO) and the American Society for Testing and Materials (ASTM),[49] which can incorporate techniques using a variety of unique man-made and even organic tissue materials.

Clinically, 3D printing in medicine is a process of translating information contained on medical images, typically in Digital Imaging and Communications in Medicine (DICOM) format, and translating that information into fabricated models for clinical use. Trainees in 3D printing need to learn the general terminology of the ISO/ASTM, differentiate among various 3D printing

TABLE 10.2
Sample Hands-On Teaching Curriculum for Medical 3D Printing.

Module	Teaching Method

1. Introduction to 3D printing
  a. General terminology and standards
  b. 3D printing technologies
  c. 3D printing materials
    i. Appearance
    ii. Mechanical properties
    iii. Chemical properties
  d. File types required for printing
	• Lectures (4)
	• Post Lecture quizzes (4)
	• Homework

2. Applications of medical 3D printing
  a. Anatomical models for
    i. Pre-op planning
    ii. Post-op analysis
    iii. Education—trainees and patient
    iv. Surgical simulations
  b. Anatomic guides (i.e., drilling guides and cutting guides)
  c. Custom-made implants
  d. Prosthetics
  e. Research
	• Lectures (5)
	• Post Lecture quizzes (5)
	• Homework

3. Radiology workflow for 3D printing
  a. Image acquisition
    i. Spatial resolution
    ii. Signal-to-noise ratio and contrast-to-noise ratio (protocols)
    iii. Artifacts
    iv. Other considerations (dual energy, metal artifact reduction, positioning, field of view)
  b. Image segmentation
    i. General techniques and overview of available software platforms
      1. Commercial versus freeware
      2. General workflow and 3D visualization techniques
      3. Export properties and quality
    ii. Image post-processing requirements for printing
  c. Image manipulation
    i. Minor changes
    ii. Major changes
    iii. Verification with CT or surface scans
	• Lectures (3)
	• Post Lecture quizzes (3)
	• Hands-on homework on image segmentation and manipulation

4. 3D printing and quality control
  a. Image acquisition and segmentation
  b. 3D printing
  c. Model cleaning and postprocessing
  d. Inspection and validation of model
	• Lectures (1)
	• Post lecture quizzes (1)
	• Homework
	• Independent study—create your own 3D printed model

5. Documentation and reimbursement
  a. Dictation and incorporation into EMR
  b. Category III CPT codes
  c. RSNA–ACR Registry for 3D printed models and guides
	• Lectures (1)
	• Post lecture quizzes (1)
	• Homework—create a full case and complete the dictation

techniques, must be able to describe differences between various 3D printing materials, and should understand which materials are biocompatible and sterilizable. They must learn the differences between medical DICOM format and formats understandable by commonly used 3D printers, typically the stereolithography (STL) format also known as the standard tessellation language or standard triangle language. Finally, trainees must understand appropriate uses for each technology and material type.

Applications of Medical 3D Printing

Trainees must be familiar with and comfortable describing the range of clinical applications of 3D printing. In addition to simply understanding how to create anatomical models for presurgical planning and post-op analysis, education, and simulation, trainees must understand how to create anatomic guides using the patient-specific imaging data. Advanced training should also incorporate the development of custom 3D printed implants and prosthetics, as well as the research applications of 3D printing. These topics have been further described in earlier chapters, and do not require further detail.

Radiology Workflow for 3D Printing

Technical and technological-related considerations form the most robust portion of a curriculum in 3D printing. Understanding the fundamental requirements of image acquisition, segmentation, post-processing techniques, and techniques for image manipulation is essential to procedure both realistic and accurate 3D models. In addition, residents must learn the technical requirements of which processing software is required to create detailed and accurate anatomical models.

CT is the most used image acquisition modality for 3D printing, though any volumetric datasets obtained from other modalities including CTA, MRA, MRI, PET, and 3D ultrasound. Structure differentiation is enhanced by high contrast, signal-to-noise ratio and spatial resolution, and minimizing partial volume effects. Slice thickness should be less than 1.25 mm to create isotropic voxels. Thicker sections decrease the accuracy, while thinner sections make segmentation process more tedious as more imaging slices must be evaluated. Depending on the organ of interest, the slice thickness requirement may be different. For example, a thickness of 0.5 mm creates sufficient accuracy for cardiac models, while orbital models may need thinner slices.[50] Similarly, depending on the organ of interest a soft or sharp reconstruction kernel may be preferred.[47] Trainees must learn about optimizing

protocols to enhance the signal and contrast in image datasets, avoid common artifacts which affect image segmentation and manipulation, and understand the effect of other commonly used clinical imaging techniques on the utility of these datasets for 3D printing.

Image Segmentation

The most challenging aspect of developing 3D anatomic models from medical imaging data is isolating the specific anatomy of interest/regions of interest (ROIs) from the primary dataset, the process of image segmentation. In the minicourse, radiology residents must learn the process of image segmentation through hands-on projects. Segmentation generally starts with importing DICOM files into a dedicated image post-processing software. The anatomical regions then need to be delineated, using automated, semi-automated, and/or manual tools.

Medical imaging software already has capabilities of automated segmentation, using region or seed-growing techniques, digital subtraction, or other techniques which begin with a defined ROI. Other segmentation techniques rely on thresholding, based on distinct contrast differences between areas (i.e., bone selection based on high density or Hounsfield Units). An in-depth discussion on image segmentation techniques is included in Chapter 3. After selecting the ROI for 3D printing, data are interpolated, smoothed, a surface-based 3D model is created, and the model is saved as a 3D file format (i.e., STL). The created model then needs to be re-evaluated against the source image for accuracy.

Although many advanced visualization and image post-processing platforms have the capability to perform segmentation and even export models in STL format, the RSNA 3D Printing SIG recommends using an FDA-cleared software for segmentation to produce 3D printed models suitable for diagnostic use.[47] Stored files should contain descriptors with standardized terminology from a consensus vocabulary,[50] should ideally include DICOM encapsulation, and should be stored in the patient archiving system.[51]

From a training perspective, developing effective image segmentation skills requires hands-on experience. Beyond having a conceptual understanding of the process, the student must be able to do it properly to have truly benefitted from the educational experience. Standardized segmenting exercises must be developed, with work checked by a qualified expert, providing ongoing and active feedback. Challenging segmentation cases should be offered, which test the students' ability to apply various segmentation techniques to anatomical structures with similar density characteristics.

3D Printing and Quality Control

Students must be capable not only to prepare medical images from 3D printing but to also create and check 3D printed models for accuracy. Students should keep a log of cases prepared to assure that they are involved in a range of printing and finishing techniques. The techniques available to the learned will vary based on equipment available; however, certain challenging applications to practice should include the printing and polishing of transparent parts, printing hollow viscera or vascular structures, and printing complex anatomic models with multiple structures.

Final image inspection and validation of models is also an important element of training in 3D printing. A systematic QA approach that includes every step of the 3D printing process is required to create valid and reliable models. Assuring that the model is accurate requires prior knowledge of the image dataset, careful understanding of the printing technique used, and attention to anatomical detail to assure that anatomical details are not distorted. Printed models need to be validated using qualitative inspection and quantitative measurement. Models can be rescanned using medical imaging equipment or surface scanning techniques and be coregistered with the reference cross sectional CT or MR.[52] Further details regarding QA can be found in Chapter 7.

A robust program will have teaching examples available which highlight prior processing errors that distort the true anatomical representation. These references are an important tool for learning QA and identifying errors. A successful QA process requires inputs from all stakeholders including ordering physician, radiologist, medical physicist, technologist, and engineer. One of the main objectives of the minicourse is to work with these parties and coordinate the 3D printing workflow with them.

Documentation and Reimbursement

One of the objectives of the 3D printing minicourse would be learning to apply a standardized lexicon for radiology reporting of 3D printing services, which aids in reimbursement. "3D printing," "additive manufacturing," and "rapid prototyping" are synonymous terms used to describe 3D printing, though expert consensus is to use the term "3D printing" in order to create a standardize lexicon.[53]

Interpretation of the 3D printed models should be documented in the patient's medical record. The interpretation should include the ROI of the printed model. 3D visualization is often required for the interpretation of the ROI. Currently, CPT codes 76376 and 76377 are used for billing purposes for 3D visualization, though the student must learn to differentiate between these two codes. CPT code 76376 should be used when 3D rendering is performed by either a radiologist or a specially trained technologist at the acquisition scanner. In contrast, CPT code 76377 is used when the 3D post-processed images are reconstructed under physician supervision on an independent workstation. Additionally, these codes are not to be used in conjunction with the new Category III CPT codes 0559T–0561T, which are temporary codes for emerging technologies.[49] As previously noted, 3D printing labs are currently supported by a combination of research and departmental funding. To be self-sustaining, 3D printing must generate ongoing revenue from its clinical service. While deep understanding of variable payer rules is beyond the scope for routine training, understanding the components of coding and billing for 3D services is a necessary element of training. Trainees must learn to develop and apply standardized reporting templates which properly incorporate description of the required elements needed to bill for 3D imaging and printing services. Fig. 10.2 provides an example of images stored in the patient's medical record along with a corresponding dictation for the 3D printed model exam.

3D printing can become reimbursed if it adds value to the patient care. The joint RSNA–American College of Radiology (ACR) 3D Printing Registry was established to try to gain information about the types of 3D printed anatomic models and guides that are being created for clinical use at hospitals and to assess what software, hardware, and time is required to generate these models.[54] In addition, the clinical benefit of the 3D printed model is being recorded. Although some case reports and small studies have shown this, more complex studies and analyses are required to develop guidelines and support reimbursement.[57] More information about reimbursement and the registry can be found in Chapter 8.

Demonstration of Competency in 3D Printing

How can a training program measure and assure competencies for each of these tasks? Formal testing can assure the student has developed a thorough knowledge base, including understanding of 3D printing technologies, techniques, materials, and image acquisition parameters. Skill level in image segmentation requires hands-on practice. Programs can require a minimum number of hours of laboratory experience for each processing stage. Alternatively, radiology residents training in manual segmentations should have multiple outputs compared against a reference standard or expert, with expectations for matched performance within a predefined standard of tolerance. Any formal program must include a hands-on practicum, in which students fully create 3D printed models from medical datasets, which are then validated and scored by expert teachers.

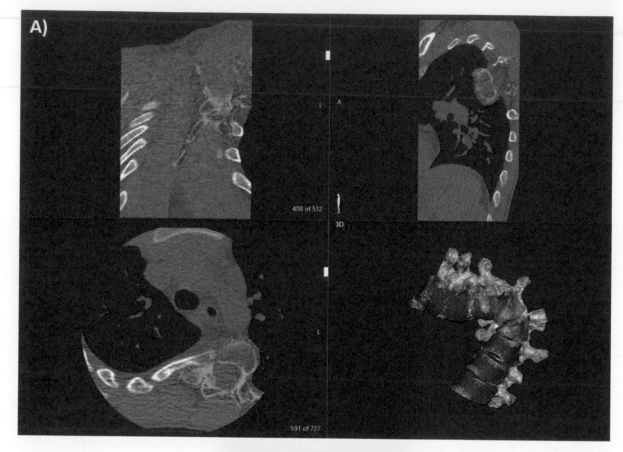

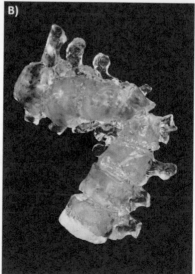

FIG. 10.2 (A) Image segmentation and 3D modeling of severe scoliosis. (B) 3D printed model printed with clear resin on the Form 3 (Formlabs, Cambridge, MA). (C) Corresponding report for the 3D printed model which is dictated and stored in the patient's medical record.

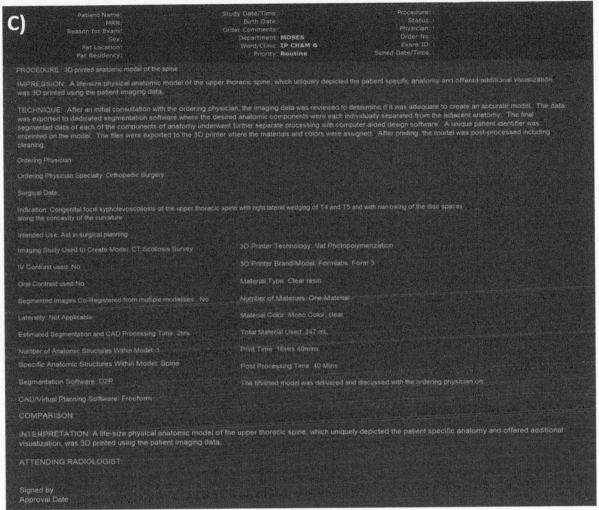

C)

Patient Name:
MRN:
Reason for Exam:
Sex:
Pat Location:
Pat Residency:

Study Date/Time:
Birth Date:
Order Comments:
Department: **MOSES**
Ward/Clinic: **IP CHAM 6**
Priority: **Routine**

Procedure:
Status:
Physician:
Order No:
Exam ID:
Sched Date/Time:

PROCEDURE: 3D printed anatomic model of the spine.

IMPRESSION: A life-size physical anatomic model of the upper thoracic spine, which uniquely depicted the patient specific anatomy and offered additional visualization, was 3D printed using the patient imaging data.

TECHNIQUE: After an initial consultation with the ordering physician, the imaging data was reviewed to determine if it was adequate to create an accurate model. The data was exported to dedicated segmentation software where the desired anatomic components were each individually separated from the adjacent anatomy. The final segmented data of each of the components of anatomy underwent further separate processing with computer-aided design software. A unique patient identifier was imprinted on the model. The files were exported to the 3D printer where the materials and colors were assigned. After printing, the model was post-processed including cleaning.

Ordering Physician:

Ordering Physician Specialty: Orthopedic Surgery

Surgical Date:

Indication: Congenital focal kypholevoscoliosis of the upper thoracic spine with right lateral wedging of T4 and T5 and with narrowing of the disc spaces along the concavity of the curvature

Intended Use: Aid in surgical planning

Imaging Study Used to Create Model: CT Scoliosis Survey

IV Contrast used: No

Oral Contrast used: No

Segmented Images Co-Registered from multiple modalities: No

Laterality: Not Applicable

Estimated Segmentation and CAD Processing Time: 2hrs

Number of Anatomic Structures Within Model: 1

Specific Anatomic Structures Within Model: Spine

Segmentation Software: D2P

CAD/Virtual Planning Software: Freeform

3D Printer Technology: Vat Photopolymerization

3D Printer Brand/Model: Formlabs, Form 3

Material Type: Clear resin

Number of Materials: One Material

Material Color: Mono Color, clear

Total Material Used: 247 mL

Print Time: 16Hrs 40mins

Post Processing Time: 40 Mins

The finished model was delivered and discussed with the ordering physician on:

COMPARISON:

INTERPRETATION: A life-size physical anatomic model of the upper thoracic spine, which uniquely depicted the patient specific anatomy and offered additional visualization, was 3D printed using the patient imaging data.

ATTENDING RADIOLOGIST:

Signed by:
Approval Date:

FIG. 10.2 cont'd.

CONCLUSIONS

Medical 3D printing is at a crossroads, with continuously improving technologies, material developments, processing techniques, and new applications and clinical use cases being shared in a technically advanced and collaborative community. Medical education should continue to harness the technology as a tool to enhance the education of students, and as a resource to advance clinical education and patient care.

In the future, alongside with 3D printing, other advanced imaging technologies such as augmented reality (AR) and virtual reality (VR) may be included in educational programs. AR and VR may be advantageous as compared to 3D printing due to the lack of time constraints to generate 3D content as well as the ability to virtually manipulate, cut (aka "dissect"), and add back layers. Students can use trial-and-error as a tool to enhance learning by either making (and learning from) mistakes, or by experimenting with multiple dissection or mock surgical approaches. Using these tools, learning complex anatomical relationships is enhanced in a manner complementary to using 3D printed models; while there is less tactile feedback, these tools offer enhanced visual clarity and more lifelike boldness to the images. Future studies will determine the added value of AR and VR as compared to 3D printing.

Physicians-in-training, particularly radiologists, need to gain hands-on experience and formal training in each step of the medical 3D printing process in order to develop practical expertise, avoid pitfalls, and position themselves as clinical leaders among a team of innovative and creative professionals. Radiologists who are clinical experts in medical 3D printing will be able to provide oversight to the biomedical engineers and radiology technologists who are involved in processing imaging data and creating 3D printed models.

For physicians, specific advantages accrue to those who become experts in 3D printing, including the opportunity to work directly with clinical counterparts, interact more with patients by actually explaining models, and potentially generate more revenue for their department. Most importantly, they can contribute to the evolution of the field and development of new learning, diagnostic, and treatment paradigm. Furthermore, physician certification for medical 3D printing may be possible through accrediting bodies such as the ACR making 3D printing even more attractive for practicing radiologists.

Sustaining an effective 3D printing program requires technical expertise, deep understanding of billing requirements, budgeting skills, understanding of the regulatory and patient safety environment, clinical and research applications, and leadership. For technically able physicians, training in all areas of 3D printing is needed to grow into future leadership roles within the specialty. Early, in-depth exposure and hands-on practice can develop radiologists and other interested physicians into future leaders in the field.

REFERENCES

1. Tejo-Otero A, Buj-Corral I, Fenollosa-Artes F. 3D printing in medicine for preoperative surgical planning: a review. *Ann Biomed Eng.* 2020;48(2).
2. Owen H. Early use of simulation in medical education. *Simul Healthc.* 2012;7(2):102—116.
3. Buck GH. Development of simulators in medical education. *Gesnerus.* 1991;48(Pt 1):7—28.
4. Lockhart RD. The art of learning anatomy. *Lancet.* 1927;2: 460—461.
5. Riederer BM. Plastination and its importance in teaching anatomy. Critical points for long-term preservation of human tissue. *J Anat.* 2014;224:309—315.
6. Lim PK, Stephenson GS, Keown TW, et al. Use of 3D printed models in resident education for the classification of acetabulum fractures. *J Surg Educ.* 2018;75:1679—1684.
7-. Anatomage. Anatomage Table. Retrieved from: https://www.anatomage.com/table/.
8. Pujol S, Baldwin M, Nassiri J, Kikinis R, Shaffer K. Using 3D modeling techniques to enhance teaching of difficult anatomical concepts. *Acad Radiol.* 2016;23:507—516.
9. Dissabandara LO, Nirthanan SN, Khoo TK, Tedman R. Role of cadaveric dissections in modern medical curricula: a study on student perceptions. *Anat Cell Biol.* 2015;48: 205—212.
10. Habbal O. The state of human anatomy teaching in the medical schools of Gulf Cooperation Council countries: present and future perspectives. *Sultan Qaboos Univ Med J.* 2009;9:24—31.
11. Huitt TW, Killins A, Brooks WS. Team-based learning in the gross anatomy laboratory improves academic performance and students' attitudes toward teamwork. *Anat Sci Educ.* 2015;8:95—103.
12. Drake RL, McBride J, Lachman N, Pawlina W. Medical education in the anatomical sciences: the winds of change continue to blow. *Anat Sci Educ.* 2009;2:253—259.
13. Elizondo-Omaña RE, Guzmán-López S, García-Rodríguez Mde L. Dissection as a teaching tool: past, present, and future. *Anat Rec.* 2005;285B:11—15.
14. McLachlan JC, Bligh J, Bradley P, Searle J. Teaching anatomy without cadavers. *Med Educ.* 2004;38:418—424.
15. Trelease RB. From chalkboard, slides, and paper to e-learning: how computing technologies have transformed anatomical sciences education. *Anat Sci Educ.* 2016;9:583—602.
16. Khot Z, Quinlan K, Norman GR, Wainman B. The relative effectiveness of computer-based and traditional resources for education in anatomy. *Anat Sci Educ.* 2013;6(4):211—215.
17. Michalski MH, Ross JS. The shape of things to come: 3D printing in medicine. *J Am Med Assoc.* 2014;312: 2213—2214.
18. Mogali SR, Yeong WY, Tan HK, et al. Evaluation by medical students of the educational value of multi-material and multi-colored three- dimensional printed models of the upper limb for anatomical education. *Anat Sci Educ.* 2018;11:54—64.
19. McMenamin PG, Quayle MR, McHenry CR, Adams JW. The production of anatomical teaching resources using three-dimensional (3D) printing technology. *Anat Sci Educ.* 2014;7:479—486.
20. Trace AP, Ortiz D, Deal A, et al. Radiology's emerging role in 3-D printing applications in health care. *J Am Coll Radiol.* 2016;13:856—862.
21. Wainman B, Wolak L, Pukas G, Zheng E, Norman GR. The superiority of three-dimensional physical models to two-dimensional computer presentations in anatomy learning. *Med Educ.* 2018;52:1138—1146.
22. Ballard D, Trace A, Ali S, et al. Clinical applications of 3D printing: primer for radiologists. *Acad Radiol.* 2018;25(1): 52—65.
23. Smith C, Tollemache N, Covill D, Johnston M. Take away body parts! An investigation into the use of 3D-printed anatomical models in undergraduate anatomy education. *Anat Sci Educ.* 2018;11:44—53.
24. Sommer A, Blumenth E. Implementations of 3D printing in ophthalmology. *Graefe's Arch Clin Exp Ophthalmol.* 2019;257:1815—1822.
25. Lim KHA, Loo ZY, Goldie SJ, Adams JW, McMenamin PG. Use of 3D printed models in medical education: a randomized control trial comparing 3D prints versus cadaveric materials for learning external cardiac anatomy: use of 3D Prints in Medical Education. *Anat Sci Educ.* 2016;9:213—221.

26. Cai B, Rajendran K, Huat Bay B, Lee J, Yen C. The effects of a functional three-dimensional (3D) printed knee joint simulator in improving anatomical spatial knowledge. *Anat Sci Educ.* 2019;12(6):610–618.

27. Javan R, Herrin D, Tangestanipoor A. Understanding spatially complex segmental and branch anatomy using 3D printing: liver, lung, prostate, coronary arteries and circle of Willis. *Acad Radiol.* 2016;23(9).1181–1189.

28. Awan O, Sheth S, Sullivan I, et al. Efficacy of 3D printed models on resident learning and understanding of common acetabular fractures. *Acad Radiol.* 2019;26(1):130–135.

29. Aldosari S, Jansen S, Sun Z. Optimization of computed tomography pulmonary angiography protocols using 3D printed model with simulation of pulmonary embolism. *Quant Imaging Med Surg.* 2019;9(1):53–62.

30. Hossien A, Gelsomino S, Maessen J. The interactive use of multi- dimensional modeling and 3D printing in preplanning of type A aortic dissection. *J Card Surg.* 2016;31(7): 441–445.

31. Sodian R, Weber S, Markert M, et al. Stereolithographic models for surgical planning in congenital heart surgery. *Ann Thorac Surg.* 2007;83:1854–1857.

32. Ngan E, Rebeyka I, Ross D, et al. The rapid prototyping of anatomic models in pulmonary atresia. *J Thorac Cardiovasc Surg.* 2006;132(2):264–269.

33. Sodian R, Weber S, Markert M, et al. Pediatric cardiac transplantation: three-dimensional printing of anatomic models for surgical planning of heart transplantation in patients with univentricular heart. *J Thorac Cardiovasc Surg.* 2008;136(4):1098–1099.

34. Potamianos P, Amis AA, Forester AJ, Mcgurk M, Bircher M. Rapid prototyping for orthopaedic surgery. *Proc Inst Mech Eng H.* 2015;212:383–393.

35. Spottiswoode BS, van den Heever DJ, Chang Y, et al. Preoperative three-dimensional model creation of magnetic resonance brain images as a tool to assist neurosurgical planning. *Stereotact Funct Neurosurg.* 2013;91(3):162–169.

36. Wake N, Rude T, Kang SK, et al. 3D printed renal cancer models derived from MRI data: application in presurgical planning. *Abdom Radiol.* 2017;42(5):1501–1509. https://doi.org/10.1007/s00261-016-1022-2.

37. Scawn RL, Foster A, Lee BW, et al. Customised 3D printing: an innovative training tool for the next generation of orbital surgeons. *Orbit.* 2015;34:216–219.

38. Park HJ, Wang C, Choi KH, Kim HN. Use of a life-size three-dimensional-printed spine model for pedicle screw instrumentation training. *J Orthop Surg Res.* 2018;13(1).

39. Clifton W, Damon A, Valero-Moreno F, et al. The Spine-Box: a freely available, open-access, 3D-printed simulator design for lumbar pedicle screw placement. *Cureus.* 2020; 12(4):e7738. https://doi.org/10.7759/cureus.7738.

40. Nickels L. World's first patient-specific jaw implant. *Met Powder Rep.* 2012;67:12–14.

41. Atalay HA, Ulker V, Alkan I, Canat HL, Ozkuvanci U, Altunrende F. Impact of three-dimensional printed pelvicaliceal system models on residents' understanding of pelvicaliceal system anatomy before percutaneous nephrolithotripsy surgery: a pilot study. *J Endourol.* 2016;30:1132–1137.

42. Ebbing J, Jaderling F, Collins JW, et al. Comparison of 3D printed prostate models with standard radiological information to aid understanding of the precise location of prostate cancer: a construct validation study. *PLoS One.* 2018;13:e0199477.

43. Blankstein U, Lantz AG, Honey RJDA, Pace KT, Ordon M, Lee JY. Simulation-based flexible ureteroscopy training using a novel ureteroscopy part-task trainer. *Can Urol Assoc J.* 2015;9:331.

44. Lerner DJ, Gifford SE, Olafsen N, Mileto A, Soloff E. Lumbar puncture: creation and resident acceptance of a low-cost, durable, reusable fluoroscopic phantom with a fluid-filled spinal canal for training at an academic program. *Am J Neuroradiol.* 2020;41(3):548–550.

45. Weinstock P, Prabhu SP, Flynn K, Orbach DB, Smith E. Optimizing cerebrovascular surgical and endovascular procedures in children via personalized 3D printing. *J Neurosurg Pediatr.* 2015;16(5):584–589.

46. July 2019 Update of the Hospital Outpatient Prospective Payment System (OPPS). CMS Manual System, Pub. 100-04, Transmittal #R4313CP, May 24, 2019, Change request 11318. Retrieved from: https://www.cms.gov/Regulations-and-Guidance/Guidance/Transmittals/2019-Transmittals-Items/R4313CP.

47. Chepelev L, Wake N, Ryan J, et al. Radiological Society of North America (RSNA) 3D printing Special Interest Group (SIG): guidelines for medical 3D printing and appropriateness for clinical scenarios. *3D Print Med.* 2018;4(11):1–38. https://doi.org/10.1186/s41205-018-0030-y.

48. Ballard DH, Wake N, Witowski J, et al. Radiological Society of North America (RSNA) 3D Printing Special Interest Group (SIG) clinical situations for which 3D printing is considered an appropriate representation or extension of data contained in a medical imaging examination: abdominal, hepatobiliary, and gastrointestinal conditions. *3D Print Med.* 2020;6(1):13.

49. Mitsouras D, Liacouras P, Imanzadeh A, et al. Medical 3D printing for the radiologist. *Radiographics.* Nov-Dec 2015; 35(7):1965–1988.

50. Leng S, McGee K, Morris J, et al. Anatomic modeling using 3D printing: quality assurance and optimization. *3D Print Med.* 2017;3(1):6. https://doi.org/10.1186/s41205-017-0014-3.

51. Noordvyk A, Ryan J, eds. *WG-17 3D;* October 10, 2019. Retrieved from: https://www.dicomstandard.org/wgs/wg-17/.

52. Chepelev L, Giannopoulos A, Tang A, et al. Medical 3D printing: methods to standardize terminology and report trends. *3D Print Med.* 2017;3:4.

53. Medcad. *CPT Codes for Surgical Planning, Guides, and 3D Models;* July 19, 2020. Retrieved from: https://medcad.net/cpt-codes-for-surgical-planning-guides-and-3d-models/.

54. ACR-RSNA 3D Printing (3DP) Registry, 2020. Retrieved from: https://www.acr.org/Practice-Management-Quality-Informatics/Registries/3D-Printing-Registry.

55. Fleming C, Sadaghiani MS, Stellon MA, Javan R. Effectiveness of three-dimensionally printed models in anatomy education for medical students and resident physicians: systematic review and meta-analysis. *J Am Coll Radiol.* 2020;17(10):1220–1229.

CHAPTER 11

3D Printing in Interventional Radiology

KAPIL WATTAMWAR, MD • NICOLE WAKE, PHD

INTRODUCTION

Interventional radiology (IR) is a subspecialty of radiology in which radiologists perform minimally invasive operations to diagnose, treat, and cure a variety of conditions. As compared to traditional surgeries, IR procedures can reduce surgical risks, operating and recovery time, costs, and at times lead to improved patient outcomes. The range of diseases and organ systems amenable to IR procedures are extensive and include vascular, oncologic, hepatobiliary, gastrointestinal, genitourinary, pulmonary, musculoskeletal, and neurologic intervention. IR procedures broadly involve angioplasty and stenting, thrombolysis, embolization, ablation, biopsy, drainage, injection, and retrieval.

Three-dimensional (3D) printing technologies are already well established in the surgical domain. In fact, even before the advent of this technology, researchers across the world were creating 3D objects for surgical planning by milling structures from foam, plastic, and other materials using a subtractive approach.[1,2] A glimpse into its role in surgical fields may substantiate parallel use cases within IR. Complex procedures require preoperative evaluation, and often, practice, to ensure a successful outcome. The role of 3D printing in surgery is usually for the purpose of illustrating anatomy in a relatable 3D method to surgeons, to create an anatomically accurate environment for hands-on simulation of a procedure, to serve as an intraoperative reference tool, to create customized equipment, and to develop tailored devices for a certain patient or procedure. This technology has been shown to reduce surgical time, increase operator confidence, and lead to improved operative results.[3–5]

There is growing evidence that physical 3D printed models aid clinicians in improving patient management and allow for improved patient outcomes.[6–9] These models can add value to clinical practice by allowing preprocedural planning or fabrication of custom devices and can have a large impact on trainee education and patient understanding. These use cases

lay the foundation for several applications of 3D printing within IR. In this chapter, we will address printing techniques and workflow relevant to IR, use cases of this technology in IR, and the future of 3D printing in IR.

3D PRINTING WORKFLOW

The general workflow to fabricate a 3D printed anatomic model involves image acquisition, segmentation, post-processing with computer-aided design (CAD) software, printing, and model post-processing, as exemplified in Fig. 11.1. As these topics have been discussed in detail in previous chapters, we will not go into depth here. However, it must be noted that a model's accuracy depends on how well the targeted structures can be clearly distinguished from surrounding tissues on the initial imaging.[10] The study of choice should provide the maximum contrast differentiation between the anatomy of interest and surrounding structures, which depends on size, shape, density, and magnetic resonance characteristics of tissue.

IR procedures vary widely by organ system, specific intervention, and age group, warranting unique imaging needs which should be considered when printing a model. For example, computed tomography (CT) may be the preferred modality when characterizing a complex inferior vena cava (IVC) filter retrieval due to the spatial resolution and ability to delineate metallic material. Certain tumors may have borders which are better defined on magnetic resonance imaging (MRI) and can aid in planning approach to a biopsy or complex ablation. Technical factors such as signal-to-noise ratio and contrast-to-noise ratio can, respectively, impact the ability to resolve fine structures such as small vessels and the ability to distinguish different materials such as pleural effusion from adjacent atelectasis.

Once an anatomic model has been segmented and prepared for printing using CAD software, the many different options for 3D printing must be considered.

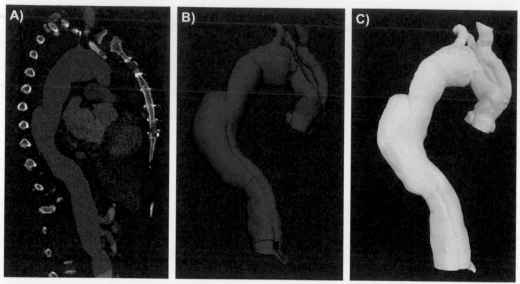

FIG. 11.1 The 3D printing workflow is demonstrated in creating a model of a dissecting aneurysm of the descending thoracic aorta. **(A)** The process begins with segmentation in which the blood pool, including both the true and false lumens, is selected. **(B)** A CAD model is created and refined. **(C)** The model is printed, in this case, on the Ultimaker S5 (Ultimaker, Utrecht, Netherlands) using polylactic acid with dissolvable polyvinyl alcohol as support.

The International Organization for Standardization and American Society of Testing and Materials have categorized these techniques under seven standardized headings including vat photopolymerization, material extrusion, directed energy deposition, powder bed fusion, binder jetting, material jetting, and sheet lamination.[11] The unique aspects of each of these techniques are discussed separately in Chapter 5 entitled "3D Printing Principles and Technologies." Techniques most relevant to use cases that arise in IR include vat photopolymerization, material extrusion, binder jetting, and material jetting. Once printing is complete, the part and the build plate are removed. The part is cleaned and support structures, if present, are removed (Fig. 11.2). For IR planning purposes, hollowed vasculature models may be required. It is important to note that for these models, technologies with dissolvable support materials are preferred.

CLINICAL USE CASES OF 3D PRINTING IN IR

Deciding when a 3D printed model can be beneficial in clinical practice based on patient outcomes is an area that is still under active investigation. Multiple studies have suggested that 3D printed models in the fields of vascular and nonvascular IR and neurointerventional radiology can bolster provider confidence and be useful

for procedural planning.[12,13] These models can be valuable for procedural planning when multiple approaches are possible, rehearsal for high-risk procedures where the margin for error is low, or even for routine procedures where operative time can be reduced. Printed models of the preoperative anatomy afford the ability to create a sophisticated procedural plan, rehearse to prevent and manage complications and reduce intraoperative radiation and anesthesia, particularly desirable in the pediatric population and in long complex cases. While multiple other modalities of advanced 3D image visualization and simulation exist, including virtual reality (VR) and augmented reality (AR), human cadaver, and live animals, 3D printing is a low-risk modality that offers unique advantages in terms of patient specificity, minimal risks to the user, and ability to integrate haptic feedback. Printed models may also be used in conjunction with imaging techniques and can accommodate use of actual interventional devices.

Vascular and Nonvascular General Interventional Procedures

Interventional treatments address a variety of pathologies in multiple organ systems through vascular, percutaneous, or natural-orifice directed routes. Printed anatomic vascular models in IR may be used for in vivo device testing, flow simulations, or presurgical planning.

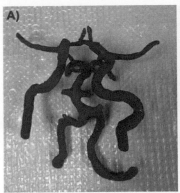 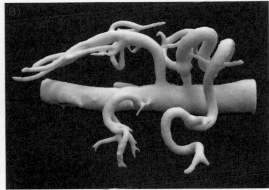

FIG. 11.2 Models of the **(A)** circle of Willis and **(B)** abdominal aorta printed with material extrusion on the Fortus 360 MC printer (Stratasys, Rehovot, Israel).

A survey-based study of common IR procedures showed that the use of 3D models for preprocedural and intraoperative guidance was feasible and low cost with promising utility in planning and execution.[12] These procedures included transarterial chemoembolization, percutaneous ablation, and splenic artery aneurysm repair. Models of relevant anatomy were printed using an affordable consumer-grade liquid resin desktop 3D printer. These included clear hollow vascular models of the aorta and target arteries and models of target organs for ablation with relevant surrounding anatomy manually denoted by painting them in different colors. The models were available prior to procedures as well as during procedures, where they were accessible in sterile bags for easy intraoperative manipulation. Interventional radiologists who performed procedures unanimously recommended the use of such models for similar cases. They rated the models favorably in terms of utility, ability to enhance spatial understanding, and ability to increase confidence in treatment approach. It should be noted that biocompatible and sterilizable surgical grade resins are available, and therefore if models are printed using these materials and appropriately sterilized preoperatively, they may be brought into the interventional suite without requiring placement in a sterile bag.

Hepatobiliary and portal vein intervention is common in IR and is an area where 3D printing may be particularly beneficial to facilitate access to the biliary or portal systems and to avoid vascular injury. For example, printed models of livers can assist in planning transjugular intrahepatic portosystemic shunt (TIPS) placement. One study postulated that reliance on 2D imaging alone may incur risk of complications such as extracapsular hemorrhage and nontarget puncture.[14] By having a model that displays the locations of hepatic

and portal vessels preoperatively, a radiologist can plan the ideal path for tract creation. In this study, hepatic parenchyma was printed with translucent acrylate polymer, containing hepatic and portal veins which were hollow and could accommodate catheters. The study noted that the complexity of printing could be reduced with a method to color vascular structures postprinting, rather than incorporating multiple colors into the raw print materials. Similar models may be advantageous in planning approach to percutaneous or transvenous liver biopsy in order to avoid complications related to vascular injury.

Portal vein stenosis is a common complication of liver transplant and often requires endovascular treatment, including balloon angioplasty and stent placement. One study used portal-phase contrast-enhanced CT data to create hollow models of portal vein stenosis for preoperative simulation of endovascular treatment and demonstrated that creating this type of 3D printed model was feasible.[15] Ten hollow models were printed using fused deposition modeling, a widely used and relatively inexpensive printing technique. The study also assessed models for reproducibility by filling them with water and obtaining T2-weighted MR images. After coregistration and binarization of the images, they were combined to create an overlap map, which demonstrated sufficient accuracy and precision in size and shape when compared to the CT mask images. Further work is required to determine the actual clinical utility of 3D printed models for portal vein stenosis.

The precision and accuracy of 3D printed models relative to the patient's anatomy is especially important for IR modeling, since many vascular structures are miniscule with intricacies and tortuosities that must be well visualized on a 3D model. Such research on model accuracy has been performed with multiple organ systems.[10] One study used 3D CT angiography data of a splenic artery aneurysm to create 10 hollow vascular models using a fused deposition modeling-type desktop 3D printer.[16] Models were filled with water and scanned with T2-weighted MRI for evaluation of the lumen. Cross-sectional areas were similar between models, reflecting high precision, and mean cross-sectional areas of the afferent artery were the same as those calculated from the original mask images, reflecting high accuracy.

3D printing has also been shown to assist with the treatment of visceral aneurysms including splenic, hepatic, gastric, epigastric, gastroduodenal, and posterior superior pancreaticoduodenal aneurysms.[16–18] Applications for 3D printing also abound in aortic and cardiovascular intervention, such as in abdominal aortic aneurysm repair[19,20] including aortic arch repair,[21,22] aortic valve replacement,[23–29] mitral valve replacement,[30–32] and pulmonary valve stent implantation.[33,34] Flow models of the abdominal vasculature may also be created to assess flow dynamics and appropriately size devices preoperatively (Fig. 11.3).

While applications for 3D printing in preoperative planning and simulation abound in IR, 3D printing also affords the creation of tools that can be used to increase efficiency and easy during IR procedures. One example is the F-Spoon, a handheld external compression device that was created to facilitate CT-guided and fluoroscopy-guided percutaneous abdominal intervention such as biopsies, drainages, and ablations.[35] The device was designed with the goal of facilitating access to targets and minimizing radiation exposure to radiologists. The design, created to accommodate a sterile cover, included a handgrip and curved armrest to allow steady control while applying continuous pressure to the abdomen. The tip of the device included a keyhole cutout which could slide around a needle embedded in the abdominal wall.

Neurointerventional Procedures

Various 3D printing techniques can be used to highlight intraoperative vascular anatomic relationships in neurointerventional radiology and neurosurgery. Multiple reports in the literature have demonstrated the feasibility of 3D printing neurovascular models using these technologies for diagnosis, preoperative planning, simulation, trainee education, and patient counseling[36–40]

At this time, the most widely utilized indication for 3D printed neurointerventional models is for the treatment of intracranial (cerebral) aneurysms. Intracranial aneurysms carry risk of rupturing, therefore must be treated using methods such as surgical clipping or endovascular coiling to seal off the aneurysm. The reported rate of intraprocedural aneurysmal rupture during coil embolization varies from 1% to 5%, significantly increasing risk of periprocedural death and disability.[41–43] The use of 3D printed models to guide approach and device selection may improve chances of successful embolization.

Several studies have shown how 3D printed intracranial aneurysm models can be useful for intervention planning.[44–47] First, in 2015, Mashiko et al. created a 3D printed vessel model which was first coated with liquid silicone and then melted leaving an outer layer as a hollow elastic model; and simulation using the elastic model was thought to be useful to understand the 3D aneurysm structure.[44] In 2015, Namba et al. also created hollowed patient-specific 3D printed aneurysm models for 10 consecutive patients undergoing endovascular coiling and these models were used for preoperative microcatheter shaping, a key factor for successful coil embolization of cerebral aneurysms which can be difficult to achieve. They found that the preplanned microcatheter shapes demonstrated stability in 9 of 10 cases.[45] A 2016 study also investigated the use of 3D printed models of intracranial arterial

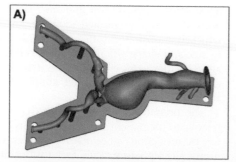 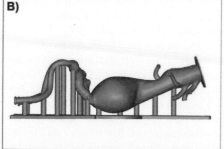

FIG. 11.3 **(A)** Superior and **(B)** lateral views of an abdominal aortic aneurysm flow model created by Materialise and available in the Mimics educational software edition (Mimics 23, Materialise, Leuven, Belgium).

aneurysms to produce optimally shaped microcatheters for coil embolization.[47] Twenty-seven aneurysms were treated using a total of 48 microcatheters shaped while referring to the 3D printed vessel model. Of the 48 catheters, only 9 (19%) required modification of the initial shape due to inappropriate positioning of the catheter and only 14 (29%) of catheter placements required repositioning due to catheter kick back. There were no procedure-related complications, including aneurysm rupture. A post-procedural questionnaire on the usefulness of the technique indicated favorability. In another study, rehearsing on 3D printed models reduced the time of operations for arteriovenous malformations (AVMs) and vein of Galen malformations.[13] It is reasonable to believe that optimal catheter shaping may be related to decreased procedure time and radiation.

3D printed negative molds typically filled with silicone can also be used to create models of aneurysms.[48] In a Japanese study, preoperative simulation of endovascular treatment for cerebral aneurysms was performed using patient-specific distensible vascular silicone models generated from 3D rotational angiographic images.[49] They demonstrated wide necks, tortuous routes of access, and hypoplastic segments. Interventions were simulated, including attempted possible methods for coil embolization, and aided in finalizing an approach and choosing the appropriate devices. The simulations were particularly useful in navigating microcatheters during the actual procedure by facilitating their shaping beforehand. One limitation noted of the silicone models was that the insertion of a catheter or guidewire did not alter vessel shapes the way they do in actuality.

Similar to above, 3D printing technology has also been used to create realistic hollowed, neurovascular models for preoperative flow simulation using clinical devices such as catheters or stents.[50–52] For example, printed models of cerebral aneurysms may be used to determine which flow diverter device is best suited for treatment and to accurately predict post-treatment flow alterations.[53,54] A case report by Sullivan et al. described rehearsal on a 3D printed model prior to treating an 8-year-old boy with a fusiform aneurysm of the supraclinoid segment of the left internal carotid artery (ICA) with a saccular component and documented growth on serial imaging.[54] Due to an increase in size of the parent vessel, attempts to use an off-label Pipeline Embolization Device (Medtronic, Dublin, Ireland) were aborted. The parent vessel was too large for any flow diverter available in the United States (US), and clip placement was not ideal due to the likely dissecting nature of the lesion. The team believed that

the patient would benefit from the SILK flow diverter device (Balt Extrusion, Montmorency, France) and US Food and Drug Administration (FDA) and local Institutional Review Board (IRB) approvals were granted. The most recent cerebral angiogram was used to 3D print the patient's cerebral vasculature. Two strategies were rehearsed using the model, including deployment of a standalone construct with the SILK device extending from the ICA terminus to the ophthalmic segment, versus a dual-device construct using the Leo + stent (Balt Extrusion, Montmorency, France) and the SILK flow diverter. The latter approach failed during simulation due to lack of ideal expansion of the Leo + device in the ICA terminus due to the sharp curvature and diameter mismatch of that segment to the more proximal carotid artery. Because of the simulation results, the patient was treated with the single construct method using the SILK flow diverter only, beginning proximal to the tortuous segment. The device was deployed uneventfully and crossed the entirety of the aneurysm neck with cone-beam CT angiogram demonstrating good wall apposition of the device without parent vessel compromise and favorable 6 month follow-up.

3D printing can also be applied to cerebral AVMs. Printed models have been found to be a useful tool for presurgical planning, allowing for shorter patient consultation time, increased acceptance of the procedure by patients and relatives, as well as shorter time between intraoperative digital subtraction angiography and start of endovascular treatment.[55] Due to the urgent nature of treatment for patients with strokes, 3D printing is not commonly utilized for preprocedure planning for thrombectomy. However, 3D printed flow models have been used to compare thrombectomy approaches and stent retriever performance in stroke models.[56–59]

3D PRINTING FOR IR TRAINING

3D printing has the potential to play a large role in IR education and training for students, residents, fellows, and any physicians looking to adopt a new procedure. The creation of 3D printed anatomical models and training phantoms can prove useful in teaching anatomy relevant to IR procedures, access techniques, and handling of wires and other devices.

Multiple studies have demonstrated 3D printed anatomy to be a more effective teaching model than the conventional cadaver model, with fewer limitations related to cost, reproducibility, and accessibility.[60–63] Repeated use of a cadaver can also destroy the normal anatomy. Meanwhile, the manufacturing of current traditional noncadaveric medical models is also costly, as well as time-consuming and complex. Models of anatomical structures can be printed with high accuracy and attention to tissue structural detail. A prospective study on veterinary students showed that students who studied using physical 3D printed models outperformed those who used textbooks or 3D computer models in aptitude tests of lower extremity anatomy.[64] In another study, a cohort of 29 medical students demonstrated significant improvement in knowledge acquisition, knowledge reporting, and structural conceptualization of ventricular septal defects after using high-fidelity 3D printed models of ventricular septal defects from MRI data.[65] Physical 3D printed liver models proved to be more effective than a traditional anatomic atlas in teaching hepatic segmental anatomy to medical students in another study.[66] VR technologies may also be useful for IR education.[67,68] Table 11.1 describes the pros and cons of each method of teaching for IR education.

The role of 3D printing in IR education goes beyond demonstrating anatomy and opens new opportunities for hands-on learning. Current resident training in endovascular techniques takes place within the fluoroscopy suite during clinical cases, potentially increasing patient and staff radiation exposure in addition to potentially negatively impacting patient outcomes. It is already well established that phantoms are valuable educational models for students and trainees to practice procedural technique and handling tools before approaching real patients, with demonstrated improvement in level of resident knowledge, confidence in technical skills, and anxiety level.[69]

Unlike in surgery where procedures are often performed under direct visualization, the image-guided nature of IR procedures poses a unique challenge to the creation of 3D printed phantoms. The ideal IR phantom must not only structurally resemble real anatomy but should also have imaging characteristics similar to tissue so that one may practice image-guided intervention, whether with fluoroscopy, CT, ultrasound, or MRI. Considerations for 3D printed imaging phantoms are discussed further in Chapter 14.

Specific to IR, one key example by Javan et al. used a 3D printed model of the liver to illustrate to key anatomical concepts in hepatobiliary intervention, such as hepatic segments and vasculature. The phantom

---

TABLE 11.1
Advantages and Disadvantages of Various Types of 3D Anatomic Models for IR Education.

Model Type	Advantages	Disadvantages
Virtual reality	• Ability to include multiple models • Patient-specific anatomy • Integration of metrics and other feedback features • Long-lasting platform • Minimal safety concerns • Imaging can be incorporated with 3D visualization	• Virtual nature may limit model fidelity and realism • Limited haptic feedback • Requires updates and maintenance
3D printed	• Patient-specific anatomy • Haptic feedback achievable • May allow use of imaging techniques and devices • Minimal safety concerns	• Costs depending on material • Time-consuming fabrication process • Limited reusability
Human cadaver	• Realistic imaging appearance and haptic feedback • Direct visualization of anatomy • Allows use of imaging techniques and devices	• High cost • Cannot customize for patient-specific anatomy/pathology • Limited reusability
Live animal	• Realistic imaging appearance and haptic feedback • Physiologic responsiveness (vital signs, hemorrhage, hemostasis) • Allows use of real imaging techniques and IR devices	• High cost • Cannot customize for patient-specific anatomy/pathology • Limited reusability

Adapted from Table 1 in Sullivan S, et al. Three-dimensional printing and neuroendovascular simulation for the treatment of a pediatric intracranial aneurysm: case report. *J Neurosurg Pediatr.* 2018;22(6):672–677.

included a simulated mass with feeding arterial supply, an abscess with a percutaneous access channel through which a trainee could practice placing a pigtail catheter, and a transhepatic channel extending to a gallbladder to demonstrate approach to cholecystostomy.[70] Another example of a fluoroscopy-compatible 3D printed phantom was created by Bundy et al. for percutaneous biliary endoscopy training. The group's phantoms had educational utility even for attending interventional radiologists who sought to add this new procedure to their repertoire.[71]

Eisenmenger et al. showed that 3D printed models compatible with angiography can provide safe and cost-effective means to develop endovascular skills and practice and plan fluoroscopic procedures without the downsides of morbidity from excessive patient radiation.[72] In this study, patient CTA data pertaining to vasculature was converted to a 3D surface rendering, the polygon count was reduced, and the resulting vascular model was printed on a standard desktop material extrusion printer, however, using dissolvable filament. Models of small diameter vasculature were cast in silicone. The printed material was then dissolved, leaving the hollow silicone models of vasculature, capable of being used under fluoroscopy. Larger diameter vessels such as the aorta and associated branch vessels were directly printed for use in training, without the need for silicone casting. Trainees used these angiographic models as cost-effective and accessible tools to improve angiography skills. The authors theorized that such 3D models could be used to compare resident abilities across years or institutions, including preprocedural assessment for angioplasty, coil deployment, stent placement, filter placement, or endovascular graft positioning. A prospective study conducted at the Memorial University of Newfoundland showed that medical students too can effectively learn vascular anatomy and basic handling skills using fluoroscopy-compatible 3D printed vascular models.[73]

3D models can also be used to simulate musculoskeletal fluoroscopic procedures. One study described a methodology for 3D printing a model of the glenohumeral joint to serve as a phantom for training in fluoroscopy-guided shoulder arthrography.[74] Osseous structures, intraarticular space, and skin surface of the shoulder were digitally extracted as separate 3D meshes from a normal CT arthrogram of the shoulder, using commercially available software. Using binder jetting, bones were 3D printed in gypsum, a mineral that is fluoroscopically radiopaque. A rubber-like material was used to print the joint capsule, using material jetting technology. The capsule was secured to the humeral head and glenoid to create a sealed intraarticular space. A polyamide mold of the skin was printed using selective laser sintering. The joint was stabilized inside the mold, and the surrounding soft tissues were cast in silicone of varying densities. The radiopaque osseous structures replicated in vivo osseous corticomedullary differentiation, with dense cortical bone and less dense medullary cancellous bone. The glenoid labrum was successfully integrated into the printed capsule. The phantom was repeatedly used to perform shoulder arthrography using anterior, posterior, and rotator interval approaches, and simulated the in vivo challenges of needle guidance. Users were also able to perform CT arthrographic imaging of the phantom.

In addition to fluoroscopy, CT is another critical modality for image guidance in IR. The groundwork to 3D print realistic CT phantoms has been laid in work which demonstrated the feasibility of creating anthropomorphic phantoms for head CT.[75] This methodology included three materials of different radiodensities to reflect the inherent differences in CT numbers between white matter, gray matter, and cerebrospinal fluid. The phantom was placed within a skull phantom and scanned on a 192-slice scanner (SOMATOM Force, Siemens Healthcare, Germany) with a routine head protocol. Although the CAD model involved a high degree of anatomic complexity, employing over 200 CAD shells, the phantom was successfully printed. On comparison of images to those of the original patient, the absolute CT numbers for tissue differed. However, the differences in CT numbers between tissue types were consistent in the two images and when viewed with similar display and different levels, the phantom and patient images displayed a similar range of gray scales and contrast levels with satisfactory similarity in anatomical structure and texture. Similar techniques can be applied to other areas of the body for preprocedural planning or education for CT-guided procedures such as drainage, ablation, or percutaneous embolization.

The realm of ultrasound compatible phantoms opens numerous opportunities for IR education related to drainages, biopsies, injections, and obtaining vascular access. Currently available commercial ultrasound phantoms are often expensive, have poor anatomic fidelity, and only exist for a limited range of procedures. Meanwhile, low-cost, do-it-yourself phantoms often consistent of gelatin castings containing embedded objects or pieces of animal tissue, therefore also with limited anatomic correlation, while also lacking robustness and requiring the use of animal tissue. A randomized study compared the use of 3D printed ultrasound compatible vascular models to readily available commercial models in training medical students to obtain femoral arterial access.[76] Contrast-enhanced CT data were segmented, processed, and printed with stereolithography. Vessels were printed using gray flexible photopolymer resin material to simulate vascular wall compliance. Bony anatomy was printed using fused deposition modeling. Trainees in neither the 3D printing arm nor the commercial arm expressed lack of confidence in performing femoral arterial access prior to the training with these models, but the post-training confidence increase exhibited by the 3D printing group was noninferior to the commercial group, suggesting that custom-made 3D printed training models could be used to instruct medical students in procedural skills.

3D printing technology can be used in combination with traditional molding techniques for ultrasound training to replicate both structural anatomical detail and textural detail to make the ultrasound appearance more realistic. One study sought to create an inexpensive ultrasound phantom for shoulder joint injection training that had a high degree of anatomic realism.[77] The study utilized open-source STL files, in which bone/muscle attachments were verified, minor adaption of muscle bodies were performed, and ligaments were created. The files were prepared for printing with a material jetting printer. The model consisted of different materials to distinguish bone from muscles, tendons, and ligaments. The skins surface file was used to create a 3-mm thick shell mold of the soft tissue. The insert and mold were assembled and filled with a gelatin mixture containing suspended psyllium husk. The model exhibited high anatomic fidelity on ultrasound for residents in training and represented a material cost of approximately $280.

The functional behavior of ultrasound phantoms can also be adapted to replicate physiologic flow dynamics. This was demonstrated in a study exploring 3D printing to convert high-resolution CT images of aortic valves with severe stenosis into life-size physical models. The dual-material models were created using material jetting 3D printing. A rigid material was used for printing regions of calcification, and a rubber-like material was used to simulate the soft tissue structures of the outflow tract, aortic root, and noncalcified valve cusps. Models were evaluated in the valve orifice area, appearance on echocardiogram, and severity of stenosis by Doppler. The models were designed to achieve strong correlation between Doppler-derived measures of peak and mean transvalvular gradient with reference standard pressure catheters across a range of flow conditions and aortic valve orifice area by Gorlin and Doppler methods.[25] These principles can be applied to creating multimaterial high-fidelity models for procedures that involve ultrasound guidance such as biopsies and drainages, embolization of pseudoaneurysms, declotting of arteriovenous grafts, and renal intervention.

3D PRINTING FOR PATIENT EDUCATION

It is vital that patients are provided with accurate and relevant knowledge that allows them to engage fully in their care. Information is often communicated to patients verbally, sometimes with the use of diagrams or the patient's own medical imaging. While physicians are trained over the course of many years to understand disease processes, patients are not. Furthermore, medical imaging can involve complex modalities where pathology is not readily apparent to the lay observer, such as in the case of multiphase contrast-enhanced CT, multisequence MRI, or ultrasound. As a result, patients often find imaging difficult to interpret[78] and they may resort to locating additional information on the Internet, where information may be of poor quality and is not always from reputable sources.[79]

Patient-specific 3D printed models are simple but effective tools that may aid patients in better comprehending their medical diagnosis, treatment options, and risks. These models thereby have the potential to improve shared decision-making and improve the patient experience. There have been several studies which show the added value of 3D printed models for patient education in pediatric cardiology,[78] posterior lumbar spinal fusion,[80] percutaneous lithotripsy,[81] endovascular aortic aneurysm repair,[82] cerebrovascular aneurysm treatment,[83] nephrectomy for suspicious renal masses and treatment of prostate cancer,[84,85] and hepatectomy for hepatic tumors.[86]

Interventional radiologists are well suited to take on the role of patient educator, especially in the growing areas of outpatient IR and interventional oncology. For example, a woman undergoing fibroid embolization may develop a better understanding of the location and bulk of her fibroids and the nature of the technique, allowing the patient to be more comfortable in decision-making when consenting to the procedure in the office, and postoperatively when dealing with pain. A patient with peripheral arterial disease may be better able to conceptualize his degree of disease and effectiveness of thrombectomy with before and after seeing 3D printed models. Patients battling malignancies require high-quality information so that they can play an active role in their treatment paradigm and maintain morale.[87] Interventional oncology typically represents part of a large multidisciplinary effort to treat cancer, offering treatments such as radioembolization, chemoembolization, and ablations. As imaging is central to the procedures as well as the source of 3D models, interventional oncology is a unique opportunity for radiology to vastly improve a patient's understanding of his or her own condition and positively impact a patient's experience.

THE FUTURE OF 3D PRINTING IN IR

3D printing has opened exciting avenues in IR for anatomical education, skill training, procedural planning, intraoperative guidance, device creation, and patient education. Use cases for 3D printing in IR continue to grow as ongoing basic research expands its capabilities.

The further development of 3D printing will include a wider range of materials leading to more durable and realistic products. The continued development of raw materials for 3D printing will expand applications for models compatible with ultrasound, fluoroscopy, CT, and MRI. In addition, the significant cost and speed of 3D printing is also expected to improve, thereby increasing the uptake of these machines at hospitals and outpatient centers, as well as willingness of the owners to fabricate prints. These advancements will benefit educators, students and trainees, patients, radiologists, and other physicians.

While current commercially available devices meet the needs of most patients, those with variant anatomy or anatomy sized outside of the traditional range may experience suboptimal treatment or even adverse effects with ready-made designs. For instance, an inappropriately sized IVC filter can cause lethal complications by migrating, embolizing fragments, or penetrating through the caval wall and resulting in bowel perforation or hemorrhage.[88] A custom printed device based on prior CT imaging can avert this problem without the cost associated with stocking large quantities of rarely used devices. Similarly, though interventional radiologists often use a select few catheters to perform most endovascular and nonvascular tasks, the potential to fabricate catheters of custom lengths, diameters, and tip configurations may reduce procedure time, radiation exposure, and risk of complications. As 3D printing develops a routine presence in radiology departments, it will offer interventional radiologists access to a limitless toolbox of devices to perform procedures more safely and efficiently.

The extrusion of bioabsorbable materials into filament can allow for the creation of short-term devices such as IVC filters, stents, and catheters which automatically dissolve over time without the need for retrieval. As 3D printing technology advances, the interventional radiologist will also be able to create customized bioactive constructs such as catheters, stents, or microspheres which can locally deliver drugs. An in vitro feasibility study used fused deposition printing to construct bioabsorbable 14 French catheters impregnated with antibiotics and chemotherapeutics.[89] Scanning electron microscope imaging showed long-lasting presence of additive powders on the catheters. Elution profiles and bacterial cultures showed sustained drug release and sizable zones of inhibition. Further work will substantiate this framework for a variety of applications, possibly related to chemotherapy, fibrinolysis, antibiotics, or antiplatelets. In theory, this innovation would allow for improved patient outcomes through tailored sizes and configurations, targeted drug delivery, custom pharmacokinetics, and improved patient adherence.

Bioprinting, which refers to the process of 3D printing using cell-encapsulating material, may also unlock possibilities in IR, such as tissue lined covered stents which mature into live vessels over time for dialysis grafts, bypass procedures in peripheral arterial disease, and TIPS placement. This technology may also improve coil embolization, as theorized by Sheth et al.[88] Inadequate coil packing can lead to recurrent bleeding, especially in patients with coagulopathy or altered dynamics. Embolization devices populated with patient-derived fibroblasts may allow for improved hemostasis through collagen matrix deposition to stability thrombus formation. Cell-laden constructs containing growth factors, immunomodulators, and antibacterial agents are also on the horizon with applications in improved wound healing.[90]

3D printing can be used in conjunction with AR and VR technologies to revolutionize the way that interventional radiologists rehearse cases and use real-time intraoperative guidance. One group used MRI-compatible and MRI-visible 3D printed models to plan and simulate safe access routes for CT- and MR-guided cryoablation of a pedicle osteoid osteoma and lamina osteoblastoma in addition to intraoperative 3D computer simulation of a theoretical ablation zone.[91] AR with the projection of rehearsal or CAD simulation onto the live operative imaging, similar to the concept of a roadmap, may facilitate quick and safe outcomes in complex cases such as this. The combination of 3D printing and AR or VR can also create a unique platform for IR education. In 2019, a group from the University of Utah reported development of a patient-specific haptic simulator to allow trainees to practice performing a TIPS.[92] They printed 3D models of liver with hollow vessels and a reusable silicone mold for liver parenchyma. Using AR and VR, trainees were able to simulate TIPS on the printed model for both anatomical reference and haptic feedback.

Trained in diagnostic imaging as well as therapeutic intervention, interventional radiologists are uniquely positioned to take a leading role in medical 3D printing for clinical use. The scope for 3D printing in IR is broad and capabilities will continue to evolve as new applications are adopted into clinical practice.

REFERENCES

1. Chareancholvanich K, Narkbunnam R, Pornrattanamaneewong C. A prospective randomised controlled study of patient-specific cutting guides compared with conventional instrumentation in total knee replacement. *Bone Jt J.* 2013;95-B(3):354–359.
2. Lambrecht JT. *3-D Modeling Technology in Oral and Maxillofacial Surgery.* Quintessence Pub. Co; 1995.
3. Mankovich NJ, Cheeseman AM, Stoker NG. The display of three-dimensional anatomy with stereolithographic models. *J Digit Imag.* 1990;3(3):200–203.
4. Brown GA, Firoozbakhsh K, DeCoster TA, Reyna Jr JR, Moneim M. Rapid prototyping: the future of trauma surgery? *J Bone Jt Surg Am.* 2003;85-A(Suppl 4):49–55.
5. Ballard DH, Mills P, Duszak Jr R, Weisman JA, Rybicki FJ, Woodard PK. Medical 3D printing cost-savings in orthopedic and maxillofacial surgery: cost analysis of operating room time saved with 3D printed anatomic models and surgical guides. *Acad Radiol.* 2020;27(8):1103–1113.
6. Diment LE, Thompson MS, Bergmann JHM. Clinical efficacy and effectiveness of 3D printing: a systematic review. *BMJ Open.* 2017;7(12):e016891.
7. Tack P, Victor J, Gemmel P, Annemans L. 3D-printing techniques in a medical setting: a systematic literature review. *Biomed Eng Online.* 2016;15(1):115.
8. Aimar A, Palermo A, Innocenti B. The role of 3D printing in medical applications: a state of the art. *J Healthc Eng.* 2019;2019:5340616.
9. Martelli N, Serrano C, van den Brink H, et al. Advantages and disadvantages of 3-dimensional printing in surgery: a systematic review. *Surgery.* 2016;159(6):1485–1500.
10. George E, Liacouras P, Mitsouras FJ, Rybicki D. Measuring and establishing the accuracy and reproducibility of 3D printed medical models. *Radiographics.* 2017;37(5):1424–1450.
11. ISO/ASTM. *Additive Manufacturing — General Principles — Terminology.* 2018.
12. Ghodadra A, Varma R, Santos E, Pinter J, Amesur N. Inexpensive 3D printed models supplement interventional radiology procedure planning. *J Vasc Intervent Radiol.* 2017;28(2):S14–S15.
13. Weinstock P, Prabhu SP, Flynn K, Orbach DB, Smith E. Optimizing cerebrovascular surgical and endovascular procedures in children via personalized 3D printing. *J Neurosurg Pediatr.* 2015;16(5):584–589.
14. Nicol K,SJ, Borrello J, Swinburne N, et al. 3D printing of a cirrhotic liver with parenchymal translucency and highlighted portal and hepatic veins for pre-TIPS planning. *J Vasc Intervent Radiol.* 2017;28(2).
15. Takao H, Amemiya S, Shibata E, Ohtomo K. Three-dimensional printing of hollow portal vein stenosis models: a feasibility study. *J Vasc Intervent Radiol.* 2016;27(11):1755–1758.
16. Takao H, Amemiya S, Shibata E, Ohtomo K. 3D printing of preoperative simulation models of a splenic artery aneurysm: precision and accuracy. *Acad Radiol.* 2017;24(5):650–653.
17. Shibata E, Takao H, Amemiya S, Ohtomo K. 3D-Printed visceral aneurysm models based on CT data for simulations of endovascular embolization: evaluation of size and shape accuracy. *Am J Roentgenol.* 2017;209(2):243–247.
18. Itagaki M. Using 3D printed models for planning and guidance during endovascular intervention: a technical advance. *Diagn Interv Radiol.* 2015;21:338–341.
19. Meess KM, Izzo RL, Dryjski ML, et al. 3D printed abdominal aortic aneurysm phantom for image guided surgical planning with a patient specific fenestrated endovascular graft system. *Proc SPIE Int Soc Opt Eng.* 2017:10138.
20. Mitsuoka H, Terai Y, Miyano Y, et al. Preoperative planning for physician-modified endografts using a three-dimensional printer. *Ann Vasc Dis.* 2019;12(3):334–339.
21. Sulaiman A, Boussel L, Taconnet F, et al. In vitro non-rigid life-size model of aortic arch aneurysm for endovascular prosthesis assessment. *Eur J Cardio Thorac Surg.* 2008;33(1):53–57.
22. Meyer-Szary J, Wozniak-Mielczarek L, Sabiniewicz D, Sabiniewicz R. Feasibility of in-house rapid prototyping of cardiovascular three-dimensional models for planning and training non-standard interventional procedures. *Cardiol J.* 2019;26(6):790–792.
23. Sodian R, Schmauss D, Markert M, et al. Three-dimensional printing creates models for surgical planning of aortic valve replacement after previous coronary bypass grafting. *Ann Thorac Surg.* 2008;85(6):2105–2108.
24. Schmauss D, Schmitz C, Bigdeli AK. Three-dimensional printing of models for preoperative planning and simulation of transcatheter valve replacement. *Ann Thorac Surg.* 2012;93(2):e31–e33.
25. Maragiannis D, Jackson MS, Igo SR, et al. Replicating patient-specific severe aortic valve stenosis with functional 3D modeling. *Circ Cardiovasc Imaging.* 2015;8(10):e003626.
26. Ripley B, Kelil T, Cheezum MK, et al. 3D printing based on cardiac CT assists anatomic visualization prior to transcatheter aortic valve replacement. *J Cardiovasc Comput Tomogr.* 2016;10(1):28–36.
27. Qian Z, Wang K, Liu S, et al. Quantitative prediction of paravalvular leak in transcatheter aortic valve replacement based on tissue-mimicking 3D printing. *JACC Cardiovasc Imaging.* 2017;10(7):719–731.
28. Hosny A, Dilley JD, Kelil T, et al. Pre-procedural fit-testing of TAVR valves using parametric modeling and 3D printing. *J Cardiovasc Comput Tomogr.* 2019;13(1):21–30.
29. Rotman OM, Kovarovic B, Sadasivan C, et al. Realistic vascular replicator for TAVR procedures. *Cardiovasc Eng Technol.* 2018;9(3):339–350.
30. Izzo RL, O'Hara RP, Iyer V, et al. 3D printed cardiac phantom for procedural planning of a transcatheter native mitral valve replacement. *Proc SPIE Int Soc Opt Eng.* 2016:9789.
31. El Sabbagh A, Eleid MF, Matsumoto JM, et al. Three-dimensional prototyping for procedural simulation of transcatheter mitral valve replacement in patients with mitral annular calcification. *Cathet Cardiovasc Interv.* 2018;92(7):E537–E549.
32. Wang DD, Eng MH, Greenbaum AB, et al. Validating a prediction modeling tool for left ventricular outflow tract (LVOT) obstruction after transcatheter mitral valve replacement (TMVR). *Cathet Cardiovasc Interv.* 2018;92(2):379–387.

33. Schievano S, Migliavacca F, Coats L, et al. Percutaneous pulmonary valve implantation based on rapid prototyping of right ventricular outflow tract and pulmonary trunk from MR data. *Radiology.* 2007;242(2):490–497.

34. Armillotta A, Bonhoeffer P, Dubini G, et al. Use of rapid prototyping models in the planning of percutaneous pulmonary valved stent implantation. *Proc Inst Mech Eng H.* 2007;221(4):407–416.

35. Epelboym Y, Shyn PB, Hosny A, et al. Use of a 3D-printed abdominal compression device to facilitate CT fluoroscopy-guided percutaneous interventions. *Am J Roentgenol.* 2017;209(2):435–441.

36. Khan IS, Kelly PD, Singer RJ. Prototyping of cerebral vasculature physical models. *Surg Neurol Int.* 2014;5:11.

37. Kondo K, Nemoto M, Masuda H, et al. Anatomical reproducibility of a head model molded by a three-dimensional printer. *Neurol Med Chir.* 2015;55(7):592–598.

38. Anderson JR, Thompson WL, Alkattan AK, et al. Three-dimensional printing of anatomically accurate, patient specific intracranial aneurysm models. *J Neurointerventional Surg.* 2016;8(5):517–520.

39. Frolich AM, Spallek J, Brehmer L, et al. 3D printing of intracranial aneurysms using fused deposition modeling offers highly accurate replications. *Am J Neuroradiol.* 2016;37(1):120–124.

40. Thawani JP, Pisapia JM, Singh N, et al. Three-dimensional printed modeling of an arteriovenous malformation including blood flow. *World Neurosurg.* 2016;90:675–683 e2.

41. Brisman JL, Niimi Y, Song JK, Berenstein A. Aneurysmal rupture during coiling: low incidence and good outcomes at a single large volume center. *Neurosurgery.* 2005;57(6):1103–1109. discussion 1103-9.

42. Pierot L, Spelle L, Vitry F, Investigators A. Immediate clinical outcome of patients harboring unruptured intracranial aneurysms treated by endovascular approach: results of the ATENA study. *Stroke.* 2008;39(9):2497–2504.

43. Elijovich L, Higashida RT, Lawton MT, et al. Predictors and outcomes of intraprocedural rupture in patients treated for ruptured intracranial aneurysms: the CARAT study. *Stroke.* 2008;39(5):1501–1506.

44. Mashiko T, Otani K, Kawano R, et al. Development of three-dimensional hollow elastic model for cerebral aneurysm clipping simulation enabling rapid and low cost prototyping. *World Neurosurg.* 2015;83(3):351–361.

45. Namba K, Higaki A, Kaneko N, et al. Microcatheter shaping for intracranial aneurysm coiling using the 3-dimensional printing rapid prototyping technology: preliminary result in the first 10 consecutive cases. *World Neurosurg.* 2015;84(1):178–186.

46. Xu Y, Tian W, Wei Z, et al. Microcatheter shaping using three-dimensional printed models for intracranial aneurysm coiling. *J Neurointerventional Surg.* 2020;12(3):308–310.

47. Ishibashi T, Takao H, Suzuki T, et al. Tailor-made shaping of microcatheters using three-dimensional printed vessel models for endovascular coil embolization. *Comput Biol Med.* 2016;77:59–63.

48. Knox K, Kerber CW, Singel SA, Bailey MJ, Imbesi SG. Stereolithographic vascular replicas from CT scans: choosing treatment strategies, teaching, and research from live patient scan data. *Am J Neuroradiol.* 2005;26(6):1428–1431.

49. Kono K, Shintani A, Okada H, Terada T. Preoperative simulations of endovascular treatment for a cerebral aneurysm using a patient-specific vascular silicone model. *Neurol Med Chir.* 2013;53(5):347–351.

50. Ionita CN, Mokin M, Varble N, et al. Challenges and limitations of patient-specific vascular phantom fabrication using 3D Polyjet printing. *Proc SPIE Int Soc Opt Eng.* 2014;9038:90380M.

51. Biglino G, Verschueren P, Zegels R, Taylor AM, Schievano S. Rapid prototyping compliant arterial phantoms for in-vitro studies and device testing. *J Cardiovasc Magn Reson.* 2013;15:2.

52. Nagesh SVS, Hinaman J, Sommer K, et al. A simulation platform using 3D printed neurovascular phantoms for clinical utility evaluation of new imaging technologies. *Proc SPIE Int Soc Opt Eng.* 2018:10578.

53. Sindeev S, Arnold PG, Frolov S, et al. Phase-contrast MRI versus numerical simulation to quantify hemodynamical changes in cerebral aneurysms after flow diverter treatment. *PLoS One.* 2018;13(1):e0190696.

54. Sullivan S, Aguilar-Salinas P, Santos R, Beier AD, Hanel RA. Three-dimensional printing and neuroendovascular simulation for the treatment of a pediatric intracranial aneurysm: case report. *J Neurosurg Pediatr.* 2018;22(6):672–677.

55. Dong M, Chen G, Li J, et al. Three-dimensional brain arteriovenous malformation models for clinical use and resident training. *Medicine.* 2018;97(3):e9516.

56. Mokin M, Ionita CN, Nagesh SV, et al. Primary stentriever versus combined stentriever plus aspiration thrombectomy approaches: in vitro stroke model comparison. *J Neurointerventional Surg.* 2015;7(6):453–457.

57. Mokin M, Nagesh SVS, Ionita CN, Levy EI, Siddiqui AH. Comparison of modern stroke thrombectomy approaches using an in vitro cerebrovascular occlusion model. *Am J Neuroradiol.* 2015;36(3):547–551.

58. Mokin M, Waqas M, Nagesh SVS, et al. Assessment of distal access catheter performance during neuroendovascular procedures: measuring force in three-dimensional patient specific phantoms. *J Neurointerventional Surg.* 2019;11(6):619–622.

59. Machi P, Jourdan F, Ambard D, et al. Experimental evaluation of stent retrievers' mechanical properties and effectiveness. *J Neurointerventional Surg.* 2017;9(3):257–263.

60. Waran V, Narayanan V, Karuppiah R, et al. Injecting realism in surgical training-initial simulation experience with custom 3D models. *J Surg Educ.* 2014;71(2):193–197.

61. AbouHashem Y, Dayal M, Savanah S, Strkalj G. The application of 3D printing in anatomy education. *Med Educ Online.* 2015;20:29847.

62. Lim KH, Loo ZY, Goldie SJ, Adams JW, McMenamin PG, et al. Use of 3D printed models in medical education: a randomized control trial comparing 3D prints versus cadaveric materials for learning external cardiac anatomy. *Anat Sci Educ.* 2016;9(3):213–221.

63. Triepels CPR, Smeets CFA, Notten KJB, et al. Does three-dimensional anatomy improve student understanding? *Clin Anat.* 2020;33(1):25–33.

64. Preece D, Williams SB, Lam R, Weller R. "Let's get physical": advantages of a physical model over 3D computer models and textbooks in learning imaging anatomy. *Anat Sci Educ.* 2013;6(4):216–224.

65. Costello JP, Olivieri LJ, Krieger A, et al. Utilizing three-dimensional printing technology to assess the feasibility of high-fidelity synthetic ventricular septal defect models for simulation in medical education. *World J Pediatr Congenit Heart Surg.* 2014;5(3):421–426.

66. Kong X, Nie L, Zhang H, et al. Do 3D printing models improve anatomical teaching about hepatic segments to medical students? A randomized controlled study. *World J Surg.* 2016;40(8):1969–1976.

67. Dankelman J, Wentink M, Grimbergen CA, Stassen HG, Reekers J. Does virtual reality training make sense in interventional radiology? Training skill-, rule- and knowledge-based behavior. *Cardiovasc Intervent Radiol.* 2004;27(5): 417–421.

68. Johnson SJ, Guediri SM, Kilkenny C, Clough PJ. Development and validation of a virtual reality simulator: human factors input to interventional radiology training. *Hum Factors.* 2011;53(6):612–625.

69. Sekhar A, Sun MR, Siewert B. A tissue phantom model for training residents in ultrasound-guided liver biopsy. *Acad Radiol.* 2014;21(7):902–908.

70. Javan R, Zeman MN. A prototype educational model for hepatobiliary interventions: unveiling the role of graphic designers in medical 3D printing. *J Digit Imag.* 2018; 31(1):133–143.

71. Bundy JJ, Weadock WJ, Chick JFB, et al. Three-dimensional printing facilitates creation of a biliary endoscopy phantom for interventional radiology-operated endoscopy training. *Curr Probl Diagn Radiol.* 2019;48(5):456–461.

72. Eisenmenger L, Ghandehari H, Jensen M, Huo E. Abstract No. 481 – Novel creation of an angiographic training model for trainees from 3D printed patient data. *J Vasc Intervent Radiol.* 2016;27(3, Supplement):S214.

73. Goudie C, Kinnin J, Bartellas M, Gullipalli R, Dubrowski A. The use of 3D printed vasculature for simulation-based medical education within interventional radiology. *Cureus.* 2019;11(4):e4381.

74. Javan R, Ellenbogen AL, Greek N, Haji-Momenian S. A prototype assembled 3D-printed phantom of the glenohumeral joint for fluoroscopic-guided shoulder arthrography. *Skeletal Radiol.* 2019;48(5):791–802.

75. Chen B, Leng SP, Vrieze TJ, et al. Design and 3D printing of an anthropomorphic brain CT phantom based on patient images. In: *Radiological Society of North America 2016 Scientific Assembly and Annual Meeting.* Radiological Society of North America; 2016. Chicago, IL.

76. Sheu AY, Laidlaw GL, Fell JC, et al. Custom 3-dimensional printed ultrasound-compatible vascular access models: training medical students for vascular access. *J Vasc Intervent Radiol.* 2019;30(6):922–927.

77. Smith B, Liacouras P, Grant G. Utilization of 3D printing to create low-cost, high fidelity ultrasound phantoms. In: *World Congress on Ultrasound in Medical Education.* 2014. Portland, OR.

78. Biglino G, Capelli C, Wray J, et al. 3D-manufactured patient-specific models of congenital heart defects for communication in clinical practice: feasibility and acceptability. *BMJ Open.* 2015;5(4):e007165.

79. Pass JH, Patel AH, Stuart S, Barnacle AM, Patel PA. Quality and readability of online patient information regarding sclerotherapy for venous malformations. *Pediatr Radiol.* 2018;48(5):708–714.

80. Liew Y, Beveridge E, Demetriades AK, Hughes MA. 3D printing of patient-specific anatomy: a tool to improve patient consent and enhance imaging interpretation by trainees. *Br J Neurosurg.* 2015;29(5):712–714.

81. Atalay HA, Canat HL, Ulker V, et al. Impact of personalized three-dimensional -3D- printed pelvicalyceal system models on patient information in percutaneous nephrolithotripsy surgery: a pilot study. *Int Braz J Urol.* 2017;43(3): 470–475.

82. Eisenmenger L, Kumpati G, Huo E. 3D printed patient specific aortic models for patient education and preoperative planning. *J Vasc Intervent Radiol.* 2016;27(3):S236–S237.

83. Wurm G, Tomancok B, Pogady P, Holl K, Trenkler J. Cerebrovascular stereolithographic biomodeling for aneurysm surgery. Technical note. *J Neurosurg.* 2004;100(1): 139–145.

84. Silberstein JL, Maddox MM, Dorsey P, et al. Physical models of renal malignancies using standard cross-sectional imaging and 3-dimensional printers: a pilot study. *Urology.* 2014;84(2):268–272.

85. Wake N, Rosenkrantz AB, Huang R, et al. Patient-specific 3D printed and augmented reality kidney and prostate cancer models: impact on patient education. *3D Print Med.* 2019;5(1):4.

86. Yang T, Tan T, Yang J, et al. The impact of using three-dimensional printed liver models for patient education. *J Int Med Res.* 2018;46(4):1570–1578.

87. van de Belt TH, Nijmeijer H, Grim D, et al. Patient-specific actual-size three-dimensional printed models for patient education in glioma treatment: first experiences. *World Neurosurg.* 2018;117:e99–e105.

88. Sheth R, Balesh ER, Zhang YS, et al. Three-dimensional printing: an enabling technology for IR. *J Vasc Intervent Radiol.* 2016;27(6):859–865.

89. Weisman JA, Ballard DH, Jammalamadaka U, et al. 3D printed antibiotic and chemotherapeutic eluting catheters for potential use in interventional radiology: in vitro proof of concept study. *Acad Radiol.* 2019;26(2):270–274.

90. Brower J, Blumberg S, Carroll E, et al. Mesenchymal stem cell therapy and delivery systems in nonhealing wounds. *Adv Skin Wound Care.* 2011;24(11):524–532. quiz 533-4.

91. Guenette JP, Himes N, Giannopoulos AA, et al. Computer-based vertebral tumor cryoablation planning and procedure simulation involving two cases using MRI-visible 3D printing and advanced visualization. *Am J Roentgenol.* 2016;207(5):1128–1131.

92. Smith TA, Eastaway A, Fine GC, et al. *Creation of a Haptic 3D Printed Simulator for TIPS Training in Augmented and Virtual Reality.* Chicago, IL: Radiological Society of North America; 2019.

CHAPTER 12

3D Printing in Nuclear Medicine and Radiation Therapy

ALEJANDRO AMOR-COARASA, PHD • LEE GODDARD, MPHYS •
PAMELA DUPRÉ, MMP • NICOLE WAKE, PHD

INTRODUCTION

Three-dimensional (3D) printing in medicine has gained increasing popularity over the past several years. In nuclear medicine and radiation therapy, where one of the main goals is to obtain quality images while keeping radiation exposure to a minimum, 3D printing is an ideal technology to help tailor many individual treatments. Additionally, 3D printing may be utilized to optimize radiopharmaceutical chemistry for nuclear medicine applications. This chapter will highlight key applications of 3D printing in nuclear medicine and radiation therapy.

NUCLEAR MEDICINE

Nuclear medicine uses radioactive substances (radiotracers, radioactive tracers, radionuclides, or radiopharmaceuticals) to diagnose, treat, and monitor a variety of diseases. A radionuclide is an atom that contains an unstable nucleus. As water runs downhill and wood burns, this nucleus will inevitably perform a rearrangement on its path to stability or, in other words, a lower energy state. As postulated by Albert Einstein in his famous $E = mc^2$ equation, where E = energy, m = mass, and c = the speed of light, energy needs to be conserved; hence, this nuclear rearrangement will produce a release of pure energy, mass, or more often both. Unlike common chemical reactions, nuclear rearrangement is independent of temperature, solvent, and pressure, and will undergo following a very predictable path regardless of the surrounding conditions. In fact, this rearrangement is so predictable that is used as a standard for time-keeping in the form of the atomic clock. These consistent emissions of mass and/or energy interact with surrounding matter and can be detected with proper instruments. Such principles form the base for the nuclear medicine applications discussed in this chapter.

Nuclear emissions may be used for different purposes depending on their nature. Energy emissions in the form of gamma packets (or quantum) are normally used for diagnosis, prognosis, therapy monitoring, and imaging (molecular imaging or MI), as well as internal and external radiation seeds and beams for treatment. Particulate emissions in the form of alpha (α, high energy $^4He^{2+}$ nuclides) and beta (β, high energy e^-) particles are used for internal radiation treatment (often called targeted radiotherapy or TRT). The different nuclear emissions can be found in Table 12.1. However, these emitters are often not suitable tools to diagnose nor treat anything on their own, and they must be consequently functionalized to increase their specificity and perform more as radiolabeled pharmaceuticals (or radiopharmaceuticals) rather than just radioisotopes. As Pharmacy is the art, practice, or profession of preparing, preserving, compounding, and dispensing medical drugs, Radiopharmacy is the same but for radiolabeled drugs use in nuclear medicine.

TABLE 12.1
Main Types of Radiation Decay.

Decay Mode	Emission Type	Composition
Alpha decay	α	Helium nucleus, $^4He^{2+}$
Beta decay	β^-	Electrons, e^-
Positron decay	β^+	Antimatter electrons, e^+
Isomeric transition	γ	Pure energy, gamma, high energy light

TABLE 12.2
Common Isotopes Used for PET Imaging.

Tracer Isotope	Half-Life	Mean Energy (MeV)	Maximum Energy (MeV)	Medical Applications
^{11}C	20.4 min	0.39	0.96	Small molecules, brain imaging
^{13}N	10 min	0.50	1.20	^{13}NH$_3$
^{15}O	2 min	0.72	1.74	H$_2^{15}$O
^{18}F	109 min	0.25	0.63	Small molecules, brain imaging
^{64}Cu	12.7 h	0.28	0.65	Medium-sized molecule labeling
^{68}Ga	68 min	0.89	1.92	Small molecules
^{89}Zr	78.4 h	0.40	0.90	Protein and antibody labeling
^{124}I	4.2 days	$\approx$0.7	1.532 (11%) and 2.435 (11%)	Protein and antibody labeling

TABLE 12.3
Common Isotopes Used for SPECT and Planar Scintigraphy Imaging.

Tracer Isotope	Half-Life	γ Energy (keV)	Medical Applications
^{67}Ga	3.26 days	93 (40%), 184 (24%), 296 (22%), 388 (7%)	Imaging/blood flow, extravasation, infection. E.g., [^{67}Ga]Ga-Citrate
^{99m}Tc	6.02 h	140.5 (89%), 18.4 (4.0%), 18.3 (2.1%)	90% of all nuclear medicine apps. E.g., [^{99m}Tc] myocardial purfusion imaging test (MIBI)
^{111}In	2.8 days	171.3 (91%), 245.4 (94%)	White blood cell labeling, octreotides
^{201}Tl	3.04 days	70.8 (46.5%), 68.9 (27.4%), 80.3 (20.5%), 167.4 (10.0%) 135.3 (2.7%)	Cardiac

From Table 12.1, it can easily be deducted that most diagnostic radiopharmaceuticals will use isomeric transition radioisotopes to trace the compound behavior and produce medical images. Subsequently, it is also easy to deduct that alpha and beta decays will have the greatest interaction with surrounding matter and should therefore be used for TRT. It is intriguing though and hard to imagine what a "positron" is or what antimatter looks like. The hard truth is we do not know for sure. These antimatter particles last for tiny fractions of a second and are hard to study due to their immediate annihilation with regular matter producing energy. Regardless of our ignorance, we know they exist because the product of such annihilation produces two gamma quanta emitted at almost exactly 180 degrees. The cumuli of these straight angled simultaneous isotropic emissions make these radioisotopes of particular interest for what is called positron emission tomography (PET), the most recent nuclear medicine imaging

technique, capable of among other things, measuring noninvasively the metabolic activity of cells in body tissues. PET allows the detection and quantification of the origin of these emissions with the highest degree of accuracy and sensitivity known to date. Common radioisotopes used in PET imaging are shown in Table 12.2.

The traditional medical imaging method utilized in nuclear medicine is called single photon emission computed tomography (SPECT) and is performed using radiopharmaceuticals labeled with pure gamma emitters (Table 12.3). This technique relies on the cumulative detection of single gamma photons emitted by disintegrating nuclei given a certain, predetermined spatial orientation. Planar scintigraphy is the simplest application for single photon emission, and normally produces two 2D images obtained as "anterior" and "posterior" poses. These poses are obtained by rotating the camera around the patient capturing the emitted gamma rays. In contrast SPECT, fundamentally a 3D

TABLE 12.4
Some Common Isotopes Used for Radiotherapy.

Tracer Isotope	Half-Life	Energy (Particle)	Medical Applications
^{90}Y	2.7 days	2.28 MeV (β^-)	Liver, neuroendocrine
^{177}Lu	6.65 days	0.497 MeV (β^-)	Prostate, neuroendocrine
^{188}Re	16.9 h	2.12 MeV (β^-)	Bone, radioimmunotherapy
^{223}Ra	11.4 days	Multiple α and β^- decays	Bone, prostate
^{225}Ac	10.0 days	Multiple α and β^- decays	Prostate, brain

imaging technique, uses a rotating camera system to obtain many projections and performs tomographic reconstruction to produce imaging slices within the body (similar to CT).

Other gamma emitting radionuclides (^{137}Cs ($t_{1/2} = 30.2$ years) and ^{60}Co ($t_{1/2} = 5.27$ years)) can be used for external beam radiation therapy because their high energy emissions can penetrate deep into human tissue. These γ-beams can be properly collimated and directed specifically to the treatment site with great accuracy. These, however, cannot be used to produce radiopharmaceuticals due to their long half-life. In contrast, internal radiation therapy or targeted radiotherapy is a treatment in which a source of radiation (normally an alpha or beta emitter) is put inside of the body (Table 12.4). The radiation source can be solid (brachytherapy) or liquid (systemic therapy). In brachytherapy, seeds, ribbons, or capsules with a radiation source are placed in or near a tumor and these solid particles give off radiation (typically gamma). In systemic therapy, the treatment is given orally or intravenously and travels through the blood or tissues, seeking out and killing cancer cells.

All these radionuclides can seldom be injected as ions without chemical modification, and they often need to be administered as part of bigger construct called **Radiopharmaceuticals**. These cannot be produced and stored for administration because of decay and the very same characteristic for which they are used: ionizing radiation and radiolysis. Therefore, radiopharmaceuticals need to be produced fresh before every administration, making this process costly and demanding of well-trained personnel. To avoid decay and radiolysis, adhere to good manufacturing pharmaceuticals guidelines, reduce costs, reduce personnel exposure to radiation, and assure drug quality and reproducibility these processes need to be automated. Several commercial automated units are available in the market, but their costs rise well above $100,000.00, and they are not optimized for a particular

synthesis. These units are what we call a "jack of all trades and master of none." To address the need to automate novel, specific reactions while lowering costs, new design and fabrication techniques must be introduced, and such is the case of 3D printing.

3D PRINTING TECHNIQUES TO OPTIMIZE RADIOPHARMACEUTICAL CHEMISTRY

The diffusion and assimilation of 3D printing technologies exemplifies ease-of-use, affordability, and versatility. Since the number of radiopharmaceuticals is bound to increase with the discovery of new molecular targets, the development of novel ligands, the availability of previously rare positron emitting radionuclides, as well as the inevitable increase of the patient population, new synthetic and reproducible techniques have to be introduced to accommodate dissimilar syntheses. The reactions that bind these radionuclides to their relevant ligands must be completed in less than one physical half-life of the radionuclide. These reactions also need to be performed with high fidelity while satisfying the regulatory concerns of administering injectable radioactive compounds to patients. These 3D printing technologies can be easily combined with recent advanced in robotics components and the reduction in their prices, to create a reliable automated synthesis unit (ASU) at a fraction of the cost (1/20th) of the commercially available ASUs.

The low cost of the ASUs achieved by 3D printing bring along a novel concept in radiopharmaceutical chemistry: "Do not accommodate the synthesis to the existing ASU, but create the ASU to fit the optimized synthesis." Such a revolutionary concept allows for true good manufacturing practices in drug production, since the process is tailored to assure quality instead of trying to build quality into existing processes. This quality is achieved by maximizing radiochemical yields and final radiochemical purities of the produced drug

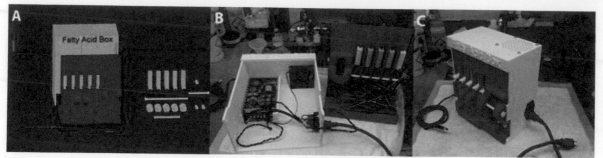

FIG. 12.1 [^{11}C] Fatty Acid ASU. **(A)**: CAD design, **(B)** Assembly, and **(C)** Final product.

products by design, and not as a result of a reaction adaptation to unfit automation.

Example 1: [^{11}C] Fatty Acid ASU

Fatty acids labeled with ^{11}C allow clinically relevant metabolic processes to be traced "in vivo." However, ^{11}C is a challenging isotope to work with since its half-life is only 20.2 min. To achieve injectable amounts of compounds post labeling and quality control, it is necessary to start with high amounts of activity (1–5 curie), which cannot be manipulated by operators. Hence, automation is a must. Fatty acids are often produced by bubbling traces of $^{11}CO_2$ carried by a stream of N_2, He, or Ar. The reasons why such methods are conceptually unfit for radiochemistry is a discussion for a different book; however, efforts to change this practice have been performed and superior yields, superior purity, and decreased synthesis times have been achieved. The major challenge for such alternative methods is the fact that such processes have never been automated, and there is not a single commercial system to accommodate them.

The combination of 3D printing, high torque servos, linear motors, and a controlling chip to which sequences can be saved and executed on demand yielded a breakthrough in automation for radiopharmaceutical production (Fig. 12.1). The ASU improved the manual syntheses by reducing synthesis time from 12 to 8 min and produced consistent decay corrected radiochemical yields. Furthermore, the ASU was capable of producing not one but three tracers of clinical interest which included [^{11}C]acetate, [^{11}C]palmitate, and [^{11}C]propionate at higher than previously reported yield, in only 8–10 min.

Example 2: [^{18}F] Dual Heater ASU

The half-life of ^{18}F ($t_{1/2} = 109$ min) is more than three times larger than that of [^{11}C]. This allows to accommodate longer synthesis times and more complex, multistep reactions. However, almost none of the commercially available ASUs are fit to perform complicated reactions, and the few that are cost more than US $150,000. Such costs are prohibitive during the testing of compounds for early agency approval for most researchers, therefore an alternative was needed. Once again, 3D printing combined with robotics solved this problem, specifically for the multistep radiosynthesis of the prostate-specific membrane antigen (PSMA) [^{18}F]RPS-040 for preclinical PET imaging which involved two separate reactions and a distillation. The total cost for developing this using 3D printing and robotics was US $7,000, approximately 5% of the commercially available ASU.

In order to perform the first automated synthesis of [^{18}F]RPS-040, an ASU was designed and assembled. To accommodate the high temperatures needed during this synthesis, the porcelain reactors' housing was 3D printed with clay using material extrusion technology. The 3D printing process of clay was optimized to account for shrinking in the kiln, and it resulted in a perfect 3D printed porcelain part with less than 1 mm error. A pierce element was used in the second reactor to cool it down to 0°C for the distillation of the intermediate and heat it up to 100°C for the following reaction steps (Fig. 12.2). The synthesis time was reduced from approximately 2 h manually to 65 min, producing a product needing only a final High-Performance liquid chromatography (HPLC) purification and reformulation for injection. Such ASU was unprecedented, and the complicated, multistep synthesis was automated, optimized, and tested without a single mechanical failure in more than 20 trials.

Example 3: [^{68}Ga] Multidrug ASU

The clinical importance of ^{68}Ga-labeled drugs ($t_{1/2} = 68$ min) is undeniable. Typically, ^{68}Ga is produced by elution of a ^{68}Ge/^{68}Ga generator, which is used directly for labeling under buffered conditions. This is a different example to the ones mentioned previously, since ASUs designed to perform this task are available

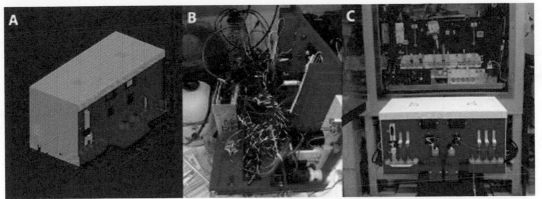

FIG. 12.2 [^{18}F] Dual Heater ASU. **(A)** CAD design, **(B)** Assembly, and **(C)** Final product (bottom) placed in comparison with the ORA Neptis commercial unit (Optimized Radiochemical Applications, Neuville, Belgium) (top).

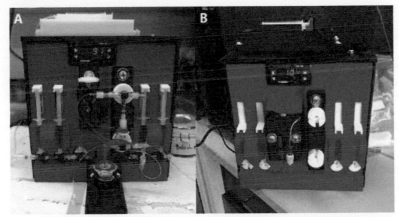

FIG. 12.3 Photographs of **(A)** [^{68}Ga] Multidrug ASU and **(B)** [^{68}Ga] Millifluidic ASU.

on the market. However, their prices oscillate from US $40,000 to $80,000, which is prohibitive for preclinical and clinical trial applications, not to mention to third-world countries that have already managed to afford the also expensive ^{68}Ge/^{68}Ga generator. This application is not as much a synthetic need as it is a financial one, therefore an ASU was produced at a value under US $2,000, and was superior to the ones commercially available by incorporating a syringe pump to elute the generator as part of the stored sequence.

The [^{68}Ga] Multidrug ASU includes a C$_{18}$ Sep-Pak Lite purification and filtration through a 0.2 μm filter membrane to provide a sterile, pyrogen-free injectable solution (Fig. 12.3A). This ASU can also be used to chelate other radiometals with many drugs used for

imaging and therapy. The list of possible drugs includes (but is not limited to) [^{90}Y]DOTATOC, [^{177}Lu]DOTA-TOC, [^{225}Ac]PSMA-617, [^{213}Bi]DOTATOC, and [^{213}Bi] PSMA-617 among many others.

Example 4: [^{68}Ga] Millifluidic ASU

This ASU was created to demonstrate the versatility of the technique and to test the boundaries of its applications. Instead of using a slow batch process for ^{68}Ga labeling, this ASU was designed to perform a continuous labeling process ending in final purification and reformulations for injection. It was demonstrated that in fast chelation reactions (e.g., [^{68}Ga]PSMA-11), similar yields to that of the Multidrug ASU are obtained but in a third of the time, saving as much as 20% of the activity lost in decay and producing a product of similar quality (Fig. 12.3B). This application also demonstrates the importance of these techniques to preliminary test revolutionary designs and evaluate their performance. Because of the low demand of these units (small radiopharmaceutical community), 3D printed ASUs can not only be used for prototyping but also for routine production of these machines.

RADIATION THERAPY

Radiation therapy, also known as radiotherapy, refers to different treatment techniques used to treat cancerous and noncancerous ailments. High doses of radiation are used to kill cancerous cells, sometimes in combination with chemotherapy or surgery. There are two broad types of radiation therapy: external beam therapy, which delivers radiation from the outside to the tumor and brachytherapy, which uses radioactive sources placed inside the patient either in or close to the tumor to deliver radiation from the inside out.

In external beam therapy, the radiation source is typically enclosed in a large gantry, able to rotate around the patient and shape the radiation beam. High energy photons, with energies approximately 100 times greater than those used in diagnostic X-rays, are the most commonly used external beam modality. Other treatment modalities include particle beam therapy where electrons, protons, neutrons, or other light nuclei are accelerated to very high energies. These photon or particle beams are then focused on the region of disease or target. Various treatment techniques are utilized to ensure that the target gets the prescribed amount of radiation, or dose, while ensuring that healthy tissues nearby are spared as much of the radiation dose as possible.

Brachytherapy techniques use radioactive sources (or isotopes) placed within the body. These radioactive materials emit alpha, beta, gamma radiation, or some combination depending on the exact radionuclide. In brachytherapy, the radiation source is a solid material that is placed either temporarily within the body, with the aid of an afterloader and applicator, or permanently within the body in the form of radioactive seeds. In systemic and/or targeted therapy, radioactive drugs, or radiopharmaceuticals, are given orally or intravenously and travel through the blood or tissue. These drugs are designed to gather in cancerous cells or specific organs where disease is present, where they emit radiation.

3D PRINTING FOR RADIATION THERAPY

As 3D printing technology has developed, the number of applications for its use has also dramatically increased. Early material extrusion printing techniques typically used rigid materials such as acrylonitrile butadiene styrene (ABS) or polylactic acid (PLA) which have been characterized for use in various external beam radiation therapy modalities.[1,2] As technologies have improved, a wider range of materials such as polyethylene terephthalate glycol and flexible materials known as thermoplastic elastomers or thermoplastic polyurethane (TPU)[3,4] have become available. Other printing technologies, such as vat photopolymerization and material jetting, have also become more widely available. These printers typically use liquid resins or photopolymers and have improved accuracy over material extrusion printers; however, material costs are typically higher and print times are longer.

There are a wide range of applications of 3D printing in radiation therapy including boluses,[1,5—11] tissue compensators,[12,13] immobilization devices,[3,14,15] brachytherapy applicators,[16—18] and anthropomorphic[19—21] and quality assurance phantoms.[22,23] Different uses of 3D printing in radiation therapy have different goals and the material chosen for each goal needs to be carefully considered because of its possible dosimetric implications. For bolus applications and tissue compensators, the goal is to add more material in the path of the therapy beam before the radiation interacts with the patient and in the case of bolus increase the dose at the surface (i.e., skin) of the patient. For these applications, the best choice of material would be one that has radiological properties that are as close as possible to water or soft tissue. Each treatment modality has specific considerations that must be taken into account when modeling the bolus material, including the physical density, electron density, and chemical composition. The printing technique, including infill density, must also be considered.

For patient immobilization devices, the goal is to keep the patient still and in the same position for each treatment but have minimal dosimetric effect on the radiation that is planned for the patient. Thus, immobilization devices should be as close to the patient as possible. For brachytherapy applications, the goal is to reduce air pockets and gaps between the applicator and surface as much as possible for a reproducible and uniform anatomy and water-like material is desired. Finally, quality assurance phantoms are used for many purposes and need to be considered separately, but an anthropomorphic phantom that mimics the human body would need to comprise different materials to mimic bone, fat, tissue, and lung in a radiologically meaningful way, i.e., a way that will interact with radiation in the same way the tissues in a human body would.

Multiple studies have been conducted looking at different uses for 3D printing in radiation therapy[24] and the way that different materials interact with radiation before they are used in patient treatment has been extensively studied.[4,25,26] It is important that each institution gather sufficient information about the material they are using prior to using it in patient treatment.

The effect of radiation on the 3D printed material must also be considered. A recent study by Wady and colleagues showed that the flexibility and mechanical strength of common 3D printed materials can be reduced by exposure to very high levels of radiation.[27] It should be noted that the amount of radiation the materials in this study was exposed to was of the order of 10^6 Gy, versus the 10s of Gy that are typically used to treat patients. Therefore, for the majority of radiation therapy applications, there should be little to no degradation in these properties over the course of treatment.

3D PRINTED BOLUS

Much of the work on 3D printing in radiation therapy has been focused on using 3D printed personalized patient boluses. A bolus is comprised of nearly tissue equivalent material directly placed on the patient's skin surface to increase surface dose deposition, or to decrease the radiation to healthy tissues adjacent to the target.[28] Conventional methods to create a bolus include cellophane wrapped wet gauze or paraffin wax that are manually shaped and placed around the treatment area. Commercial boluses made of preformed gel sheets with synthetic gel oil are also available;[29] however, these sheets can be of limited use in nonuniform areas due to the lack of conformality to the patient surface. This can lead to sizable air gaps between the bolus and the skin which may affect the skin sparing effect and cause unwanted high and/or low dose areas.[30] Thermoplastic sheets are also commercially available;[31] these are

heated until they become malleable, they are then formed against the patient surface. Once cooled they solidify and hold their shape unless reheated. Both gel and thermoplastic sheets are available in a range of sizes and thicknesses depending on the energy of the treatment radiation. Thermoplastics and wax can be molded to the patient surface to create patient-specific boluses that retain their shape and improve repositioning accuracy between treatment fractions. Thermoplastic material can help reduce any air gaps but can lead to nonuniform bolus thickness causing discrepancies between the planned and delivered radiation doses. The formation process on a patient's skin can also be anxiety provoking, especially if performed on the head and neck, or other sensitive regions.[32] Manual formation of wax boluses or pressing warm thermoplastic material against a sensitive area until it cools can also be painful for the patient if the area is tender to the touch.

3D printing allows for the fabrication of boluses with geometries that can be customized to fit each patient. The use of 3D printing techniques allows for the production of complex patient-specific boluses which can improve the uniformity of the radiation dose to the desired area and decrease the radiation dose to surrounding tissues. A patient-specific 3D printed bolus can be designed from pre-treatment planning volumetric imaging datasets such as treatment planning CTs, without the need for manual shaping of the device on the patient. Boluses can be made in a range of rigid and flexible materials to ensure good conformality to the patient, while maintaining patient comfort. Fig. 12.4 shows a range of bolus materials that could be used to treat a nasal lesion including a cut-out Superflab sheet (4A), a molded Aquaplast sheet (4B), and both flexible (4C) and rigid (4D) 3D printed boluses. 3D printed boluses can also be designed to fit around patient immobilization devices to improve positioning reproducibility as shown in Fig. 12.5. The radiation dose treatment planning system (TPS) typically has bolus design tools that allow for the creation of radiation therapy structure files which can then be converted into printable file types. 3D printed boluses have been utilized for many types of cancer treatments including head and neck or facial cancers[33] and breast cancer.[11]

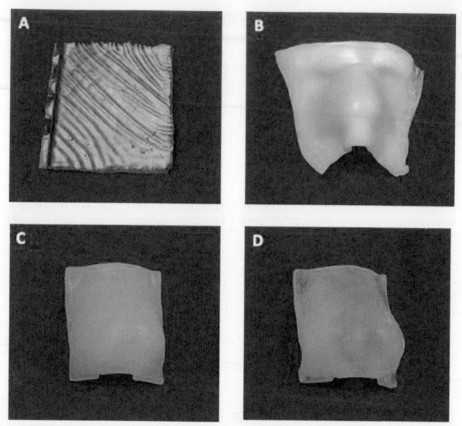

FIG. 12.4 **(A)** Superflab™ vinyl gel bolus **(B)** Aquaplast™ thermoplastic bolus **(C)** flexible 3D printed bolus printed with VisiJet M2 ENT material **(D)** rigid 3D printed bolus printed with VisiJet M2R-CL material. Both 3D printed bolus models were printed using material jetting (MJP2500, 3D Systems, Rock Hill, SC).

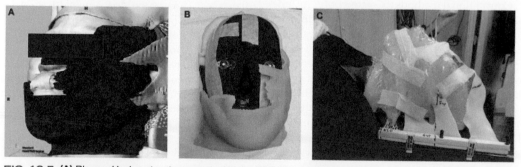

FIG. 12.5 **(A)** Planned bolus structure created in the TPS (Aria Eclipse v15, Varian Medical Systems Inc. Palo Alto, California, US). **(B)** Printed model shown on a head phantom model. **(C)** 3D printed model shown taped onto the patient prior to treatment.

3D PRINTED TISSUE COMPENSATORS

Some external beam passive scattering particle therapy techniques are limited in that the energy used to treat the target is fixed. This can lead to unwanted radiation dose deposited beyond the target area. Tissue compensators are used in particle beam therapy to manipulate the dose deposition within the patient. They can be used to compensate for both the irregular patient

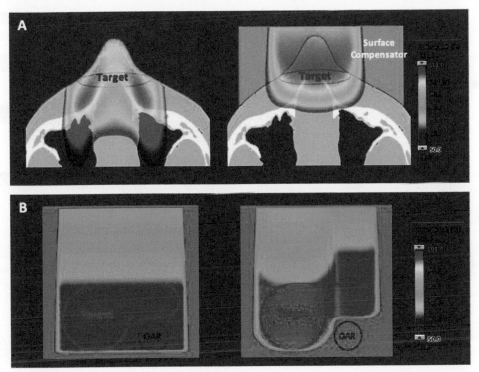

FIG. 12.6 **(A)** Dose distribution for electron therapy treatment of a nose/nasal target without (left) and with (right) the use of an irregular surface compensator **(B)** Dose distribution for proton therapy treatment in a water phantom without (left) and with distal edge compensation (right).

surface shape and the nonuniform distal target shape to improve dose deposition geometry. They can either be placed directly on the patient surface or away from the patient, but still in the beam path, depending on the particle beam being utilized.

Fig. 12.6A shows an example irregular surface compensator sometimes used for electron beam therapy. Here a milled, tissue equivalent plastic is placed directly onto the patient surface, this idealized case shows the improved uniformity of dose across the target and minimization of excess dose deposition distal to the target. Fig. 12.6B shows the effect of a distal edge compensator used in passive scattering proton therapy. These compensators are placed in the beam path away from the patient surface. Here an example organ at risk (OAR) is positioned distally to the target, compensators can be used to spare dose to OAR's distal to the target, but increases the dose proximally to the target.

Tissue compensators can be made from a range of materials, such as brass, plexiglass, or other plastics, but are typically milled from solid blocks of material using computer numerical control (CNC) milling machines. The compensator material needs to be characterized in the TPS, similarly to bolus materials. For passive scattered proton beam therapy each treatment field for each patient will require patient-specific compensators and blocks. Proton facilities typically have onsite facilities to create these devices due to this requirement. Electron surface compensation is not required for every patient and so many institutions may not have the necessary equipment on site to allow for the accurate creation of these devices, so external manufacturers are used. This can lead to delays in treatment depending on the manufacturing and shipping times involved. 3D printers are available at a lower cost than CNC machines allowing smaller facilities to create tissue compensators onsite.

3D PRINTED IMMOBILIZATION DEVICES

Immobilization devices such as molds, casts, and headrests are used in radiation therapy to make sure that the patient stays in the correct position over the course of treatment. If a patient is not immobilized properly, then he/she is at risk for improper treatment and unwanted side effects. Immobilization is especially important for head and neck tumors that reside close to organs at risk such as the brain stem or spinal cord.[34] Commercially available immobilization devices such as the HeadSTEP iFRAME, BreastSTEP, and WingSTEP immobilization systems (Elekta, Stockholm, Sweden) are available. In addition, personalized immobilization devices can be created using traditional methods such as casting or thermoforming. These masks are available in a range of formations and rigidities for different treatment types from a number of vendors. However, these methods can be stressful and cause significant discomfort to the patient, especially when being performed around the face.[35,36]

3D printing personalized immobilization devices can ease the production process and improve comfort for the patient. Studies have shown that personalized 3D printed immobilization devices have highly repeatable positional accuracy[37,38] and they can decrease damage to surrounding tissue.[39] Any 3D printed immobilization devices should be included in the treatment planning scan to ensure that the effects on the dose deposition within the target are accurately calculated.

3D PRINTING FOR BRACHYTHERAPY

Two types of brachytherapy treatments are used for disease treatment: low dose rate (LDR) and high dose rate (HDR). As all 3D printing applications are used with HDR brachytherapy, LDR will not be discussed.

HDR brachytherapy involves the temporary placement of highly radioactive sources within the patient for short periods of time. A machine called an afterloader allows for the remote positioning of the radioactive source at varying distances within a sealed applicator. These applicators can be placed within the body cavities for the treatment of gynecological cancers, intraluminal for the treatment of esophageal cancers, or within surgically placed catheters. Commercial HDR brachytherapy applicators are available for a range of disease sites. Recently, manufacturers have made large improvements in allowing for the customization of dose deposition within the patient. However, there are still limitations, either with the size of the applicator available or the fit of the applicator to the patient.

Cylindrical applicators for the treatment of vaginal cancers typically come in a fixed range of diameters. 3D printing has been explored as a method to create

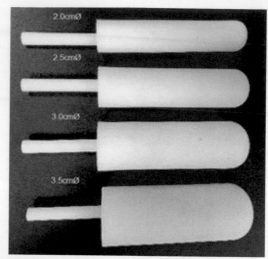

FIG. 12.7 3D printed cylinder set with diameters ranging from 2.0 cm to 3.5cm printed with VisiJet M2R-WT materials using a MJP2500 printer (3D Systems, Rock Hill, SC).

more individualized sizes to improve patient comfort and dose deposition within the patient.[17,18] These applicators typically have a single central channel and/or a ring of peripheral channels for the brachytherapy source to travel within. In addition to customizable sizing, channel placement can also be customized to optimize dose deposition. Commercially available applicators have a limited shelf life, for centers that have a low volume of such treatments 3D printed cylinders allow for a cost-effective alternative. Fig. 12.7 shows a set of 3D printed cylinders, each with a central channel to allow the placement of a needle catheter through which the source will travel.

SURFACE TREATMENTS

Brachytherapy can also be used to treat surface/skin diseases. In these treatments catheters for the brachytherapy source are either surgically implanted under the skin or placed in external applicators. These can take the form of hand formed molds typically formed from thermoplastics or other materials[40,41] or flexible applicators such as the Freiburg flap (Elekta, Stockholm, Sweden). These applicators hold the catheters a fixed distance from the surface. While this can be advantageous in areas of limited curvature it can be difficult to fit to highly curved surfaces. 3D printing allows for the printing of custom surface applicators. These can have custom spacing between channels or differing distances from the patient surface for different channels. They can also be designed to better fit the patient surfaces. Challenges in creating these devices include, but are not limited to, accurate channel sizing and curvature to ensure that the source can travel within the applicator. 3D printed holders can also be designed for use with existing applicators to ensure consistent placement for repeated treatments. Before clinical use, 3D printed applicator materials should be studied to ensure that they are sufficiently water-like and do not interact differently than commercially available applicators.

3D PRINTING OF ANTHROPOMORPHIC PHANTOMS

Phantoms for use in radiation therapy typically take the form of flat slabs of a single material or more complex configurations of different materials. Anthropomorphic phantoms that mimic the human body are also commercially available. These phantoms are typically designed for use with specific ion chambers or other radiation measurement devices such as radiochromic film, thermoluminescent dosimeters, optically stimulated luminescent dosimeters, or solid-state detectors. Anthropomorphic phantoms are costly and generally cannot be customized easily. 3D printing allows for the design and fabrication of phantoms for a specific purpose at a relatively low cost.

Where suitable materials are available, 3D printers can be used directly to create anthropomorphic phantoms. If printer materials are not suitable for the desired purpose, 3D printers may still be used to create shell structures which can then be filled with suitable materials. Fig. 12.8 shows an example of such a structure. Here a pelvis structure was generated using a 2 mm shell which was then filled with a liquid silicone and chalk mixture that creates a structure of similar radiographic density to bone.[42]

Fig. 12.9 shows another structure created using a similar methodology. In this model the ribs and vertebral bodies were used to generate a shell structure that was printed in a dissolvable material. Once filled with the silicone/chalk mixture and allowed to cure, the shell was dissolved, resulting in a flexible phantom that could then be placed around another shell created in the shape of a lung. This was then covered in Aquaplast tissue equivalent material.

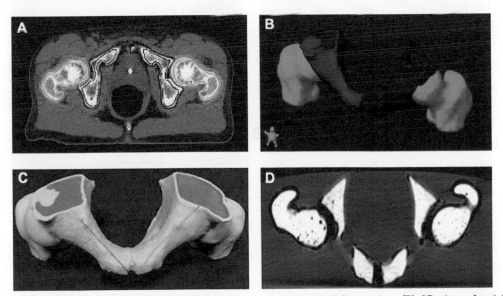

FIG. 12.8 **(A)** Axial CT slice showing the shell structure generated for printing, **(B)** 3D view of pelvis structures, **(C)** superior view of the 3D printed pelvic shell filed with silicone rubber, and **(D)** CT image of the pelvic phantom shown in a water bath.

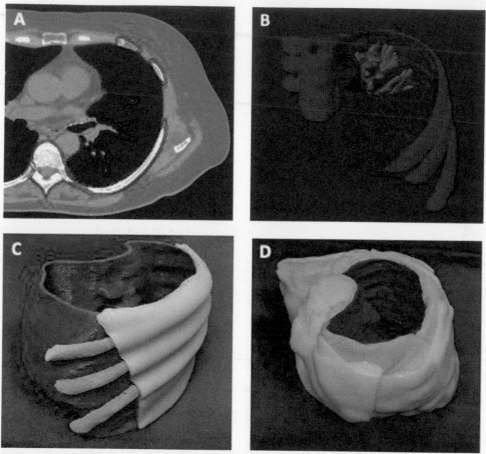

FIG. 12.9 **(A)** Axial CT slice showing contours of the shell structure generated for printing, **(B)** 3D visualization of segmented lung structures, **(C)** partial 3D printed phantom model showing individual materials, and **(D)** final phantom model with aquaplast covering.

CONCLUSION

3D printing provides practical and affordable solutions for nuclear medicine and radiation therapy treatments. By allowing for optimized radiopharmaceutical chemistry development and tailoring cancer therapies to each individual, 3D printing can truly enhance patient care. Despite major recent advances in the field, there is a need for more printing materials with a wider range of properties suitable to tailor treatments and for new phantoms that allow for testing of different equipment. 3D printing technologies allow for the prototyping and formation of new phantoms to quickly meet clinical and research needs. For further information on considerations for 3D printed phantoms please see Chapter 14. As treatment modalities, printing technologies, and printing materials evolve, further developments and even more patient-specific treatments will be seen.

REFERENCES

1. Burleson S, Baker J, Hsia AT, Xu Z. Use of 3D printers to create a patient-specific 3D bolus for external beam therapy. *J Appl Clin Med Phys*. 2015;16(3):5247.
2. Su S, Moran K, Robar JL. Design and production of 3D printed bolus for electron radiation therapy. *J Appl Clin Med Phys*. 2014;15(4):194–211.
3. Michiels S, D'Hollander A, Lammens N, et al. Towards 3D printed multifunctional immobilization for proton therapy: initial materials characterization. *Med Phys*. 2016;43(10):5392.
4. Markovic A. 3D printed bolus with flexible materials: treatment planning accuracy and practical aspects. *Int J Radiat Oncol Biol Phys*. 2017;99(2):E696.
5. Kim SW, Shin HJ, Kay CS, Son SH. A customized bolus produced using a 3-dimensional printer for radiotherapy. *PLoS One*. 2014;9(10):e110746.
6. Su S, Moran K, Robar JL. Design and production of 3D printed bolus for electron radiation therapy. *J Appl Clin Med Phys*. 2014;15(4):4831.

7. Zou W, Fisher T, Zhang M, et al. Potential of 3D printing technologies for fabrication of electron bolus and proton compensators. *J Appl Clin Med Phys.* 2015;16(3):4959.

8. Canters RA, Lips IM, Wendling M, et al. Clinical implementation of 3D printing in the construction of patient specific bolus for electron beam radiotherapy for non-melanoma skin cancer. *Radiother Oncol.* 2016;121(1):148–153.

9. Park SY, Choi CH, Park JM, Chun M, Han JH, Kim JI. A patient-specific polylactic acid bolus made by a 3D printer for breast cancer radiation therapy. *PLoS One.* 2016;11(12):e0168063.

10. Lukowiak M, Jezierska K, Boehlke M, et al. Utilization of a 3D printer to fabricate boluses used for electron therapy of skin lesions of the eye canthi. *J Appl Clin Med Phys.* 2017;18(1):76–81.

11. Yang K, Park W, Ju SG, et al. Heart-sparing radiotherapy with three-dimensional printing technology after mastectomy for patients with left breast cancer. *Breast J.* 2019;25(4):682–686.

12. Craft DF, Balter P, Woodward WA, Kry S, Salehpour MR, Howell RM. Design and feasibility of 3D printed tissue compensators for postmastectomy radiation therapy. *Int J Radiat Oncol Biol Phys.* 2018;102(3):S184.

13. Brancaccio R, Bettuzzi M, Casali F, Cornacchia S, Morigi M, Pasini A. Real-time system for dosimetry in IORT (intra operative radiation therapy). In: *Paper presented at: 14th IEEE-NPSS Real Time Conference, 4–10 June 2005.* 2005.

14. Briggs M, Clements H, Wynne N, Rennie A, Kellett D. 3D printed facial laser scans for the production of localised radiotherapy treatment masks – a case study. *J Vis Commun Med.* 2016;39(3–4):99–104.

15. Laycock SDHM, Scrase CD, Tam MD, et al. Towards the production of radiotherapy treatment shells on 3D printers using data derived from DICOM CT and MRI: pre-clinical feasibility studies. *J Radiother Pract.* 2015;14(01):92–98.

16. Laan RC, Nout RA, Dankelman J, van de Berg NJ. MRI-driven design of customised 3D printed gynaecological brachytherapy applicators with curved needle channels. *3D Print Med.* 2019;5(1):8.

17. Cunha JAM, Mellis K, Sethi R, et al. Evaluation of PC-ISO for customized, 3D printed, gynecologic HDR brachytherapy applicators. *J Appl Clin Med Phys.* 2015;16(1):246–253.

18. Xu Y, Lin SC, Hamilton RJ, Watchman CJ, Dougherty ST. Improved dose distribution with 3D printed vaginal cylinder applicator for VariSource HDR afterloader. *Int J Radiat Oncol Biol Phys.* 2018;102(3):e480–e481.

19. Gear JI, Cummings C, Craig AJ, et al. Abdo-Man: a 3D-printed anthropomorphic phantom for validating quantitative SIRT. *EJNMMI Phys.* 2016;3(1):17.

20. Hernandez-Giron I, den Harder JM, Streekstra GJ, Geleijns J, Veldkamp WJH. Development of a 3D printed anthropomorphic lung phantom for image quality assessment in CT. *Phys Med.* 2019;57:47–57.

21. Zhang F, Zhang H, Zhao H, et al. Design and fabrication of a personalized anthropomorphic phantom using 3D printing and tissue equivalent materials. *Quant Imag Med Surg.* 2019;9(1):94–100.

22. O'Halloran J, Gilligan P, Cleary S, et al. A 3D printed phantom for image quality assessment in cone-beam CT. *Phys Med.* 2018;52:170.

23. Woods K, Ayan AS, Woollard J, Gupta N. Quality assurance for a six degrees-of-freedom table using a 3D printed phantom. *J Appl Clin Med Phys.* 2018;19(1):115–124.

24. Tino R, Yeo A, Leary M, Brandt M, Kron T. A systematic review on 3D-printed imaging and dosimetry phantoms in radiation therapy. *Technol Cancer Res Treat.* 2019;18, 1533033819870208.

25. Bassi S, Langan B, Malone C. Dosimetry assessment of patient-specific 3D printable materials for HDR surface brachytherapy. *Phys Med.* 2019;67:166–175.

26. Ju SG, Kim MK, Hong C-S, et al. New technique for developing a proton range compensator with use of a 3-dimensional printer. *Int J Radiat Oncol Biol Phys.* 2014;88(2):453–458.

27. Wady P, Wasilewski A, Brock L, et al. Effect of ionising radiation on the mechanical and structural properties of 3D printed plastics. *Addit Manuf.* 2020;31:100907.

28. Vyas V, Palmer L, Mudge R, et al. On bolus for megavoltage photon and electron radiation therapy. *Med Dosim.* 2013;38(3):268–273.

29. CNMC+. http://www.teambest.com/CNMC_docs/treatment/position/CNMC_TA_Superflab_Bolus_05292015.pdf. Accessed 13 June 2020.

30. Butson MJCT, Yu P, Metcalfe P. Effects on skin dose from unwanted air gaps under bolus in photon beam radiotherapy. *Radiat Meas.* 2000;32(3):201–204.

31. https://www.rpdinc.com/aquaplast-rt-custom-bolus-140. Accessed 15 June 2020.

32. Sharp L, Lewin F, Johansson H, Payne D, Gerhardsson A, Rutqvist LE. Randomized trial on two types of thermoplastic masks for patient immobilization during radiation therapy for head-and-neck cancer. *Int J Radiat Oncol Biol Phys.* 2005;61(1):250–256.

33. Zhao Y, Moran K, Yewondwossen M, et al. Clinical applications of 3-dimensional printing in radiation therapy. *Med Dosim.* 2017;42(2):150–155.

34. Cacicedo J, Perez JF, Ortiz de Zarate R, et al. A prospective analysis of inter- and intrafractional errors to calculate CTV to PTV margins in head and neck patients. *Clin Transl Oncol.* 2015;17(2):113–120.

35. Oultram SFN, Clover L, Ponman L, Adams C. A comparison between patient self-report and radiation therapists' ability to identify anxiety and distress in head and neck cancer patients requiring immobilization for radiation therapy. *J Radiother Pract.* 2012;11:74–82.

36. Goldsworthy SDTK, Latour JM. A focus group consultation round exploring patient experiences of comfort during radiotherapy for head and neck cancer. *J Radiother Pract.* 2016;15:143–149.

37. Haefner MF, Giesel FL, Mattke M, et al. 3D-Printed masks as a new approach for immobilization in radiotherapy - a study of positioning accuracy. *Oncotarget.* 2018;9(5):6490–6498.

38. Sato KTK, Dobashi S, Kishi K, et al. Positional accuracy valuation of a three dimensional printed device for head and neck immobilisation. *Radiother Oncol.* 2016;119:S126–S127.

39. Chen THCM, Tien DC, Wang RY, et al. Personalized breast holder (PERSBRA): a new cardiac sparing technique for left-sided whole breast irradiation. *Int J Radiat Oncol Biol Phys.* 2017;99(2):E646.

40. Liebmann A, Pohlmann S, Heinicke F, Hildebrandt G. Helmet mold-based surface brachytherapy for homogeneous scalp treatment: a case report. *Strahlenther Onkol.* 2007;183(4):211–214.

41. Boman EL, Paterson DB, Pearson S, Naidoo N, Johnson C. Dosimetric comparison of surface mould HDR brachytherapy with VMAT. *J Med Radiat Sci.* 2018;65(4):311–318.

42. Abu Arrah A. An easily made, low-cost, bone equivalent material used in phantom construction of computed tomography. *Int J Appl Eng Res.* 2018;13:7604–7609.

CHAPTER 13

3D Printing in Forensic Radiology

JONATHAN M. MORRIS, MD • R. ROSS REICHARD, MD • KIARAN P. MCGEE, PHD

INTRODUCTION

Forensic radiology has been described as the use of imaging in both the antemortem and postmortem setting in order to detect and document various pathologies for medicolegal purposes.[1] While considered small in comparison to other subspecialties within radiology, the field's origins date back over 120 years within the United States (US) with the first reported case of X-rays being used as illustrative/demonstrative evidence in 1896.[2] Since that time, advances in radiologic imaging, most notably the development and widespread adoption of cross-sectional imaging along with advanced post-processing techniques such as multiplanar reconstruction and surface rendering techniques, have been integrated into this subspecialty.[3] The application of cross-sectional imaging in combination with advanced visualization techniques allows forensic radiology to provide unique and additional information, particularly in the postmortem setting in which a traditional autopsy may not be practical such as when presented with a severely decomposed body.[3]

In 2010, Jeffery[4] identified five major areas in which radiology is utilized by forensic radiologists including identification of bodies which are not identifiable by other means, firearm deaths in which the location (entry, exit wounds) and identification of residual fragments is required, nonaccidental injury and child abuse in which radiographic signatures are used to differentiate between recent and historical musculoskeletal trauma, barotrauma in which air embolisms are identified, and the identification of traumatic subarachnoid hemorrhage.

The application and integration of three-dimensional (3D) printing technologies to create accurate, precise, and realistic 3D anatomical models is thus consistent with the historical development and adaptation of new technologies in forensic radiology. In addition, victim-specific 3D anatomic modeling poses many advantages that are both complimentary to and create new opportunities in both the antemortem and postmortem settings including but not limited to the ability to sanitize gruesome human injuries thereby allowing previously inadmissible evidence to be presented to a jury, the ability to provide physical life size replication of injuries, the preservation and reproduction of human remains long after their disposal, and the ability to explain complex injury patterns that while clear to the expert radiologist remain confusing to the nonmedical professional.

The purpose of this chapter is to provide an overview of the relatively nascent application of 3D printed anatomic models in forensic radiology; describe, through illustrative examples, the various applications; and to provide context for both the strength and limitations of this technology as applied to forensic radiology.

HISTORICAL OVERVIEW

Since the discovery of the X-ray by Wilhelm Röntgen in 1895, the forensic sciences have long appreciated the importance of imaging. Lichtenstein[5] described the first medicolegal use of X-rays in which a radiograph was first used to localize a bullet lodged between a male gunshot victim's fibula and tibia on Christmas Eve of 1895 in Canada and then later presented as evidence in the assailant's trial. The result of which led to a conviction and 14-year jail term. Due to the high contrast between foreign metal objects compared to bone and soft tissue, X-rays found their initial application in the investigation and location of gunshot wounds and associated shrapnel. Over the course of the next 125 years, conventional plane film radiography has been demonstrated to be an invaluable forensic tool as witnessed by its use in a diverse range of applications including malpractice investigations both as a method of documentation and protection against it, fatality investigation, the identification of victims through forensic dental identification, multiple victim fatalities, injury investigation such as abuse, and in nonviolent crimes.[5,6]

3D Printing for the Radiologist. https://doi.org/10.1016/B978-0-323-77573-1.00004-X

Most recently, the advent of cross-sectional imaging techniques, in particular computed tomography (CT) and magnetic resonance imaging (MRI), has allowed forensic radiology to noninvasively diagnose a range of injuries and crimes in both the premortem and postmortem settings. In fact, several institutions throughout the world, recognizing the utility of these imaging modalities, require whole-body imaging prior to traditional autopsy with the majority of cases undergoing postmortem CT.[1]

FORENSIC RADIOLOGIC IMAGING

As of 2020, autopsy remains the gold standard for establishing cause of death. There are multiple reasons for this including historical precedent—this is the primary method taught to and practiced by medical examiners, the relatively low technology and cost of performing an autopsy, and the ubiquity of the traditional autopsy suite. By contrast, imaging, and in particular cross-sectional imaging (MRI, CT), remain adjunct tools that rely on access to and interpretation of imaging data generated by them. Interpretation of radiologic findings is further complicated by the need to have access to radiologists with expertise in identifying injuries associated with death.[1,6−11] This is especially true in the postmortem setting in which injuries sustained are not typically encountered in the outpatient radiologic imaging setting (e.g., drowning) or tissue undergoes gross alteration due to the violent nature of the injury or delay from the time of expiration to imaging (e.g., drowning or putrification).

It is important to appreciate that performing an autopsy is not automatic in the determination of death or as part of a death investigation. Instead, its primary use is to determine unequivocally the true cause of death when the circumstances of the decedent's death remain unclear based on physical examination of the body and death scene. In addition, autopsy, while hopefully establishing causality, does have limitations. For example, by its very nature it is unable to preserve the injury, traumatic fractures to bones and/or soft tissue damage due to lacerations and penetrating trauma are removed, and some pathologies such as early cardiac ischemia[12] or intracranial vascular injuries[13] are poorly visualized when compared to imaging findings. In this setting, imaging can and is playing an increasing role in not only providing unequivocal evidence on the cause of death thereby eliminating the need for autopsy but also to increase the quality of the pathologist's advice to a coroner when determining if an autopsy should be performed.[14]

As a result of the advantages and application of imaging in the forensic sciences, the use of postmortem CT and MR (PMCT, PMMR, sometimes referred to as the virtual autopsy or virtopsy[15]) has grown significantly. The concept of PMCT was first proposed in Israel in 1994 in response to certain religious communities as an alternative to invasive postmortem procedures.[16] In 1997, in response to similar requests, a PMMR service was established in the United Kingdom.[17] Since that time, further evolution of the application of PMCT has occurred resulting in the establishment of a mobile CT scanner for on scene assessment of mass casualties[18] and more recently the development of an entire mass casualty imaging system including acquisition, reporting, secure data transfer, and storage known as Fimag.[19] Weustink et al.[12] also reported on the use of both PMCT and PMMR in combination with ultrasound guided biopsy as a method for minimally invasive autopsy to either substitute or augment a conventional autopsy. Hoey et al.[20] described the use of PMCT which they referred to as CATopsy for the prediction of death in trauma patients, while Rutty et al.[21] have described the utility of PMCT as an investigative tool in the case of an intentional neonatal upper airway obstruction. Jackowski et al.[22] have reported on the use of PMCT for the identification of venous air embolism. Similarly, the use of both PMCT and PMMR has been described in the postmortem assessment of massive gas embolism following severe decompression sickness resulting from a diving accident.[23] PMCT has also been widely used in injuries related to foreign metal objects including handgun and rifle injuries[24] as well as knife wounds to multiple organs such as the aorta[25] and brainstem.[13] Within the medicolegal context, PMCT has also been described as a method for establishing the cause of fatal outcomes following medical intervention in the hospital setting.[26]

An obvious question is that if PM imaging—most notably PMCT and PMMR—is to replace conventional autopsy, what is the diagnostic accuracy of this approach? Several studies have indicated that rather than replace conventional autopsy, PM imaging serves to augment information provided by either approach thereby increasing the yield of information provided by either. That is, information obtained from either is complimentary. For example, Donchin et al.[16] reported that in a blinded study involving 25 trauma victims in which autopsy findings were compared to PMCT radiologic findings, PMCT identified 70.5% pathologic states compared to 74.8% detected by autopsy. Farkash et al.[27] used PMCT in fatal military penetrating trauma; and although they found it useful, the authors noted that PMCT is not without limitation including limits in detecting superficial injuries of the extremities and the exact route of fragments. Levy et al.[28] noted that in the case of gunshot-related fatalities, PMCT underestimated the number of gunshot wounds (78 detected by autopsy vs. 68 by PMCT). Similarly, Cirielli et al.[29] described the use of PMCT in 23 postmortem investigations in which virtual autopsy matched the findings of traditional autopsy in 15 (65%) of cases, whereas traditional autopsy was needed in the remaining 8(35%) but that validity of virtual autopsy was highest for traumatic deaths.

From the studies described above it is apparent is that PM imaging diagnostic accuracy can be improved by the use of multiple PM imaging modalities. For example, Rutty et al.[30] have reported that PMCT when combined with PM coronary angiography (PMCTA) was able to identify the cause of death, as established by autopsy, in 92% of the 241 cases reviewed. The use of multiple PM imaging modalities provides the ability to more completely asses the spectrum of injuries that may occur such as the identification of subarachnoid hemorrhage in which PMMR has proven to be more sensitive than PMCT.[31] To further illustrate the synergistic nature of both modalities, Bollinger et al.[32] reported on the use of PMCT and PMMR in the determination of death by hanging in a car. In this report the authors noted that data obtained from both imaging techniques identified the cause of death being cerebral hypoxia as opposed to a brainstem lesion induced by a hangman fracture.[32] In addition, PMMR identified soft tissue damage including hemorrhage and bleeding. Similarly, Oesterhelweg et al.[33] described how both PMCT and PMMR provide complimentary information that in combination improve the accuracy of the diagnosis of the cause of death in the presence of laryngeal foreign bodies. Finally, Durnhofer et al.[15] provided an excellent review of the use of both PMCT and PMMR as a virtual autopsy tool across a range of causes of death including natural causes, accident, suicide, homicide, or iatrogenic causes.

3D ANATOMICAL MODELING IN FORENSIC RADIOLOGY

As 3D printing and anatomical modeling technologies evolve, their application in forensic radiology is similarly growing. The most obvious of which is the use of 3D models in the courtroom as demonstrative evidence. The presentation of real evidence, particularly in situations involving a violent death that results in dismemberment or severe trauma, is often either illegal or deemed too graphic for presentation to a jury thereby biasing their ability to render an appropriate and fair verdict. In addition, actual evidence may not be permissible or practical due to the fact that it is in an advanced state of decay or putrification.[34] Traditionally, photographic evidence is typically presented as an alternative; however, this technology is not without limitation including the fact that the subject material can undergo distortion either as a photograph or a 3D virtual model, photographic representation results in the loss of all depth information, and the presentation of an object does not necessarily provide a true representation of the physical dimensions of the object.[3] The use of 3D printed models alleviates all of these problems by providing life size representations of the actual subject/anatomical information that is deemed admissible as evidence and sufficiently sanitized thereby rendering them acceptable to a lay jury. In addition, the use of color printing technologies allows accurate representation of multiple anatomic structures and injuries such as bone fractures, vessels, cardiac infarction, ruptured organs, and bite wounds.[35]

Several case studies demonstrate the value of 3D printing in the courtroom and point to the emerging and increasingly important role of this technology in the judicial process. Baier et al.[36] have described the use of micro-CT to identify the circumstances of an assault that resulted in the death of the victim. By creating a 3D model of the skull, the pathologist was able to determine the number of assault weapons and perpetrators. This evidence, along with an actual 3D model, was used as part of evidence resulting in the conviction of two defendants who were sentenced to life in prison. A second case illustrates the use of 3D printing in particularly gruesome circumstances that involved the discovery of a dismembered corpse within a suitcase submerged in a canal in the United Kingdom.[37] In this situation, a submerged suitcase was discovered by canal workers. Suspicious of the contents, police were called followed by a CT scan at a local hospital revealing a severed head, left lower leg, and arms of an individual. Subsequent searching of the canal revealed a second suitcase with the remainder of the victim. 3D printing allowed the virtual fitting of the suitcase remains to a third set of charred remains located at the crime scene linking the two sites. While the use of 3D printing provided a more complete description of the crime, the combined evidence when presented to the suspect resulted in a full confession.[37] The third and final example involves the presentation of 3D printed models associated with the death of a female subject due to strangulation and blunt force trauma.[38] The perpetrator of the crime in this situation was the boyfriend and biological father of the female victim's children. Fig. 13.1 shows the 3D models that were used as demonstrative evidence in the court case that resulted in the conviction of the suspect and a sentence of life in prison.

Outside of the courtroom, 3D printed anatomic models are being used for a variety of applications including accidental deaths and traumatic injuries. Eckhardt et al.[39] described the use of 3D surface scanning and printing in the case of accidental death due to autoerotic asphyxia not only as a method for identifying and illustrating the method of death but also as an effective method of digitally preserving the evidence prior to alteration due to histologic sampling and autopsy. 3D anatomic models have also been used in the antemortem setting in which the initial trauma can be identified based on presurgical CT imaging of the subject.[40] 3D printing of cranial bones in traumatic head injuries has also been reported[41] in which 3D printed versions of the recomposed bony structures are fitted to the cadaver thereby assisting in the postmortem identification of the victim by means of facial recognition. Lastly, Barrera et al.[42] have described the use of 3D printing in

nonaccidental rib cage factures in children. When presented to members of the Child Protection Team of the author's institution, the authors reported on the instant and spontaneous physical manipulation of the models illustrating the importance of understanding the size of the actual model.

The use of 3D models in the forensic sciences raises the question of accuracy both in terms of spatial fidelity of the data and the accurate representation of injury/pathology. Spatial fidelity is in large part determined by the resolution of the data used to create the model as well as the various processes including segmentation, smoothing, and cropping of data that are part of the 3D modeling process. While CT data are generally considered superior when compared to MR in terms of spatial fidelity, the accuracy of the final model is also determined by acquisition parameters used, for example, in the case of a postmortem CT scan. Slice thickness and in plane pixel dimensions are the ultimate limiting factors in determining the degree of spatial accuracy the final model will have. If a CT scan is performed with slice thicknesses of 5 mm or greater, it is unreasonable to envision a model in which objects less than this dimension can be accurately reproduced.

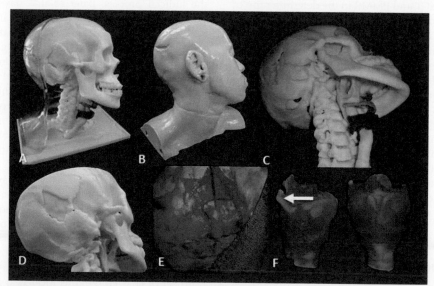

FIG. 13.1 Images of 3D printed anatomic forensic models from a postmortem CT scan. Female victim who was beaten, strangled, and later discarded in a watering trough. Autopsy revealed severe blunt force trauma, including a massive skull fracture, and strangulation.[38] **(A)** 3D printed model of skull, trachea, hyoid bone, and fractured larynx manufactured with material jetting (Connex 500, Stratasys, Eden Prairie, MN). Skin surface has been printed as a cut away and in clear material to show relationships. **(B)** 3D model with flesh tone opaque material demonstrating posterior scalp laceration and indentation from neckless impression. **(C)** 3D model allows relationships of bone trauma and fractured cartilage to be viewed from multiple angles. **(D)** Magnified view of skull fractures allows preservation of trauma before autopsy. **(E)** Autopsy photo of skull fracture. **(F)** Autopsy photo of fractured superior horn of the laryngeal cartilage (*white arrow*).

Given these limitations, several reports of the spatial accuracy of 3D models in forensics have already been published indicating that their accuracy is between −0.4 mm and 1.2 mm[3] and 2 mm.[43]

Accurate reproduction of the object being printed is also affected by the correct identification and segmentation of the anatomic structures comprising the model. This requires additional expertise necessary to identify structures that are either distorted or corrupted due to injury or by postmortem changes. Forensic radiologists hence provide unique expertise necessary to perform this task. Post-processing operations commonly performed as part of the model creation process such as smoothing and interpolation can also distort the original imaging data further verifying the essential role of the forensic radiologist in ensuring the authenticity of the final product.

FORENSIC 3D PRINTING USE CASE SCENARIOS

The use and application of 3D anatomic models in the forensic sciences is as diverse as the types of injuries and traumas. To that end, the following includes illustrative examples of 3D anatomic models in forensics and is by no means to be considered exhaustive.

BLUNT TRAUMA

Blunt force trauma is the injury resulting from the use of blunt force to an individual either intentionally (transportation related, blast injuries or impact with a solid object, etc.) or by accident, are categorized into four categories including contusion, abrasion, laceration, and fracture, and are the most commonly seen in forensic practices.[44]

3D printed forensic models are proving to be particularly helpful in describing the often complex injuries that are encountered in blunt trauma, particularly in pediatric cases where there is the added emotional toll of the loss of life. Fig. 13.2 illustrates this in the case of a 2-month-old who suffered a cranial cervical dissociation following a motor vehicle accident. Fig. 13.2A,E, and F shows computer-aided design (CAD) volume rendered images derived from the whole body CT scan performed prior to autopsy, while Fig. 13.2B,C,

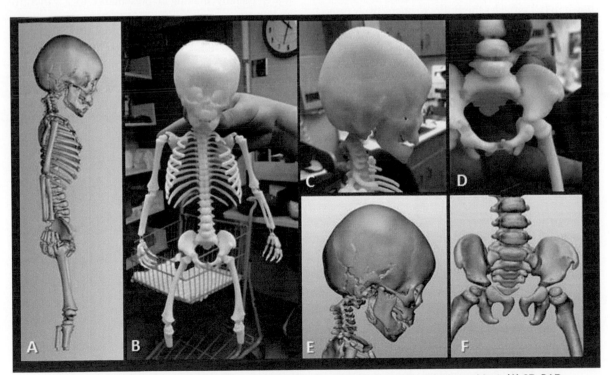

FIG. 13.2 Cranial cervical dissociation in a 2-month-old secondary to motor vehicle accident. **(A)** 3D CAD full-body reconstruction from postmortem CT scan allows full-body assessment before autopsy. **(B)** 3D printed full body reconstruction showing numerous osseous injuries in life size. **(C)** 3D printed and **(E)** CAD magnified view craniocervical dissociation. **(D)** 3D printed and **(F)** CAD magnified view iliac wing fracture. (CT data provided courtesy of the University of New Mexico.)

and D are photographs of the 3D model for the corresponding 3D rendered images. Note that unlike the volume rendered images, the scale of the model is immediately communicated to the observer with the presence of the adult hand holding the model in Fig. 13.2B and D. The model also shows additional fracture of the iliac wing as shown in Fig. 13.2D and F. As traumatic as these injuries are, it is unlikely that actual accident scene or autopsy photos could be shown to the general public due to potential psychologic injury or bias of the jury. 3D forensic models therefore provide the opportunity to bridge this gap by sanitizing such a traumatic and emotionally disturbing injury.

As illustrated in Fig. 13.3, 3D forensic modeling can be applied not only to pediatric blunt force trauma but to any trauma, independent of age. In this instance, the model is reproduced from a CT scan of an 83-year-old female with bilateral distal femur fractures which were suspected to be the result of elder abuse. While the CT scan (A) and volume rendered image (B) communicate the extent of the injury, neither provide the opportunity for the observer to physically inspect bony anatomy. In contrast, the 3D model as shown in (C) provides the ability to interactively inspect the injury thereby providing a spatial context that cannot be communicated by digital means.

PENETRATING TRAUMA

While less common than blunt trauma, penetrating trauma describes the result of impact with an external object resulting in piercing of the skin causing underlying tissue damage and an open wound.[45]

Gunshot Wounds

According to statistics published by the US National Vital Statistics System, there are 32,000 deaths and 67,000 injuries from firearms in the US[46] per year with the highest being due to self-harm followed by assault-related injuries. In addition, those most disproportionately affected are males, racial/ethnic minority populations, and young Americans.[46] Of those injuries that were intentional (i.e., self-inflicted), 51.4% of nonfatal wounds were to the head or neck.[47] Fig. 13.4 shows the typical projectile trajectories as a result of a gunshot wound to the head. Given the variety and complexity of injuries, as well as their extremely destructive nature, 3D printing provides a unique opportunity to effectively communicate these characteristics while simultaneously sanitizing the injury thereby making it presentable to a variety of audiences.

Two examples of gunshot wounds and the corresponding anatomic models are shown in Fig. 13.5

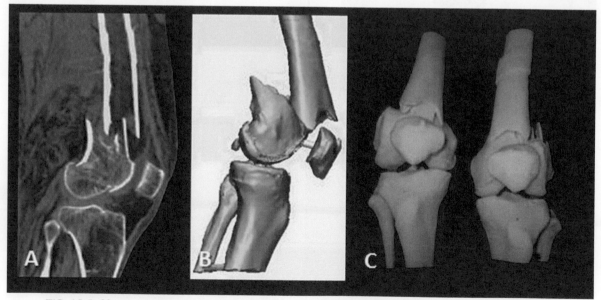

FIG. 13.3 83-year-old female with bilateral distal femur fractures investigated as being a victim of elder abuse **(A)**. Sagittal reconstruction from antemortem CT scan **(B)**. 3D CAD reconstruction demonstrating comminuted distal femur fracture of the left leg **(C)**. 3D printed model of both knees allowing victim-specific life size models. The models were used by lay members of the investigation to understand the directional force of injury and correlate with reported trauma.

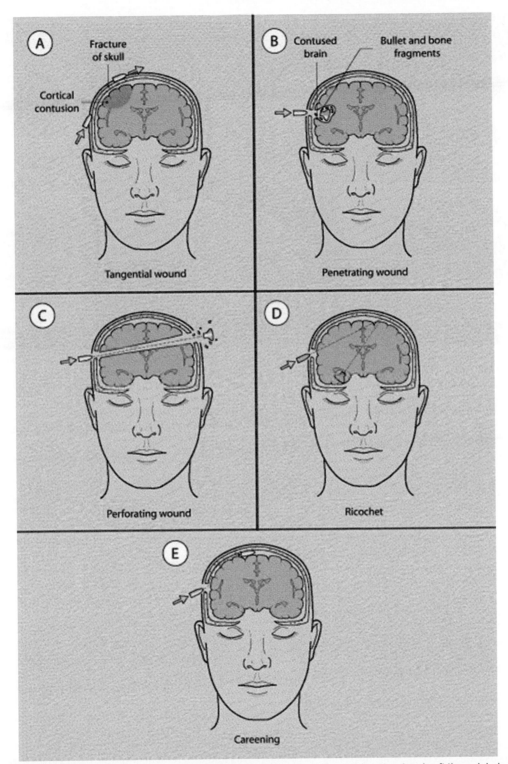

FIG. 13.4 Various trajectories of a projectile (bullet) to the head and the resultant hard and soft tissue injuries. (Reproduced with permission from Blissitt PA. Care of the critically ill patient with penetrating head injury. *Crit Care Nurs Clin* 2006;18(3):321–332. doi: https://doi.org/10.1016/j.ccell.2006.05.006[48].)

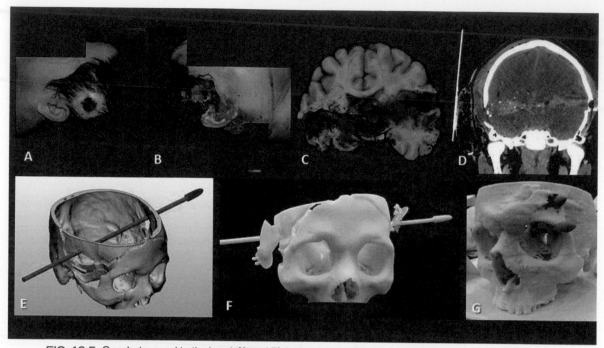

FIG. 13.5 Gunshot wound to the head. **(A and B)** Autopsy photographs from bullet entrance and exit wound. **(C)** Autopsy photograph of coronal slice though victim's brain demonstrating bullet trajectory. **(D)** Coronal CT scan postmortem demonstrating hemorrhagic bullet trajectory. Internal beveling is seen at bullet entrance site on the right and external beveling on the left. **(E)** 3D CAD reconstruction of the fractured calvarium with the bullet trajectory made from the CT scan entrance and exit wounds **(F)**. 3D printed model demonstrating fractures beveling and bullet trajectory. **(G)** 3D printed model from a separate gunshot case demonstrating bullet fragmentation and two exit paths through calvarium from a single entrance wound.

and 13.6. Fig. 13.5 shows a self-inflicted gunshot wound to the head that resulted in the death of the subject. Graphic postmortem photographs Fig. 13.5A–C show the entrance (A) and exit wounds (B) as well as the trajectory of the bullet through the brain (C), while (D) shows a coronal reformatted CT image taken prior to death. Fig. 13.5E shows the segmented 3D image of the bony anatomy of the subject identifying the bullet trajectory as shown by the blue rod. A 9-mm bullet has been added to the tip of the trajectory to indicate the direction of the bullet and is not intended to represent the true bullet. Fig. 13.5F shows the 3D printed model. Note that the figure demonstrates a challenge of creating such a model in the presence of bone fragments that are not physically attached to other bony structures. In this instance several thin disks were added to create the connections and hence demonstrate fragment locations. Fig. 13.5G shows a second, unrelated case demonstrating fragmentation of the bullet as well as beveling and fracturing of bony anatomy.

3D forensic models of bullet wounds outside of the head provide unique challenges as well as opportunities as shown in Fig. 13.6 which illustrates a gunshot wound through the chest resulting in pneumothorax, rib fractures, and intraparenchymal hemorrhage. The complex anatomy of the heart, lung, and rib cage as well as the soft tissue damage resulting from the bullet means that additional time and effort is required in the segmentation and modeling steps necessary to create the 3D anatomic model. Segmentation and separation of arteries and veins as well as airways and lung parenchyma from a single noncontrast CT scan pose unique challenges during segmentation and illustrate the value of having input and oversight by a forensic radiologist. The creation of life-like models as shown in (C) and (E), however, illustrate the value of higher end (i.e., industrial) 3D printers with sufficient build volume necessary to print such a large model as well as a color pallet large enough to provide a spectrum of colors needed to identify and differentiate multiple tissues and objects within a single printed model.

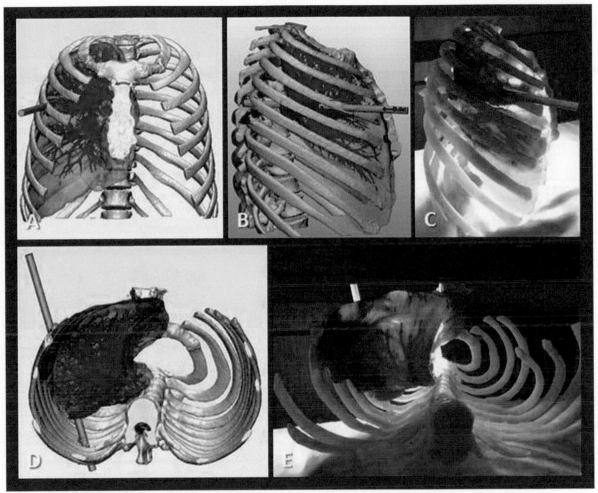

FIG. 13.6 37-year-old male gunshot wound through the chest resulting in pneumothorax, rib fractures, and intraparenchymal hemorrhage. **(A)** Coronal, **(B)** Sagittal, and **(D)** Superior views of 3D CAD files segmented from victims posttraumatic chest CT. Bullet Trajectory (Blue Rod), Lung (Transparent Light Pink) Pulmonary vasculature (Red), and Intraparenchymal hemorrhage (Blue) **(C)** Sagittal and **(E)** Superior views of the life-sized 3D printed multimaterial thorax allows the lung to be printed in clear to highlight the course of the bullet, the intraparenchymal hemorrhage, and the fractures of the ribs. 3D printed model allows viewing the model from any angle in an easy to understand simple manner.

Fig. 13.7 illustrates the use of 3D forensic models for an extremity gunshot wound which in this instance was in a 48-year-old male traveling abroad shot through the left lower extremity with bullet lodging into the right ankle beneath the talus. While photographic (Fig. 13.7A), X-ray (Fig. 13.7B), and reformatted CT data(Fig. 13.7C) identify the entrance, exit, and bullet location, the 3D forensic model (Fig. 13.7D and E) provides both contextual information by showing the direction of the bullet as indicated by the rod as well as the extent of the injury to both left and right ankle joints.

Rifle Bolt

The following example illustrates the use of 3D modeling in accidental penetrating trauma as well as highlights some of the limitations and advantages of this technology. The victim, an amateur gunsmith, was firing a homemade antique rifle. During the discharge of the weapon, the rifle bolt was ejected backwards along the barrel axis striking the subject in the left cheek. Fig. 13.8 shows the victim upon presentation to the emergency room with the bolt in place. Notice that the bolt exited the subject slightly anterior to the left ear.

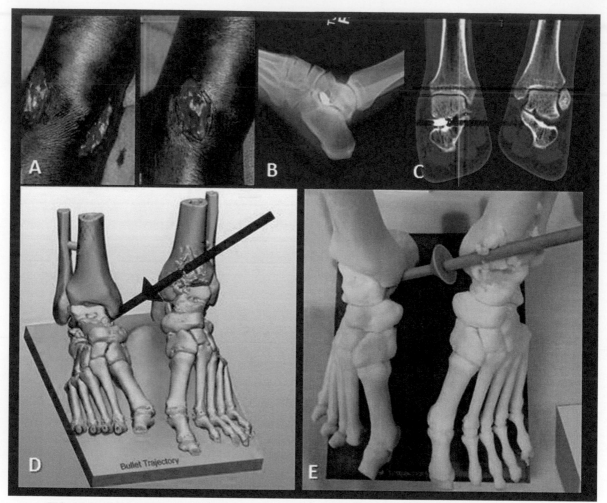

FIG. 13.7 48-year-old male traveling abroad was shot though the left lower extremity with bullet lodging into the right ankle beneath the talus. **(A)** Photograph of the lower extremities demonstrating the soft tissue injury. **(B)** X-ray of the right ankle demonstrating bullet. **(C)** Coronal CT scan demonstrating both ankles with the bullet in a subtalar location. Note the streaking artifact produced by the bullet obscuring its exact location. **(D)**. 3D CAD reconstruction of both lower extremities with bullet trajectory (*blue arrow*) CAD element added. CAD allows custom stands to be created for victim-specific data to rest on (light blue stand). **(E)**. 3D printed model allows viewing the model from any angle in an easy to understand simple manner.

The graphic nature of the injury identifies the challenges with presenting such material either to the victim or their family members. At the time of presentation, a CT scan was performed that was used to reconstruct the volume rendered images of the injury. Note the loss of resolution of the rifle bolt in the volume rendered images. This is due to both a relatively large slice thickness used in the acquisition of the CT data (3 mm) and artifacts resulting from the large differences in Hounsfield units between the metal of the rifle bolt and surrounding bone and soft tissue. Such artifacts are common on CT scans in the presence of foreign metal objects and can result in distortion of both the metal object and surrounding tissue thereby compromising the fidelity of the 3D anatomic forensic model. Finally, the figure also shows the reconstructed 3D forensic models. Note that the same loss of resolution of the rifle bolt, particularly along the grooves of the bolt (arrow), is seen in the model as described with the volume rendered images illustrating that spatial fidelity and resolution of the model is affected by both the resolution of the dataset used as well as the

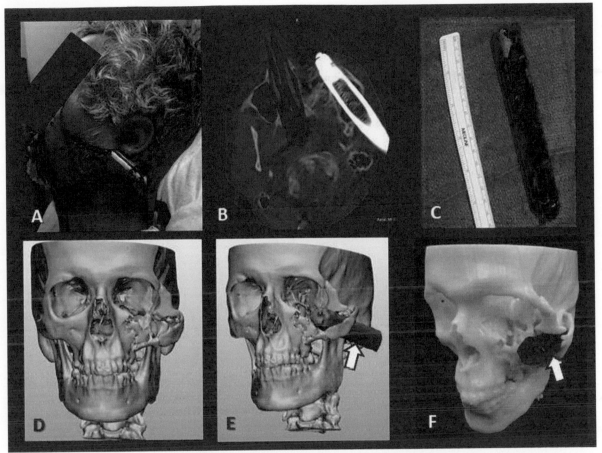

FIG. 13.8 55-year-old male with an accidental penetrating trauma. A rifle bolt malfunctioned exiting the rear of the rifle striking the victim in the left cheek exiting anterior to the left ear. **(A)** The photograph shows the subject at the time of presentation to the emergency room. **(B)** Axial CT images demonstrate beam hardening artifacts due to the presence of the foreign metal. These artifacts pose significant problems when segmenting and contouring both the anatomy of the subject as well as the foreign object. This is one limit of foreign body reconstruction in 3D printing without surface scanning. **(C)** Photograph of removed rifle bolt. 3D CAD reconstruction of skeletal injury **(D)** with the bolt subtracted and **(E)** in place to guide reconstruction. **(F)** 3D printed anatomic model not only illustrates the projectile and its path through the subject but also illustrates limitations imposed both in terms of resolution and artifacts in the final model.

resolution limits of the 3D printer used to create the final model.

BLUNT FORCE POLYTRAUMA

Fig. 13.9 illustrates the utility of 3D forensic models in situations in which multiple (poly) traumas occur in a single victim. In this situation, a 52-year-old male working at an automotive experienced a crush injury that resulted in multiple rib and spine fractures, torn inferior vena cava (IVC) resulting in pericardial effusion and cardiac tamponade. Due to the extent of the

injuries, the subject died in the hospital several days later. The models presented demonstrate the versatility of 3D printing by allowing multiple models of the same injury to be printed. By judicious selection of printing technologies including vat photopolymerization (Form 2, Formlabs, Cambridge, MA), binder jetting (Projet 660, 3D Systems, Rock Hill, SC) and material jetting (Objet Connex 500, Stratasys, Eden Prairie, MN), anatomic regions and colors, individual injuries can be highlighted. For instance, Fig. 13.9A and B show the bony anatomy of the entire spinal column and pelvis as well as the heart, aorta, and vena cava.

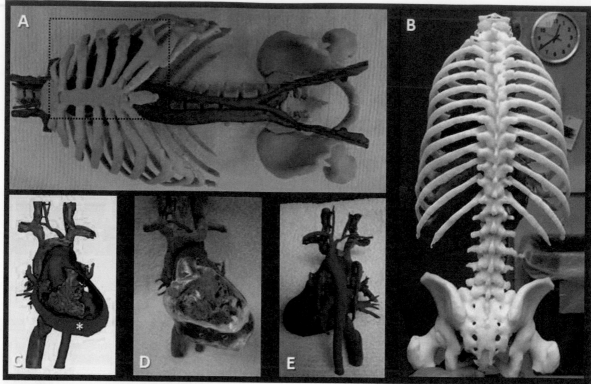

FIG. 13.9 52-year-old male who died in hospital secondary to a crush injury at an automobile plant resulting in multiple rib and spine fractures, torn IVC resulting in pericardial effusion and cardiac tamponade. Model used in trial as demonstrative evidence with the jury. **(A)** Whole torso and pelvic 3D printed model of the victims osseous structures, chest cartilage, aorta, IVC, and heart. Black dashed box demonstrates numerous fractures. **(B)** Posterior whole torso and pelvis view demonstrating additional fractures. **(C)** 3D CAD reconstruction of the heart demonstrating relationship of the torn IVC to the pericardium which is thickened (white asterisk) secondary to effusion. **(D)** Multimaterial 3D printed model with detachable anterior clear pericardium to show ventricle cavity and effusion. **(E)** Posterior view of 3D printed heart shows relationship of torn IVC to pericardium.

The use of different colors to represent the spine, ribs, and pelvis can be used to draw attention to or away from specific injuries in order to highlight a given injury. Smaller models of specific organs, in this case the heart as shown in Fig. 13.9D and E, highlight important clinical findings, in this case a pericardial effusion, that may be masked by the entire model.

NONACCIDENTAL (PENETRATING AND BLUNT) TRAUMA

Nonaccidental trauma describes injuries resulting from direct intent such as homicide, intentional vehicular injury, suicide, and abuse. Due to the diversity of etiologies, these injuries include either or both penetrating and blunt traumas.

As noted previously, 3D forensic models can play an important role in pediatric trauma cases given the often overwhelming secondary emotional trauma that is inflicted not only on family members but also the general public. This latter effect can have significant impact of the judicial process and the need for both procedural and retributive justice. To illustrate this, consider the blunt trauma sustained by a 25-month-old following maternal aunt dropping a television on the child's head causing skull base calvarial dissociation, brain herniation, and death as seen in Fig. 13.10. 3D forensic models of the victim's skull as shown in Fig. 13.10D–F allow communication of the extent of injury that would likely be intolerable if the information was presented in a different format (i.e., photographs). The introduction of these models during legal proceedings has the potential to allow the prosecutor

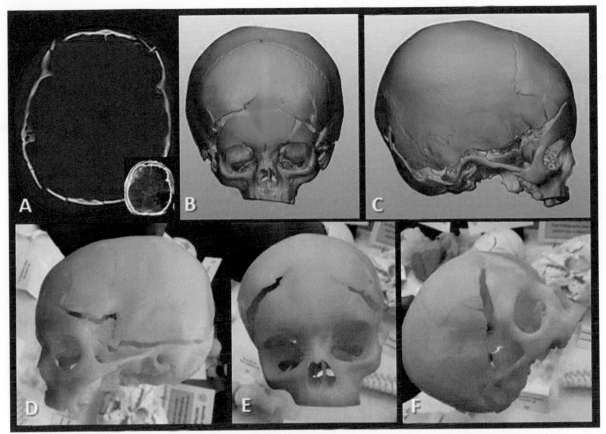

FIG. 13.10 Blunt trauma secondary to maternal aunt dropping a TV on 25-month-old head causing skull base calvarial dissociation, brain herniation, and death. **(A)** Premortem noncontrast axial head CT demonstrating fractures, subdural and intraparenchymal hemorrhage, and diffuse hypoxia (inset). **(B)** Anterior and **(C)** Lateral 3D reconstruction (3-matic, Materialise, Leuven, Belgium) exported as STL file for printing. **(D)** Left lateral, **(E)** Anterior, and **(F)** Right lateral photographs of the 3D printed skull which allows law enforcement, social workers, courtroom exhibitors, and lay jury to understand the injury in a victim-specific life size manner.

to present crime scene data without prejudicing the jury (procedural justice) against the accused. Similarly, allowing members of the jury to hold and manipulate the models would allow them to grasp the true extent of the injuries sustained while potentially minimizing the emotional impact of the death of a child during deliberations (retributive justice). While not shown, images of the victim either prior to or following the injury as well as autopsy photos would unlikely be admissible during legal proceedings due to their overwhelming emotional response by members of a jury.

HOMICIDE

As described previously, probably the most common application of 3D anatomic models in the forensic sciences to date is for the reproduction of both evidence pertaining to and victims of homicide. To illustrate the utility and versatility of these models consider the following case study in which an 86-year-old male was assaulted by his 46-year-old son resulting in, among other injuries, a severe blunt force injury to the head. The assailant was pursued by police who died as a result of loss of control of his automobile. The victim was reported dead at the scene as was transferred to our institution subsequently undergoing a whole-body CT scan before traditional autopsy. Autopsy photographs (Fig. 13.11A and E) illustrate two points: first, the graphic nature of the injuries sustained (Fig. 13.11A) and the fact that autopsy is by its nature destructive (Fig. 13.11E). It is unlikely that such photos could be presented as part of any legal proceedings or as

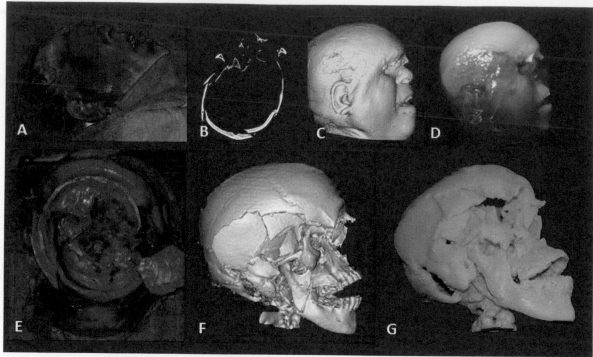

FIG. 13.11 86-year-old male with marked facial skeletal trauma and brain herniation secondary to stomping injury from son. **(A)** Autopsy photo of victims head showing marked bruising and facial asymmetry. **(B)** Postmortem CT demonstrating innumerable fractures. **(C)** 3D reconstruction and **(D)** 3D printed multimaterial clear and white model of the overlying skin sanitizes the autopsy photos while maintaining relationship to underlying skeletal trauma. **(E)** Autopsy photo demonstrating the destructive nature of autopsy as the soft tissues and bones are removed the original trauma is not able to be recreated. **(F)** 3D CAD reconstruction and **(G)** 3D printed skeletal model demonstrate the relationship of the markedly deformed calvarium and facial bones of the victim.

evidence during a jury trial. By contrast, both skin segmentation (Fig. 13.11C) and bone segmentation (Fig. 13.11F) allow a sanitized visualization of the massive and fatal injuries endured by the victim. The versatility of forensic 3D printed models is shown in (Fig. 13.11D and G) and illustrates how specific features such as the external skin contour of the subject in relation to the multiple bone fractures can be identified and highlighted as well as isolating specific injuries which in this instance are the multiple and extensive fractures of the skull. An axial CT scan of the subject obtained prior to autopsy is shown in (Fig. 13.11B). While multiple fractures are seen in the CT scan, the true extent of these injuries would require interpretation by a forensic radiologist. By comparison, no such expertise is needed when reviewing the 3D model presented in either (Fig. 13.11D or G).

FUTURE DIRECTIONS AND CHALLENGES

It is likely that the use of 3D printed anatomic models will see continued growth in forensic radiology. Evidence for this exists in both our own practice as well as the community at large. For example, in an 8-year period the number of 3D printed anatomic models generated at the Mayo Clinic has grown from a single model in 2006 to over 100 in 2014.[49] Similar growth can be seen based on the PubMed search of the term "3D printing radiology" which listed a single publication in the year 1996 to 420 publications in 2019. Hence, it is not unreasonable to predict similar growth trends within the forensic radiology space. This growth will most likely be driven by a range of factors including but not limited to the scientific accuracy of the model at depicting a given injury or cause of death, the ability to introduce models as demonstrative evidence in legal proceedings thereby making evidence admissible that would previously not been so, rapid communication of complex anatomic structures and injuries to non (i.e., lay) personnel, and finally the ability to rapidly and cost-effectively produce such models for broad dissemination. A driver for such growth will be the education of the larger forensics community through increased reports of the use of 3D printing in academic and peer-reviewed journals. As more and more of the community begin to appreciate the advantages of 3D anatomic models in the forensic sciences, the demand for this service will similarly grow.

Despite the foreseeable growth on the use of 3D anatomic models in the forensic sciences, several challenges remain. The first is the cost and expertise associated with generating anatomically accurate 3D models. While small desktop 3D printers can be purchased with limited capital expenditure, establishing a reliable and large-scale volume service requires a significant investment in both equipment and personnel and which can easily exceed several millions of dollars depending upon the size of the facility. The expense of establishing and running such a program must be passed on to the customer in the form of the printed model. In the legal context, if the cost of such a model is deemed too expensive, it is unlikely to be used. While high profile legal cases can generate significant financial payments to victims, these cases are rare by comparison to the majority of legal proceedings. Another limitation is the access to both antemortem and postmortem cross-sectional imaging necessary to create the 3D models. Unless these imaging modalities are easily accessible at the time of autopsy, it is unlikely that they will be performed on a routine basis. Although several countries including Australia[14] and the United Kingdom[19] have established PMCT services, the practice is not widespread as it is likely that, at least within the US will be limited to academic hospitals with easy access to postmortem imaging facilities or have dedicated imaging facilities within their mortuary such as the Radiology—Pathology Center for Forensic Imaging (CFI) at the University of New Mexico School of Medicine. In addition to cross-sectional imaging access, availability of trained forensic radiologists remains a limitation. In general, forensic radiology remains a small subspecialty within radiology. Given the need for expertise in 3D printing and modeling, the number of highly skilled and trained radiologists will remain small and therefore inhibit growth of the field. Finally, as with all developing fields, there remain no nationally or internationally accepted standards for the appropriate use and application of 3D printing in forensic radiology. What is needed is standardization of procedures and protocols

overseen by some type of national and/or international governing body. It is expected that as the field grows, there will be guidance for appropriate use as well as standard protocols for the creation of 3D printed anatomic forensic models.

REFERENCES

1. Decker SJ, Braileanu M, Dey C, et al. Forensic radiology: a primer. *Acad Radiol.* 2019;26(6):820—830. https://doi.org/10.1016/j.acra.2019.03.006.
2. Golan T. The authority of shadows: the legal embrace of the X-ray. *Hist Reflexions-reflexions Historiques.* 1998;24:437—458.
3. Carew RM, Morgan RM, Rando C. A preliminary investigation into the accuracy of 3D modeling and 3D printing in forensic anthropology evidence reconstruction. *J Forensic Sci.* 2019;64(2):342—352. https://doi.org/10.1111/1556-4029.13917.
4. Jeffery AJ. The role of computed tomography in adult post-mortem examinations: an overview. *Diagn Histopathol.* 2010;16(12):546—551. https://doi.org/10.1016/j.mpdhp.2010.08.017.
5. JF I. Forensic radiology. In: RA C, ed. *A History of the Radiological Sciences.* Reston, VA: American College of Radiology Radiology Centennial; 1996:579—605.
6. Eckert WG, Garland N. The history of the forensic applications in radiology. *Am J Forensic Med Pathol.* 1984;5(1):53—56. https://doi.org/10.1097/00000433-198403000-00010.
7. DiPoce J, Guelfguat M, DiPoce J. Radiologic findings in cases of attempted suicide and other self-injurious behavior. *Radiographics.* 2012;32(7):2005—2024. https://doi.org/10.1148/rg.327125035.
8. Flach PM, Thali MJ, Germerott T. Times have changed! Forensic radiology—a new challenge for radiology and forensic pathology. *Am J Roentgenol.* 2014;202(4):W325—W334. https://doi.org/10.2214/AJR.12.10283.
9. Messmer JM, Fierro MF. Radiologic forensic investigation of fatal gunshot wounds. *Radiographics.* 1986;6(3):457—473. https://doi.org/10.1148/radiographics.6.3.3685503.
10. Ruder TD, Thali MJ, H GM. Essentials of forensic post-mortem MR imaging in adults. *Br J Radiol.* 2014;87(1036):20130567. https://doi.org/10.1259/bjr.20130567.
11. Wilson AJ. Gunshot injuries: what does a radiologist need to know? *Radiographics.* 1999;19(5):1358—1368. https://doi.org/10.1148/radiographics.19.5.g99se171358.
12. Weustink AC, Hunink MG, van Dijke CF, Renken NS, Krestin GP, Oosterhuis JW. Minimally invasive autopsy: an alternative to conventional autopsy? *Radiology.* 2009;250(3):897—904. https://doi.org/10.1148/radiol.2503080421.
13. Nathoo N, Boodhoo H, Nadvi SS, Naidoo SR, Gouws E. Transcranial brainstem stab injuries: a retrospective analysis of 17 patients. *Neurosurgery.* 2000;47(5):1117—1122. https://doi.org/10.1097/00006123-200011000-00018. discussion 1123.

14. Lynch MJ, Woodford NW. The role of post-mortem imaging in preliminary examinations under the Coroners Act 2008 (Vic): a forensic pathologist's perspective. *J Law Med.* 2014;21(4):774−779.

15. Dirnhofer R, Jackowski C, Vock P, Potter K, Thali MJ. VIRTOPSY: minimally invasive, imaging-guided virtual autopsy. *Radiographics.* 2006;26(5):1305−1333. https://doi.org/10.1148/rg.265065001.

16. Donchin Y, Rivkind AI, Bar-Ziv J, Hiss J, Almog J, Drescher M. Utility of postmortem computed tomography in trauma victims. *J Trauma.* 1994;37(4):552−555. https://doi.org/10.1097/00005373-199410000-00006. discussion 555-556.

17. Bisset RA, Thomas NB, Turnbull IW, Lee S. Postmortem examinations using magnetic resonance imaging: four year review of a working service. *Br Med J.* 2002;324(7351):1423−1424. https://doi.org/10.1136/bmj.324.7351.1423.

18. Rutty GN, Robinson CE, BouHaidar R, Jeffery AJ, Morgan B. The role of mobile computed tomography in mass fatality incidents. *J Forensic Sci.* 2007;52(6):1343−1349. https://doi.org/10.1111/j.1556-4029.2007.00548.x.

19. Rutty GN, Robinson C, Morgan B, Black S, Adams C, Webster P. Fimag: the United Kingdom disaster victim/forensic identification imaging system. *J Forensic Sci.* 2009;54(6):1438−1442. https://doi.org/10.1111/j.1556-4029.2009.01175.x.

20. Hoey BA, Cipolla J, Grossman MD, et al. Postmortem computed tomography, "CATopsy", predicts cause of death in trauma patients. *J Trauma.* 2007;63(5):979−985. https://doi.org/10.1097/TA.0b013e318154011f. discussion 985-976.

21. Rutty GN, Jeffery AJ, Raj V, Morgan B. The use of postmortem computed tomography in the investigation of intentional neonatal upper airway obstruction: an illustrated case. *Int J Leg Med.* 2010;124(6):641−645. https://doi.org/10.1007/s00414-010-0438-4.

22. Jackowski C, Thali M, Sonnenschein M, et al. Visualization and quantification of air embolism structure by processing postmortem MSCT data. *J Forensic Sci.* 2004;49(6):1339−1342.

23. Ozdoba C, Weis J, Plattner T, Dirnhofer R, Yen K. Fatal scuba diving incident with massive gas embolism in cerebral and spinal arteries. *Neuroradiology.* 2005;47(6):411−416. https://doi.org/10.1007/s00234-004-1322-z.

24. Oehmichen M, Meissner C, König HG, Gehl HB. Gunshot injuries to the head and brain caused by low-velocity handguns and rifles. A review. *Forensic Sci Int.* 2004;146(2−3):111−120. https://doi.org/10.1016/j.forsciint.2004.06.023.

25. Thali MJ, Schwab CM, Tairi K, Dirnhofer R, Vock P. Forensic radiology with cross-section modalities: spiral CT evaluation of a knife wound to the aorta. *J Forensic Sci.* 2002;47(5):1041−1045.

26. Heinemann A, Vogel H, Heller M, Tzikas A, Püschel K. Investigation of medical intervention with fatal outcome: the impact of post-mortem CT and CT angiography. *Radiol Med.* 2015;120(9):835−845. https://doi.org/10.1007/s11547-015-0574-5.

27. Farkash U, Scope A, Lynn M, et al. Preliminary experience with postmortem computed tomography in military penetrating trauma. *J Trauma.* 2000;48(2):303−308. https://doi.org/10.1097/00005373-200002000-00018. discussion 308-309.

28. Levy AD, Abbott RM, Mallak CT, et al. Virtual autopsy: preliminary experience in high-velocity gunshot wound victims. *Radiology.* 2006;240(2):522−528. https://doi.org/10.1148/radiol.2402050972.

29. Cirielli V, Cima L, Bortolotti F, et al. Virtual autopsy as a screening test before traditional autopsy: the verona experience on 25 Cases. *J Pathol Inf.* 2018;9(1):28. https://doi.org/10.4103/jpi.jpi_23_18.

30. Rutty GN, Morgan B, Robinson C, et al. Diagnostic accuracy of post-mortem CT with targeted coronary angiography versus autopsy for coroner-requested post-mortem investigations: a prospective, masked, comparison study. *Lancet.* 2017;390(10090):145−154. https://doi.org/10.1016/s0140-6736(17)30333-1.

31. Añon J, Remonda L, Spreng A, et al. Traumatic extra-axial hemorrhage: correlation of postmortem MSCT, MRI, and forensic-pathological findings. *J Magn Reson Imag.* 2008;28(4):823−836. https://doi.org/10.1002/jmri.21495.

32. Bolliger S, Thali M, Jackowski C, Aghayev E, Dirnhofer R, Sonnenschein M. Postmortem non-invasive virtual autopsy: death by hanging in a car. *J Forensic Sci.* 2005;50(2):455−460.

33. Oesterhelweg L, Bolliger SA, Thali MJ, Ross S. Virtopsy: postmortem imaging of laryngeal foreign bodies. *Arch Pathol Lab Med.* 2009;133(5):806−810. https://doi.org/10.1043/1543-2165-133.5.806.

34. Errickson D, Thompson TJU, Rankin BWJ. The application of 3D visualization of osteological trauma for the courtroom: a critical review. *J Forensic Radiol Imag.* 2014;2(3):132−137. https://doi.org/10.1016/j.jofri.2014.04.002.

35. Ebert LC, Thali MJ, Ross S. Getting in touch—3D printing in forensic imaging. *Forensic Sci Int.* 2011;211(1):e1−e6. https://doi.org/10.1016/j.forsciint.2011.04.022.

36. Baier W, Warnett JM, Payne M, Williams MA. Introducing 3D printed models as demonstrative evidence at criminal trials. *J Forensic Sci.* 2018;63(4):1298−1302. https://doi.org/10.1111/1556-4029.13700.

37. Baier W, Norman DG, Warnett JM, et al. Novel application of three-dimensional technologies in a case of dismemberment. *Forensic Sci Int.* 2017;270:139−145. https://doi.org/10.1016/j.forsciint.2016.11.040.

38. Morris JM, McGee KP, Reichard RR, O'Laughlin JD, MacLean JD. Substantive admissibility of 3D forensic medical graphics and models. *Am J Trial Advocacy.* 2020;44(1).

39. Eckhardt M, Shah K, Bois M, Maleszewski J, Moore K, Lin P. Healed fracture of superior horn of thyroid cartilage in autoerotic asphyxia: an indication of prior activity? A case report utilizing 3D scanning and printing of the larynx. *Acad Forensic Pathol.* 2018;8(1):170−179. https://doi.org/10.23907/2018.012.

40. Woźniak K, Rzepecka-Woźniak E, Moskała A, Pohl J, Latacz K, Dybała B. Weapon identification using

antemortem computed tomography with virtual 3D and rapid prototype modeling—a report in a case of blunt force head injury. *Forensic Sci Int.* 2012;222(1): e29–e32. https://doi.org/10.1016/j.forsciint.2012. 06.012.

41. Urbanová P, Vojtíšek T, Frišhons J, Šandor O, Jurda M, Krajsa J. Applying 3D prints to reconstructing postmortem craniofacial features damaged by devastating head injuries. *Leg Med.* 2018;33:48–52. https://doi.org/10.1016/j.legalmed.2018.05.005.

42. Barrera CA, Silvestro E, Calle-Toro JS, et al. Three-dimensional printed models of the rib cage in children with non-accidental injury as an effective visual-aid tool. *Pediatr Radiol.* 2019;49(7):965–970. https://doi.org/10.1007/s00247-019-04368-7.

43. Edwards J, Rogers T. The accuracy and applicability of 3D modeling and printing blunt force cranial injuries. *J Forensic Sci.* 2018;63(3):683–691. https://doi.org/10.1111/1556-4029.13627.

44. Simon LV, Lopez RA, King KC. *Blunt Force Trauma.* Treasure Island (FL): StatPearls Publishing Copyright © 2020, StatPearls Publishing LLC.; 2020.

45. Blank-Reid C, Reid PC. Penetrating trauma to the head. *Crit Care Nurs Clin.* 2000;12(4):477–487.

46. Fowler KA, Dahlberg LL, Haileyesus T, Annest JL. Firearm injuries in the United States. *Prev Med.* 2015;79:5–14. https://doi.org/10.1016/j.ypmed.2015.06.002.

47. Gotsch KE, Annest JL, Mercy JA, Ryan GW. *Surveillance for Fatal and Nonfatal Firearm-Related Injuries — United States, 1993–1998;* 2001. https://www.cdc.gov/mmwr/preview/mmwrhtml/ss5002a1.htm.

48. Blissitt PA. Care of the critically ill patient with penetrating head injury. *Crit Care Nurs Clin.* 2006;18(3):321–332. https://doi.org/10.1016/j.ccell.2006.05.006.

49. Matsumoto JS, Morris JM, Foley TA, et al. Three-dimensional physical modeling: applications and experience at Mayo clinic. *Radiographics.* 2015;35(7):1989–2006. https://doi.org/10.1148/rg.2015140260.

CHAPTER 14

3D Printed Imaging Phantoms

NICOLE WAKE, PHD • CARLOTTA IANNIELLO, MS • RYAN BROWN, PHD •
CHRISTOPHER M. COLLINS, PHD

INTRODUCTION

To reproducibly and precisely characterize the ability of a medical imaging system to safely produce accurate images, it is useful to image objects which have properties similar to human tissues for the imaging method being tested, have geometries and compositions that are known exactly, and can remain in an exact location in the imaging system for indefinite periods of time. For this purpose, imaging phantoms are produced for every method (or modality) of medical imaging.

Today, imaging phantoms typically consist of materials (liquids, gels, semisolids, and/or solids depending on the tissue being mimicked and the imaging modality being evaluated) with desired properties and known geometries arranged in glass or plastic containers, sometimes also with glass or plastic inclusions of known dimensions. A variety of phantoms made with a range of shapes, purposes, and methods are commercially available; however, these phantoms are typically costly and often feature simplified geometries. Many applications may require customizable and anatomically realistic configurations, which are not typically achievable with traditional manufacturing technologies. For reference, Table 14.1 includes a number of vendors and links to sites displaying medical imaging phantoms designed for a wide range of purposes.

Three-dimensional (3D) printing promises new methods and possibilities for the production of medical imaging phantoms, ranging from rapid and accurate production of new designs through accurate reproduction of complex, anatomical shapes based on data from medical images. The number of works incorporating 3D printing in the production of phantoms is growing rapidly.[1] Consequently, it is difficult to give a comprehensive review, and so we rather present an introduction highlighting the variety of materials and approaches with reference to numerous examples. Here, after a brief discussion of material properties pertinent to each major medical imaging modality, we introduce a variety of methods demonstrated to date for all major medical imaging modalities, arranged according to the role of the 3D printed material in phantom production.

MATERIAL PROPERTIES PERTINENT TO MAJOR MEDICAL IMAGING MODALITIES

In all forms of medical imaging, some form of energy or matter is administered to the human body. For medically useful information to be produced, tissues must respond differently to the energy or matter applied.

In planar X-ray imaging, computed tomography (CT), magnetic resonance imaging (MRI), and ultrasound imaging, energies of various types are applied to all tissues in the region of interest, and after tissue-specific interactions through space and time, the detected energy has a signature which can be used to map tissue characteristics based on location. For single-photon emission computed tomography (SPECT) and positron emission tomography (PET), radioactive chemicals (or radiotracers) are introduced into the body, accumulating to different degrees in different regions depending on the tissue-specific affinity to the chemical introduced. High-energy photons resulting from radioactive decay (SPECT) or interaction of an emitted positron with a nearby electron (PET) pass through the body to external detectors so that a map of the distribution of the source radiotracers can be generated. Though not desired, these photons may interact with tissue on their way out of the body, which can adversely affect the data acquisition and final image. Generally, phantoms for SPECT and PET are not designed to mimic the accumulation of radiotracer in different tissues but to characterize the ability to accurately quantify the concentration of radiotracer throughout space despite both (1) limitations in system resolution and accuracy (due to a combination of system limitations and the random nature of radioactive decay) and (2) alterations in detected energy due to interactions with matter it passes through.

3D Printing for the Radiologist. https://doi.org/10.1016/B978-0-323-77573-1.00007-5

TABLE 14.1
General Overview of Commercially Available Imaging Phantoms.

Manufacturer	Website	Modalities
Biodex Medical Systems	https://www.biodex.com/nuclear-medicine/products/phantoms	- Nuclear medicine - PET/CT
Carville Limited	https://www.carvilleplastics.com/products/imaging-phantoms/	- X-ray - CT - MRI
Computerized Imaging Reference Systems, Inc. (CIRS)	https://www.cirsinc.com/products/	- CT - Mammography - MRI - Radiation therapy - Ultrasound - X-ray/Fluoro
Gold Standard Phantoms	https://www.goldstandardphantoms.com/	- MRI - MRS
Kyoto Kagaku	https://www.kyotokagaku.com/	- X-ray - CT - Ultrasound - Nuclear medicine - Mammography
Leeds Test Objects	https://www.leedstestobjects.com/#	- Fluoroscopy - X-ray - Mammography - CT - MRI - Nuclear medicine - Radiotherapy - Preclinical
Modus Medical Devices	https://modusqa.com/	- MRI - Radiation therapy - Optical CT
PTW Freiburg	https://www.ptwdosimetry.com/en/	- Radiation therapy
Radcal Corporation	https://radcal.com/	- CT - Fluoroscopy - X-ray
Radiology Support Devices, Inc.	http://rsdphantoms.com/	- X-ray - CT - Nuclear medicine - Radiation therapy

X-ray imaging, CT, PET, and SPECT all rely on detection of high-energy photons after they pass through all or part of the body. These photons may be scattered or absorbed in various interactions with objects (primarily electrons) in matter they pass through, resulting in an attenuation of the signal intensity. For this reason, electron density is a key characteristic of materials meant to mimic tissues in these modalities. However, how a photon interacts with a given electron depends on the energy of the photon and the affinity of the given electron to its associated nucleus. Therefore, a material with a composition designed to mimic a particular tissue for mammography (breast imaging), where photon energies are low (~20 keV), might not mimic the same tissue well for CT, where photon energies are typically above 100 keV, and would likely mimic that same tissue even less well for PET, which relies on source photons with an energy of 511 keV. To be clear, X-rays (used in X-ray imaging and CT) and gamma rays (used in SPECT and PET) all consist of high-energy photons, with X-rays for medical purposes being produced by an X-ray tube and gamma rays being a product of radioactive decay of an unstable nuclear isotope. The rate of attenuation through tissue (μ) relates directly to the "radiopacity" of the tissue, which is most commonly characterized on a scale relative to the values for air and water, resulting in "Hounsfield units" (HU) ranging from -1000 for air, 0 for pure water, to (approximately) 1000 for bone.

In ultrasound imaging, a beam of acoustic waves generated in a multielement piezoelectric transducer is steered through the tissue and the waves reflected back to the transducer are detected and translated into an image based on the time the reflection was detected in each element of the transducer. For ultrasound, key material characteristics include density, stiffness (related to speed of sound in a given material), backscattering, and attenuation (μ_{us}, related to both backscattering and absorption in a given material). Together, these material characteristics will affect the propagation speed of the sound waves within the tissues (with the speed being higher in tissues such as bone with increased density and stiffness), and how bright a tissue appears in an image (with tissues having greater backscattering appearing brighter). In addition to backscattering of a given tissue, reflections are produced at interfaces between materials

of different stiffnesses. For this reason, most energy is reflected at the interface between soft tissue and bone and it is difficult to see beyond these interfaces. In diagnostic medical ultrasound, frequencies from 3 to 10 MHz are most commonly used, and the ability of a given material to mimic a given tissue depends to some degree on the specific frequency used.

In MRI, three different magnetic fields are applied in any number of strategic sequences through time to interrogate tissues as to their spatial density, rate of return to resting state (T_1 relaxation or spin—lattice relaxation rate), and rate of signal decay (T_2 or spin—spin relaxation rate). By far, the most common nucleus used is that of hydrogen (a single proton), though it is possible to interrogate other nuclei as well. Importantly, the human body itself can alter the distribution of the applied magnetic fields and affect the images. In particular, the static magnetic field (B_0) is altered by the distribution of magnetic susceptibility (χ_m) through tissue, and the radiofrequency magnetic field (B_1) is altered by both tissue electric permittivity and tissue electric conductivity. Importantly, the B_1 field can induce electrical currents in the body that result in unintended heating of tissues. While phantoms can be designed to represent distortions of the fields caused by the human body and even resultant heating, in MRI the tissue properties that are more pertinent to signal and contrast between tissues are proton density (ρ), T_1, and T_2. Except for ρ and χ_m, all of these properties listed above are dependent on B_0. Therefore, phan-

TABLE 14.2
Summary of Material Properties Pertinent to Various Common Imaging Modalities.

Modality	Detected Energy	Pertinent Material Properties
Planar X-ray imaging	Photons with energies 15—140 keV	Attenuation μ (scattering, absorption)
CT	Photons with energies 100—140 keV	Attenuation μ (scattering, absorption)
SPECT	Photons with energies 140—364 keV	Attenuation μ (scattering, absorption)
PET	511 keV photons	Attenuation μ (scattering, absorption)
Ultrasound	Ultrasonic vibrations at frequencies 3—10 MHz	Stiffness (speed of sound), backscattering, and attenuation μ_{us}
MRI	Radiofrequency magnetic field with frequencies 20—300 MHz (corresponding to B_0 field strengths 0.5 to 7 T)	Proton density ρ, T_1, and T_2 relaxation rates, magnetic susceptibility χ_m, electric permittivity, electric conductivity

tom properties must be matched according to tissue properties for given B_0, which ranges from about 0.5 to 7 T for diagnostic systems.

Due to the time-dependent nature of sequences, physiological processes (including blood flow, perfusion, respiration, and variations in metabolic rate) and physical phenomena (such as diffusion) can also be characterized with medical imaging, and phantoms can be designed to represent these time-dependent characteristics as well. In this chapter, we will focus primarily on phantom material properties with only brief allusion to approaches to simulate physiology in phantoms. Also, while we limit this table to physical interaction as described above, it is also possible to design phantoms to mimic tissues in many other physical properties pertinent to medical imaging, such as directional diffusion for MRI.[2]

Table 14.2 contains a summary of material properties and ranges of photon energy, field strength, or frequency (depending on the modality) relevant to each modality.

IMAGING PHANTOMS WITH CONVENTIONAL MATERIALS IN 3D PRINTED CONTAINERS

Due to decades of research into tissue-mimicking materials for creating imaging phantoms with a wide range of purposes and, in contrast, the relatively limited range of materials currently available as media for 3D printing, an obvious first step to producing useful imaging phantoms with 3D printing is to print containers (and inclusions) to hold (and displace) conventional materials already known to effectively mimic tissues in the configuration desired. Two very different examples from the literature are shown in Figs. 14.1 and 14.2.

Fig. 14.1 shows a 3D printed version of a commercial phantom used to examine resolution, attenuation, and concentration in PET-CT.[3] The 3D printed cylindrical container has many cylindrical holes of different diameter and spacing. The holes are filled with a radioactive fluid with known concentration of the given radioisotope of interest. This fluid can also contain predetermined concentrations of CT contrast agent (in this case containing iodine) designed to increase attenuation of CT photon beams. Images of a plane passing through the phantom show high intensity corresponding to the radioactive fluid—filled sources in the PET images and also high intensity corresponding to the high-attenuation fluid-filled cylinders in the CT images. (Note that for historical reasons related to use of film exposure and examination of what would be considered a "negative" exposure for diagnostic purposes, materials

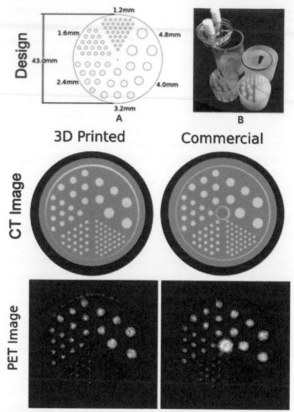

FIG. 14.1 Top: **(A)** Diagram and **(B)** photograph of the 3D printed and commercial micro deluxe phantoms. The 3D printed micro deluxe phantom is on the right of the photograph, and the commercial micro deluxe phantom is on the left. Middle: CT cross sections of each micro deluxe phantom filled with iodine contrast agent. Bottom: PET cross sections of each micro deluxe phantom filled with a solution containing 333 kBq/mL (9 µCi/mL) F-18. (Reproduced with permission, from reference Bieniosek MF, Lee BJ, Levin CS. Technical note: characterization of custom 3D printed multimodality imaging phantoms. *Med Phys.* 2015;42(10): 5913–5918.)

such as bone with high attenuation and which cast a low-signal shadow by blocking photons are shown as having a high intensity in planar X-ray and CT images.)

Fig. 14.2 shows images of a 3D printed anthropomorphic head phantom with four chambers designed to hold tissue-mimicking fluids or gels.[4] In this application, the four chambers were filled with gels designed to have electrical properties relevant to different tissue types for the purpose of measuring radiofrequency-induced heating and consequent temperature increase during MRI. CT of the empty phantom shows relatively high attenuation (high image intensity) from the 3D printed material and low attenuation in the empty chambers. Once the

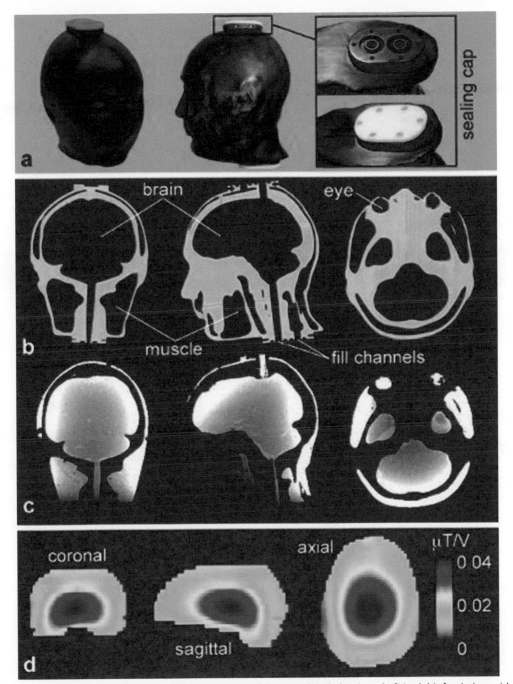

FIG. 14.2 Constructed phantom. **(A)** Photographs of the completed phantom. Left to right: front view, side view, and details of the mechanical sealing: o-ring indentations surrounding filling channels and small holes for screws (top) and screwed on sealing cap (bottom). **(B)** CT scan of the empty phantom. **(C)** MRI of completed phantom filled with gel. **(D)** B1+ map (magnitude) of the gel-filled phantom at 7T. (Reproduced with permission, from reference Graedel NN, Polimeni JR, Guerin B, Gagoski B, Bonmassar G, Wald LL. An anatomically realistic temperature phantom for radiofrequency heating measurements. *Magn Reson Med*. 2015;73(1):442–450.)

chambers are filled, MR images show high-signal intensity from the gel-filled chambers and low-signal intensity from the 3D printed material. Because tissues with low water content (such as fat and bone) also have low electric permittivity and electric conductivity, the chambers were only used to represent tissues with high water content, including brain, muscle, and the vitreous humor within the eyes. These tissues were mimicked by combining water with agar as a gelling agent, sodium azide to prohibit bacterial growth, sodium chloride to control electrical conductivity, and polyethylene to control electric permittivity.

As mentioned above, using 3D printing methods to produce containers for more conventional tissue-mimicking materials can make use of decades of research

into such materials. Since many tissue-mimicking materials are water based (as are many tissues), it is important to ensure that 3D printed containers are waterproof. Depending on the 3D printed material being used, methods of waterproofing may be necessary and can range from applying acetone to bond the outer material layer into a continuous waterproof surface, or coating (by dipping, spraying, or painting) the material with waterproofing substance.[4]

The composition of a conventional tissue-mimicking material is highly dependent on the imaging modality, application, and tissue of interest. Table 14.3 summarizes a number of representative approaches to mimicking tissue with conventional materials for various modalities and purposes.[3–20] Given the wide

TABLE 14.3
Examples of Approaches to Mimic Desired Material Properties with Conventional Methods.

Desired Material Property	Material Composition(s)	Reference(s)
Increase scatter and attenuation of high-energy photons (X-ray, CT, SPECT, PET)	- Water, silicone, or wax-based liquids, gels, or semisolids with differing amounts of liquid contrast agents (often containing iodine or barium) or powders with mineral or metallic content (W, Ti, $CaCO_3$)	3,5,6
	- Solid matrix of polystyrene/polypropylene mix with various amounts of metallic and mineral powders (TiO_2, MgO, $CaCO_3$, graphite)	7
	- Plaster to represent bone	8
Increase backscatter of ultrasonic waves	Incorporate microscopic glass spheres into liquid, silicone, or wax-based gel	9,10
Alter material stiffness and speed of ultrasonic waves	Adjust number of freeze/thaw cycles for PVA-C (cryogenic PVA)	11,12
Increase attenuation of ultrasonic waves	Adjust concentration of condensed milk compared to water in gel	10
Decrease T_1 (MRI)	- Gd-based contrast agent or Cu-EDTA with water-based liquid or gel	10,13,14
	- Increase concentration of glycerol	15
	- Increase concentration of nickel	16
	- Increase concentration of copper sulfate	17
	- Use oil, wax, or lipid-based material	18
Decrease T_2 (MRI)	- Increase agarose content in water-based liquid or gel	9,14–17
	- Add superparamagnetic iron oxide (SPIO)	18
	- Use oil, wax, or lipid-based material	18
Increase electrical conductivity	Increase concentration of NaCl in liquid or gel	4,21
Decrease electrical permittivity	- Increase concentration of sugar, polyethylene powder, or PVP	4,19,20
	- Use oil, wax, or lipid-based material	19

range of approaches used, the list is by no means comprehensive, but only representative.

Table 14.4 shows examples from the literature where 3D printed containers and inclusions are used to hold and shape or displace conventional phantom materials, with the 3D printed material being part of the final phantom, but not itself mimicking tissue.[3,4,22–26]

IMAGING PHANTOMS WITH CONVENTIONAL MATERIALS FORMED IN 3D PRINTED MOLDS

In many applications, a challenge for using 3D printed containers is that the container walls themselves may add an unrealistic partition between neighboring materials or unrealistic boundary around the phantom.

TABLE 14.4
Examples of Phantoms Where 3D Printed Materials Are Used to Contain and/or Displace Conventional Tissue-Mimicking Materials.

Phantom type	Printing technology and material(s)	Filling material(s)	Imaging modality	References
Geometric rods	Material jetting - VisitJet M3 (3D Systems, Rock, Hill, NC)	- Iodine contrast agent (CT) - 200uCi of FDG solution (MR)	- PET/CT - PET/MR	3
Cylindrical phantom with inserts	Material extrusion - Acrylonitrile butadiene styrene (ABS) P430 (Stratasys, Eden Prairie, MN)	- Radioactive solution of water and ^{18}FDG	- Radiation therapy	22
Anthropomorphic multimodality head phantom	Vat photopolymerization - Epoxy resin (brand information not available)	- Dipotassium phosphate to mimic bone - Agarose powder and distilled water to mimic brain - Distilled water for the ventricles - BANG®3-proTM Gel for the tumor surrogate	- CT - MRI - Radiation therapy - Proton therapy	20
Anthropomorphic MRI head phantom	Material extrusion - Polycarbonate and ABS (Stratasys, Eden Prairie, MN)	- Agar gels with polyethylene powder and NaCl to adjust electrical properties	MRI	4
Shepp–Logan phantom	Material extrusion - ABS (Stratasys, Eden Prairie, MN)	- Solutions consisting of various concentrations of common brain metabolites including N-acetyl-L-aspartic acid, choline chloride, creatine, and sodium L-lactate prepared in phosphate-buffered saline containing 0.02% sodium azide - Corn oil	MRS	24
Breast	Material extrusion - ABS (Stratasys, Eden Prairie, MN)	- Oil, water - Polyvinyl chloride (PVC) based and 3D printed inserts for quality assessment	MRI	25 26

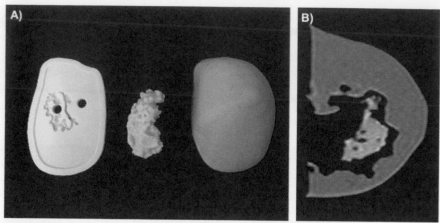

FIG. 14.3 3D Printed Breast Phantom model[25] showing **(A)** 3D printed breast phantom compartments printed with material extrusion (Fortus 360mc, Stratasys) with the base (left), FGT (middle), and breast (right). **(B)** Sagittal view of the 3D printed breast phantom acquired on a 7T magnet.

Fig. 14.3 shows a two-compartment 3D printed breast phantom, printed with material extrusion using polycarbonate, sealed with a watertight paint, and filled to mimic the dielectric properties of human breast tissue.[25] Herein, the fatty compartment was filled with peanut oil and the fibroglandular tissue (FGT) compartment was filled with a polyvinylpyrrolidone-based phantom material.[20] Note that the 3D printed material separating the compartments appears black in between the fat and FGT.

Many of the materials listed above can retain their shape. 3D printed molds can be used to shape conventional materials and then be removed, chemically or physically, once the tissue-mimicking material gels or hardens. Fig. 14.4 shows ultrasonic images of anthropomorphic kidney phantoms made of three different materials where the phantom was made by pouring the desired material into an outer 3D printed photopolymer mold partially filled with a previously 3D printed wax mold.[27] After the desired material solidifies, it is removed from the outer mold mechanically and the inner mold is dissolved with ethanol.

Table 14.5 provides examples of cases where 3D printing was used to create a mold and then the 3D printed component was removed after the compartment was filled.[28–32]

3D PRINTING FOR VASCULAR FLOW PHANTOMS

Patient-specific 3D printed vascular models allow for precise and repeatable flow experiments to be

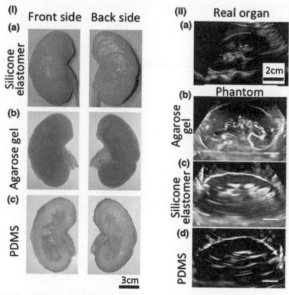

FIG. 14.4 Left: Photographs of the kidney phantoms made of different materials (front and back side): **(Ia)** Silicone elastomer, **(Ib)** Agarose gel, **(Ic)** PDMS. Right: Ultrasound images of **(IIa)** the human kidney in comparison to ultrasond images of the three models composed of **(IIb)** Agarose gel, **(IIc)** Silicone elastomer, and **(IId)** PDMS. The agarose model outperforms the other types of materials in terms of replicating the outer shape and tissue of the kidney, especially the appearance of the collection system, when compared to the real organ. (Reproduced with (open access) permission from reference Adams F, Qiu T, Mark A, et al. Soft 3D-printed phantom of the human kidney with collecting system. *Ann Biomed Eng.* 2017;45(4):963–972.)

TABLE 14.5

Examples of Publications with 3D Printed Molds Which Were Filled with Tissue-Mimicking Materials and Then the Mold Removed.

Phantom type	Printing Technology and Material(s)	Filling Material(s)	Imaging Modality	References
Neck	Material jetting - VeroClear (Stratasys, Eden Prairie, MN)	- Various agar solutions	- Ultrasound	28
Brain phantom	Material jetting - TangoPlus (Stratasys, Eden Prairie, MN)	- Polyvinyl alcohol	- CT - Ultrasound - MRI	29
Vascular phantom	Material extrusion - ABS	- Polyvinyl alcohol, dimethyl sulfide, and water	- MRI - Cone beam CT	30
Neck phantom including the trachea, skin, and vasculature	Binder jetting - Gypsum (3D Systems, Rock Hill, SC) Vat photopolymerization - Prime gray resin (iMaterialise, Materialise, Leuven, Belgium) Powder bed fusion - Polyamide (brand information not available)	- High concentration gelatin	- CT - Ultrasound	31
Pelvic phantom	Material jetting - VeroClear (Stratasys, Eden Prairie, MN)	- Gadolinium-based contrast agent and NaF - Vegetable oils - Vaseline and K_2HPO_4 - Agarose - Silicone	- CT and MRI	32

performed with simulated physiological blood flow conditions.[33,34] Vascular flow models of any vascular anatomy may be created, with most cases utilizing contrast-enhanced CT or MRI. 3D printed vascular phantoms may be used to simulate interventional procedures,[35] to determine flow-induced vascular remodeling,[36] to test thrombectomy devices and approaches,[37,38] and to assist with planning for cardiac valve replacement.[39] The use of 3D printed vascular models enables surgeons to better predict problems prior to performing the procedure. An example of a 3D printed vascular model is shown in Fig. 14.5.

MIMICKING TISSUE WITH 3D PRINTED MATERIALS

Although currently available 3D printing materials have a narrower range of imaging properties than

what can be achieved with other means, some 3D printed materials can effectively mimic tissue properties. For example, for X-ray imaging, Veneziani et al. created geometric plates of varying thicknesses using acrylonitrile butadiene styrene (ABS) and polylactic acid (PLA), two common types of plastics for material extrusion printing technologies,[40] and found that the attenuation coefficient ranged from 0.014 to 0.020 mm^{-1} for ABS and from 0.017 to 0.024 mm^{-1} for PLA, which corresponds to a range for soft tissues from fat to muscle. ABS, PLA, and a combination of PLA and stainless steel powder have also been evaluated with CT imaging, with the HU measuring -36, 160, and 810, resembling fat, muscle, and bone, respectively.[41] For CT, various material jetting materials have been evaluated at varying tube potentials, with the HU ranging from approximately 40 to 130

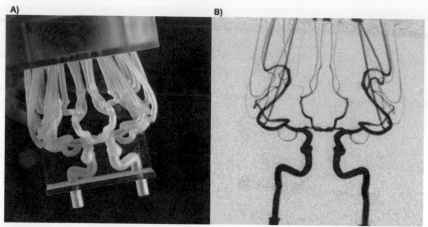

FIG. 14.5 **(A)** 3D printed anterior neurovascular phantom printed with a J750 (Stratasys, Eden Prairie, MN) using VeroClear material for the support and Agilus for the vascular structures. **(B)** Angiogram demonstrating flow simulation using the 3D printed model, smaller arteries are 300 microns diameter. (Figures courtesy of Ciprian Ionita, PhD, University of Buffalo.)

HU.[42] This HU range corresponds to that in some soft tissues and fats.

The MRI properties of the RGD-525 material jetting material (Stratasys, Rehovot, Israel) have also been evaluated using a 3 T magnet, with T_1 and T_2 relaxation times equal to 193.5 ± 2.2 and 32.8 ± 0.2 ms, respectively.[43] For clinical MRI, it is difficult to match true tissue characteristics, since these materials must be rich in hydrogen having relatively long relaxation rates, which is uncommon for most commercially available 3D printing materials that are plastic (rich in hydrogen but in a solid form), powder, or metal based.

In regard to ultrasound imaging, sound waves must be able to propagate through, and be backscattered by, the printed material in a manner similar to tissue. While conventional materials have been developed to mimic ultrasonic properties of tissue (Table 14.3, Fig. 14.4), readily available 3D printed materials have yet to demonstrate appropriate wave propagation or wave backscattering (Fig. 14.6).[44]

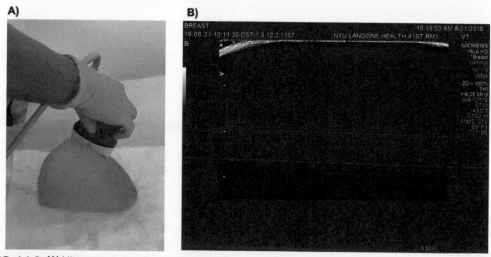

FIG. 14.6 **(A)** Ultrasound of a 3D printed breast phantom printed on the Stratasys J750 with a combination of tissue matrix and VeroClear materials. **(B)** Corresponding ultrasound image demonstrating no signal in the 3D printed model.

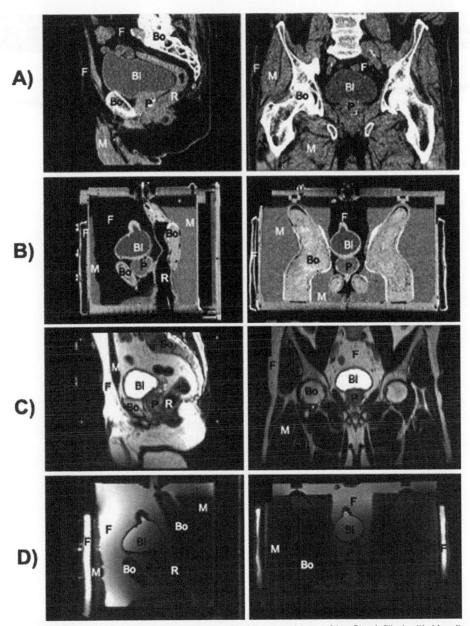

FIG. 14.7 3D printed pelvis phantom prototype with 3D printed bone (VeroClear) filled with Vaseline and K_2HPO_4 for marrow; Agar gel–based organs made with 3D printed molds. **(A)** Patient CT at 120 kVp, **(B)** CT of the phantom at 120 kVp, **(C)** T_2-weighted MRI of patient, **(D)** T_2-weighted MRI of phantom all with the sagittal views (left) and coronal views (right). The muscle-simulating gel surrounds the bone inside the phantom. A 3D printed placeholder in the center of the phantom is used to create the cavity for the organs and oil, when the gel is poured into the cylinder. *Bl*, bladder; *Bo*, bone; *F*, fat; *M*, muscle; *P*, prostate; *R*, rectum; *S*, syringe. (Reproduced with permission, from reference Niebuhr NI, Johnen W, Güldaglar T, et al. Radiological properties of tissue surrogates used in a multimodality deformable pelvic phantom for MR-guided radiotherapy. *Med Phys*. 2016;43(2):908–916.)

TABLE 14.6
Examples Where a 3D Printed Material Represents Tissue Directly in the Image.

Phantom Type	Printing Technology and Material(s)	Filling Material(s)	Imaging Modality	References
Breast	Material jetting - VeroClear, TangoPlus, Tissue Matrix (Stratasys, Eden Prairie, MN)	None	Ultrasound	44
Thorax (lung, liver), deformable with air inflating and deflating lungs	Material extrusion - Flexible thermoplastic polyurethane (Jinhua Xinke 3D Technology Co, Ltd Zhejiang, China)	Polyorganosiloxane gel with flexible plastic structures for liver (molded)	CT, MRI	45
Lung	Material jetting - Visijet EX200 (Projet HD 3000, 3D Systems, Rock Hill, SC)	None	CT	46
Head	Material extrusion - PLA (Ninjabot NJB-300 W)	Plaster (for bone)	CT	8
Radioactive sphere	Material jetting - Visijet FTX (3D Systems, Rock Hill, SC) Green doped with ^{99}Tc	None	SPECT	47
Neurovascular phantom	Material jetting - Vero White and Tango Black (Stratasys, Eden Prairie, MN)	ICG—bovine blood mixture with 3.2 µM of ICG (Pulsion Medical Inc., Powell, OH, USA), and IR800—bovine blood mixture with 50 nM of IR800 (IRDye800 800CW Carboxylate, LI-COR, Lincoln, NE, USA)	Near-infrared fluorescence imaging	48
Pelvic phantom	Material jetting - VeroClear (Stratasys, Eden Prairie, MN)	- Gadolinium-based contrast agent and NaF - Vegetable oils - Vaseline and K_2HPO_4 - Agarose - Silicone	- CT and MRI	32
Breast phantom	Material jetting - TangoPlus and Vero PureWhite (Stratasys, Eden Prairie, MN) - Jf Flexible (Molecule Digital LLC, Concord, CA) - Jf Flexible with tungsten doping (US Research Nanomaterials Inc., Houston, TX)	None	X-ray mammography	49

TABLE 14.6
Examples Where a 3D Printed Material Represents Tissue Directly in the Image.—cont'd

Phantom Type	Printing Technology and Material(s)	Filling Material(s)	Imaging Modality	References
Cortical bone	Vat photopolymerization, photopolymer resin (Prismlab China Ltd, Shanghai, China) for bone	Gd-doped water is used to mimic soft tissues	MRI	60
Three types: 1. Distortion model 2. Solid tumor model 3. Test object for textural analysis	Material jetting - Material 1: RGD-525, Material 2: Objet Vero white plus (RGD-325), Material 3: Objet support (SUP-705) (Stratasys, Eden Prairie, MN)	None	CT, MRI	51

Due to the limitations of using printed materials themselves to mimic human tissue properties, in many cases the 3D printed material is included in a phantom with conventional tissue-mimicking materials, and even acting as a container of these materials at the same time. For example, a 3D printed material can represent bone tissue in a 3D printed skull that at the same time contains conventional material used to represent brain tissue. Fig. 14.7 shows a phantom where a 3D printed material is used to represent bone, the 3D printed bone contains a material to represent bone marrow, and soft-tissue materials are created by filling 3D printed molds with other materials.[32] Table 14.6 includes examples where a 3D printed material represents tissue directly in the image.

SUMMARY

Just as 3D printing is developing and spreading rapidly, so are its applications in medical imaging, including its use in producing imaging phantoms. Here, we present a survey of methods and materials used until now in producing phantoms for major medical imaging modalities. To be sure, this survey includes only a small portion of the work on this subject, and new methods and materials are constantly being introduced. We also only included the most well-known medical imaging methodologies utilized today, while 3D phantoms can also be produced for new imaging methods that may well be more common in the future including, for example, Optical Coherence Tomography.[52] Nonetheless, we hope this provides a starting point for those new to the concept

and a resource reflecting a variety of the approaches to 3D printing imaging phantoms used today. Finally, despite the large amount of work that has been done attempting to characterize the imaging properties of 3D printed materials, there is a large unmet need for printable materials that are truly compatible with multimodality imaging. In the future, by customizing printing mediums with inclusion of additives, it can be possible to mimic tissues more closely than with standard manufacturer-issued media.

REFERENCES

1. Filippou V, Tsoumpas C. Recent advances on the development of phantoms using 3D printing for imaging with CT, MRI, PET, SPECT, and ultrasound. *Med Phys*. 2018;45(9):e740–760.
2. Fieremans E, De Deene Y, Delputte S, Özdemir MS, Achten E, Lemahieu I. The design of anisotropic diffusion phantoms for the validation of diffusion weighted magnetic resonance imaging. *Phys Med Biol*. 2008;53(19):5405.
3. Bieniosek MF, Lee BJ, Levin CS. Technical note: characterization of custom 3D printed multimodality imaging phantoms. *Med Phys*. 2015;42(10):5913–5918.
4. Graedel NN, Polimeni JR, Guerin B, Gagoski B, Bonmassar G, Wald LL. An anatomically realistic temperature phantom for radiofrequency heating measurements. *Magn Reson Med*. 2015;73(1):442–450.
5. Lee M-Y, Han B, Jenkins C, Xing L, Suh T-S. A depth-sensing technique on 3D-printed compensator for total body irradiation patient measurement and treatment planning. *Med Phys*. 2016;43:6137–6144.
6. Hokamp NG, Obmann VC, Kessner R, et al. Improved visualization of hypodense liver lesions in virtual monoenergetic images from spectral detector CT: proof of concept

in a 3D-printed phantom and evaluation in 74 patients. *Eur J Radiol;*109:114—123.

7. Homolka P, Gahleitner A, Prokop M, Nowotny R. Optimization of the composition of phantom materials for computed tomography. *Phys Med Biol.* 2002;47(16): 2907.

8. Kadoya N, Abe K, Nemoto H, et al. Evaluation of a 3D-printed heterogeneous anthropomorphic head and neck phantom for patient-specific quality assurance in intensity-modulated radiation therapy. *Radiol Phys Tech.* 2019;12(3):351—356.

9. Maneas E, Xia W, Nikitichev DI, et al. Anatomically realistic ultrasound phantoms using gel wax with 3D printed moulds. *Phys Med Biol.* 2018;63(1):015033.

10. D'Souza WD, Madsen EL, Unal O, Vigen KK, Frank GR, Thomadsen BR. Tissue mimicking materials for a multi-imaging modality prostate phantom. *Med Phys.* 2001; 28(4):688—700.

11. Morais P, Tavares JM, Queirós S, Veloso F, D'hooge J, Vilaça JL. Development of a patient-specific atrial phantom model for planning and training of inter-atrial interventions. *Med Phys.* 2017;44(11):5638—5649.

12. Laing J, Moore JT, Vassallo R, Bainbridge D, Drangova M, Peters TM. Patient-specific cardiac phantom for clinical training and preprocedure surgical planning. *J Med Imaging.* 2018;5(2):021222.

13. Sasaki M, Shibata E, Kanbara Y, Ehara S. Enhancement effects and relaxivities of gadolinium-DTPA at 1.5 versus 3 Tesla: a phantom study. *Magn Reson Med Sci.* 2005;4(3): 145—149.

14. Ikemoto Y, Takao W, Yoshitomi K, et al. Development of a human-tissue-like phantom for 3.0-T MRI. *Med Phys.* 2011;38:6336—6342.

15. Blechinger JC, Madsen EL, Frank GR. Tissue-mimicking gelatin-agar gels for use in magnetic resonance imaging phantoms. *Med Phys.* 1988;15:629—636.

16. Christoffersson JO, Olsson LE, Sjoberg S. Nickel-doped agarose-gel phantoms in MR imaging. *Acta Radiol.* 1991; 32:426—431.

17. Mitchell MD, Kundel HL, Axel L, Joseph PM. Agarose as a tissue equivalent phantom material for NMR imaging. *Magn Reson Imaging.* 1986;4:263—266.

18. Hines CD, Yu H, Shimakawa A, McKenzie CA, Brittain JH, Reeder SB. T1 independent, T2* corrected MRI with accurate spectral modeling for quantification of fat: validation in a fat-water-SPIO phantom. *J Magn Reson Imag.* 2009; 30(5):1215—1222.

19. Duan Q, Duyn JH, Gudino N, et al. Characterization of a dielectric phantom for high-field magnetic resonance imaging applications. *Med Phys.* 2014;41(10):102303.

20. Ianniello C, de Zwart JA, Duan Q, et al. Synthesized tissue-equivalent dielectric phantoms using salt and polyvinyl-pyrrolidone solutions. *Magn Reson Med.* 2018;80(1): 413—419.

21. Neves AL, Leroi L, Cochinaire N, Abdeddaim R, Sabouroux P, Vignaud A. Mimicking the electromagnetic distribution in the human brain: a multi-frequency MRI head phantom. *Appl Magn Reson.* 2017;48:213—226.

22. Cerviño L, Soultan D, Cornell M, et al. A novel 3D-printed phantom insert for 4D PET/CT imaging and simultaneous integrated boost radiotherapy. *Med Phys.* 2017;44(10): 5467—5474.

23. Gallas RR, Hünemohr N, Runz A, Niebuhr NI, Jäkel O, Greilich S. An anthropomorphic multimodality (CT/MRI) head phantom prototype for end-to-end tests in ion radiotherapy. *Zeitschrift fuer Medizinische Physik.* 2015;25(4):391—399.

24. Kasten JA, Vetterli T, Lazeyras F, Van De Ville D. 3D-printed shepp-logan phantom as a real-world benchmark for MRI. *Magn Reson Med.* 2016;75(1):287—294.

25. Wake N, Ianniello C, Brown R, et al. 3D printed patient-specific dual compartment breast phantom for validating MRI acquisition and analysis techniques. *Trans Addit Manuf Meets Med.* 2019;1(1).

26. He Y, Liu Y, Dyer BA, et al. 3D-printed breast phantom for multi-purpose and multi-modality imaging. *Quant Imaging Med Surg.* 2019;9(1):63—74. https://doi.org/10.21037/qims.2019.01.05.

27. Adams F, Qiu T, Mark A, et al. Soft 3D-printed phantom of the human kidney with collecting system. *Ann Biomed Eng.* 2017;45(4):963—972.

28. Baba M, Matsumoto K, Yamasaki N, et al. Development of a tailored thyroid gland phantom for fine-needle aspiration cytology by three-dimensional printing. *J Surg Educ.* 2017;74(6):1039—1046.

29. Chen SJ, Hellier P, Marchal M, et al. An anthropomorphic polyvinyl alcohol brain phantom based on Colin27 for use in multimodal imaging. *Med Phys.* 2012;39(1):554—561.

30. Chueh JY, Van Der Marel K, Gounis MJ, et al. Development of a high resolution MRI intracranial atherosclerosis imaging phantom. *J Neurointerventional Surg.* 2018;10(2):143—149.

31. Javan R, Cho AL. An assembled prototype multimaterial three-dimensional—printed model of the neck for computed tomography—and ultrasound-guided interventional procedures. *J Comput Assist Tomogr.* 2017;41(6):941—948.

32. Niebuhr NI, Johnen W, Güldaglar T, et al. Radiological properties of tissue surrogates used in a multimodality deformable pelvic phantom for MR-guided radiotherapy. *Med Phys.* 2016;43(2):908—916.

33. O'Hara RP, Chand A, Vidiyala S, et al. Advanced 3D mesh manipulation in stereolithographic files and post-print processing for the manufacturing of patient-specific vascular flow phantoms. *Proc SPIE Int Soc Opt Eng.* 2016:9789.

34. Sommer K, Izzo RL, Shepard L, et al. Design optimization for accurate flow simulations in 3D printed vascular phantoms derived from computed tomography angiography. *Proc SPIE Int Soc Opt Eng.* 2017:10138.

35. Kaschwich M, Dell A, Matysiak F, et al. Development of an ultrasound-capable phantom with patient-specific 3D-printed vascular anatomy to simulate peripheral endovascular interventions. *Ann Anat.* 2020;232:151563.

36. Tutino VM, Rajabzadeh-Oghaz H, Chandra AR, et al. 9.4T magnetic resonance imaging of the mouse circle of Willis enables serial characterization of flow-induced vascular remodeling by computational fluid dynamics. *Curr Neurovasc Res.* 2018;15(4):312—325.

37. Mokin M, Ionita CN, Nagesh SV, Rudin S, Levy EI, Siddiqui AH. Primary stentriever versus combined stentriever plus aspiration thrombectomy approaches: in vitro stroke model comparison. *J Neurointerventional Surg.* 2015;7(6):453–457.

38. Mokin M, Setlur Nagesh SV, Ionita CN, Mocco J, Siddiqui AH. Stent retriever thrombectomy with the cover accessory device versus proximal protection with a balloon guide catheter: in vitro stroke model comparison. *J Neurointerventional Surg.* 2016;8(4):413–417.

39. Izzo RL, O'Hara RP, Iyer V, et al. 3D printed cardiac phantom for procedural planning of a transcatheter native mitral valve replacement. *Proc SPIE Int Soc Opt Eng.* 2016:9789.

40. Veneziani GR, Correa E, Potiens PA, Campos LL. Attenuation coefficient determination of printed ABS and PLA samples in diagnostic radiology standard beams. *J Phys: Conf Ser.* 2016;733.

41. Abdel-Magid BVD, Vrieze T, Leng S. Composite materials for 3D printing of medical phantoms. *Paper Presented at: 5th Annual Composites and Advanced Materials Expo, CAMX 20182018; Dallas.*

42. Leng S, Chen B, Vrieze T, et al. Construction of realistic phantoms from patient images and a commercial three-dimensional printer. *J Med Imaging.* 2016;3(3):033501.

43. Mitsouras D, Lee TC, Liacouras P, et al. Three-dimensional printing of MRI-visible phantoms and MR image-guided therapy simulation. *Magn Reson Med.* 2017;77(2):613–622.

44. Ali A, Wahab R, Huynh J, Wake N, Mahoney M. Imaging properties of 3D printed breast phantoms for lesion localization and core needle biopsy training. *3D Print Med.* 2020;6(1):4.

45. Colvill E, Krieger M, Bosshard P, et al. Anthropomorphic phantom for deformable lung and liver CT and MR imaging for radiotherapy. *Phys Med Biol.* 2020;65(7):07NT02.

46. Hernandez-Giron I, den Harder JM, Streekstra GJ, Geleijns J, Veldkamp WJ. Development of a 3D printed anthropomorphic lung phantom for image quality assessment in CT. *Phys Med.* 2019;57:47–57.

47. Läppchen. *3D Printing of Radioactive Phantoms for Nuclear Medicine Imaging.* 2020.

48. Liu Y, Ghassemi P, Depkon A, et al. Biomimetic 3D-printed neurovascular phantoms for near-infrared fluorescence imaging. *Biomed Optic Express.* 2018;9(6):2810–2824.

49. Rossman AH, Catenacci M, Zhao C, et al. Three-dimensionally-printed anthropomorphic physical phantom for mammography and digital breast tomosynthesis with custom materials, lesions, and uniform quality control region. *J Med Imaging.* 2019;6(2):021604.

50. Rai R, Manton D, Jameson MG, et al. 3D printed phantoms mimicking cortical bone for the assessment of ultrashort echo time magnetic resonance imaging. *Med Phys.* 2018;45(2):758–766. https://doi.org/10.1002/mp.12727.

51. Rai R, Wang YF, Manton D, Dong B, Deshpande S, Liney GP. Development of multi purpose 3D printed phantoms for MRI. *Phys Med Biol.* March 29, 2019;64(7):075010. https://doi.org/10.1088/1361-6560/ab0b49.

52. Dong E, Zhao Z, Wang M, et al. Three-dimensional fuse deposition modeling of tissue-simulating phantom for biomedical optical imaging. *J Biomed Optic.* 2015;20(12):121311.

CHAPTER 15

Considerations for Starting a 3D Printing Lab in the Department of Radiology

NICOLE WAKE, PHD

INTRODUCTION

Medical three-dimensional (3D) printing provides essential services within the modern hospital system. Patient-specific 3D printed anatomic models are used clinically to provide improved understanding of anatomy, more exact pathology evaluation, and more precise surgical intervention. 3D printed anatomic models can be used for many applications including presurgical planning, intraoperative guidance, trainee education, and patient counseling. Furthermore, 3D printed anatomic guides created from the patient's imaging data can positively impact patient care by improving procedural accuracy.[1,2] By allowing for improved understanding of anatomy, enabling precontouring of implants, and providing real-time guidance in the operating room (OR), 3D printed anatomic models and guides can reduce OR costs secondary to shortening procedure times.[3–7]

Surgeons have a low margin of error when providing care. Their goal is to obtain the best outcome on the first attempt, which may be challenging for high-complexity cases, even for the most experienced surgeons. Although both radiologists and surgeons are skillful at interpreting two-dimensional (2D) images, errors in interpretation may occur.[8] Furthermore, mentally reconstructing 2D images into 3D representations is challenging. In the operative setting, surgeons are frequently conflicted in both their assessment of 2D images as well as their 3D interpretation where having an incorrect understanding of the true anatomy may potentially lead to an inappropriate surgical approach, increased operative times, and complications which all may impair patient outcomes.[9,10] Putting a physical 3D printed model of the anatomy in the hands of the surgeons allows them to see the true anatomy first-hand, thereby minimizing the chance of interpretation error and allowing them to be better prepared for the procedure.[9]

In order to create patient-specific 3D printed anatomic models and guides, Digital Imaging and Communication in Medicine (DICOM) images are first acquired from any volumetric imaging modality (see Chapter 2). Computed tomography (CT) is the most common modality due to the ease of post-processing CT data, but magnetic resonance imaging (MRI) and ultrasound imaging are also utilized. Using the DICOM images, the desired anatomical regions of interest (ROIs) are then segmented, and the segmented ROIs are converted to a computer-aided design (CAD) format in preparation for printing (see Chapters 3 and 4). Since the source data for these 3D printed models are the volumetric radiological imaging data, it is logical for a point of care 3D printing lab to be housed in the radiology department. However, collaboration across specialties is necessary and perhaps even having a synergistic partnership with related departments will be key to a successful lab.

Many hospitals already have a 3D Imaging Lab within their Department of Radiology that produces 3D volume renderings of anatomy to assist with visualization and surgical planning. This type of 3D visualization on a 2D display is limited though and does not provide the same depth as actually seeing the anatomy in 3D. The human visual system is highly dependent on visualization spatial relationships in 3D. Compared to 2D displays, 3D displays have been demonstrated to improve depth perception, decrease surgical times, and decrease perceived workflow for laparoscopic surgeries.[11]

The timing for expanding an existing 3D Imaging Lab to include 3D printing services or opening a dedicated radiology-centered 3D printing lab is ideal based on the academic landscape, technological advances in image processing and 3D printing, and the emerging regulatory and reimbursement environments surrounding

3D Printing for the Radiologist. https://doi.org/10.1016/B978-0-323-77573-1.00002-6

3D printing–based technologies. Including 3D printing in-house at the point of care will enhance best practices by making 3D printing more accessible for the end user, ultimately leading to improved patient care, increased patient satisfaction, and cost savings for the healthcare system.[12,13]

3D printing technology is impacting the practice of medicine in almost every way imaginable. High-profile cases like the separation of conjoined twins and face transplant have been in the media's eye.[14–17] More day-to-day applications such as planning for orthopedic tumor surgery, facial reconstruction, and total knee replacement are on the rise, impacting at least tens of thousands of patients across the United States. By providing 3D anatomical models, doctors gain an insight that cannot be replicated by any form of medical diagnostics. In addition, medical student and surgeon training programs across specialties can benefit from use of the latest digital and physical training tools, in many cases offsetting or augmenting cadaveric practice sessions.

In the past, as mentioned in Chapter 6, 3D printing was available only through outside vendors, resulting in expensive costs (Table 15.1). Recent innovations have made this technology accessible to many hospitals. Insourcing this work in a centralized 3D printing and advanced visualization facility can enhance patient care by shortening the time between ordering a model and holding it. A dedicated 3D printing lab will also enhance trainee education, support cutting-edge research, and will bring increased revenue and grant funding to the institution. This chapter will discuss considerations for starting a 3D Printing Lab within a Department of Radiology.

FINANCIAL PLAN

Establishing a dedicated hospital-based 3D printing lab requires administrative support, physician leadership and guidance, biomedical engineers and technologist champions, and printing technicians. The financial plan for the 3D printing lab must include personnel costs as well as expenses for the construction or renovation of physical space, hardware and software expenses including maintenance costs, and potential revenue for 3D printed models (including clinical revenue via Category III CPT codes and research revenue).

In regard to staffing, determining the number of full-time equivalent staff will be based on the anticipated case volume. It is likely that most labs will start out small and will grow over time. To start out with, a lab could have one physician who serves as the medical director, performing image segmentation of complex

TABLE 15.1

List of Commercially Available 3D Printing Services and Types of 3D Printed Models.

Model Type	Vendors

ANATOMIC MODELS (RADIOLOGY FOCUSED)	- 3D Systems Healthcare (Littleton, CO)
	  - *On-demand anatomical models*
	- Materialise (Leuven, Belgium)
	  - *HeartPrint and other*
	- TeraRecon (Durham, NC)
	  - *Partnership with WhiteClouds*
	- Vital Images (Minnetonka, MN)
	  - *Partnership with Stratasys (Eden Prairie, MN)*

ANATOMIC MODELS (SURGERY FOCUSED) AND GUIDES/TEMPLATES/VIRTUAL SURGICAL PLANNING	
- Craniomaxillofacial (CMF)	- DePuy Synthes (West Chester, PA) and Materialise (Leuven, Belgium) - KLS Martin (Tuttlingen, Germany) - Osteomed (Addison, TX) and MedCad (Dallas, TX) - Stryker (Kalamazoo, MI) and 3D Systems Healthcare (Littleton, CO) - Zimmer-Biomet (Warsaw, IN)
- Spine	- K2M (Leesburg, VA) - Medtronic (Minneapolis, MN) - Mighty Oak Medical (Denver, CO)
- Orthopedic	- Zimmer-Biomet (Warsaw, IN)
PERSONALIZED IMPLANTS	
- Craniomaxillofacial (CMF)	- DePuy Synthes (West Chester, PA) and Materialise (Leuven, Belgium) - KLS Martin (Tuttlingen, Germany) - Osteomed (Addison, TX) and MedCad (Dallas, TX) - Stryker (Kalamazoo, MI) and 3D Systems Healthcare (Littleton, CO) - Zimmer-Biomet (Warsaw, IN)
- Orthopedic/Other	- 4Web (Frisco, TX) - K2M (Leesburg, VA) - Onkos (Parsippany, NJ) - Ossis (Christchurch, New Zealand)

anatomy and overseeing the printing process, as well as one technologist who performs basic image segmentation, runs the printers, and post-processes the models. Over time, based on the needs of the lab, this would expand to include more physicians, more technologists, biomedical engineers to carry out the design work especially for anatomic guides, and potentially could include printer technicians to run and maintain the printing hardware.

For the first few years, it is expected that the 3D printing lab will not generate significant revenue. However, over time this is expected to change, especially once Category I CPT codes are established for 3D printed anatomic models and anatomic guides. Until there is full reimbursement for 3D printed models, in order to cover some of the costs of running the lab, it is possible that surgical departments requesting 3D printed models will contribute money for image postprocessing and material cost based on the number of models requested. Grant or donor funds may also be utilized to help sustain the costs of running the lab.

At the time of writing, the price of a 3D printed anatomic reference model could range from approximately $1,000 to $5,000 USD depending on the printing technologies and materials used, and 3D printed guides and templates could range from approximately $1,500 to $10,000 USD per case. Although there is an up-front cost to purchase software and hardware, over time the cost of 3D printing at the point of care is expected to be much more cost-effective than outsourcing to vendors. Indirect benefits of 3D printing for the hospital include decreased operation times, decreased complications, improved patient outcomes, and improved patient and physician satisfaction. Future work will be performed to evaluate which case types are created in-house, to quantitatively measure how these models can positively impact patient care, and to determine the actual cost savings.

TRAINING

There are currently no formal training programs for physicians interested to take the lead on medical 3D printing, therefore physicians must self-train to become proficient in the 3D printing process. For technologists interested in medical 3D printing, there is now a certificate program through Clarkson College which prepares imaging professionals to be knowledgeable and proficient in the medical 3D printing process.[18] However, most established technologists, especially those already doing 3D image post-processing in dedicated 3D imaging labs, would most likely not return to school at this

time. Technologists such as those who are proficient in 3D image post-processing may learn to perform image segmentation and CAD work as an extension of their current 3D visualization methods. Biomedical engineers may also be interested to perform some of this work and specific training will depend on their knowledge of medical imaging modalities as well as anatomy.

Once a 3D printing technologist or biomedical engineer is hired, the learning curve for performing adequate image segmentation, CAD, and printing is generally steep. An organized training program with defined and measurable objectives for each step of the process will help to set clear expectations. In order to build the optimized workflow and to integrate in the hospital infrastructure, the employee will become proficient in the following: (1) Understanding of diagnostic medical image acquisition techniques required for advanced visualization techniques and 3D modeling, (2) Mastering 3D image post-processing methods including segmentation, registration, and creation of 3D surface meshes, (3) Proper documentation and storage of design files, (4) Printing processes and materials, (5) Working with clinical teams to deliver and view models, and (6) Quality Assurance (QA) of 3D models.

SOFTWARE CONSIDERATIONS

Many hospitals and hospital systems may have institution-wide licenses for 3D image post-processing and these software packages might have the capability to export segmented ROIs into CAD file formats. Examples of commonly used 3D image post-processing platforms with these capabilities include the Intellispace Portal (Philips, Amsterdam, Netherlands), Aquarius (Terarecon, Durham, NC), Advanced Workstation (GE Healthcare, Waukesha, WI), and Vitrea (Vital Images, Minnetonka, MN). If possible, these platforms, which many technologists are already familiar with, could be utilized to create 3D printed anatomic models. Specific 3D printing software packages are also available and may provide added benefits in regard to ease of segmentation as well as CAD modeling following the segmentation process. It is also important to note that for 3D printed medical models used at the point of care, it is recommended that FDA-cleared software is utilized.[19] Costs for this type of software are approximately $10,000–$20,000 USD per license and may be perpetual or yearly licenses. Floating licenses may also be available for an increased cost. Note that for certain software there are minimum hardware requirements.

The stereolithography (STL) file format and other file formats utilized to create 3D printed models do not contain DICOM information, which is important in order to properly store this information in a patient's medical record. At this time, DICOM Working Group-17 has worked to establish the DICOM 2018b standard where 3D file information in an STL format is contained within a DICOM Information Object.[20] To date, one vendor has incorporated the new DICOM-encapsulated STL standard into their image segmentation platform.[21] Integration of the DICOM format will allow for STL files to be traceable and properly integrated into a patient's medical record. It is expected that more image post-processing platforms and Picture Archiving and Communication System (PACS) vendors will support these file types in the future. Until then, in order to properly archive these files, the files should be stored on a secure, backed-up network, and limited representative images of the segmentation and model may be sent to PACS systems to be stored in the patient medical record.

3D PRINTING OPERATIONAL CONSIDERATIONS

Herein, five 3D printing technologies have been introduced as potential workhorses for the medical 3D printing laboratory: material extrusion, polymer powder bed fusion, binder jetting, material jetting, and vat photopolymerization. It is important to plan and anticipate the operational requirements and specifications for these different process types. As an aid to understanding these, five representative printers are identified with specific characteristics and requirements of each type (Table 15.2).

Space Planning

Sufficient space must be provided in the 3D lab to house the printers, storage cabinet(s), post-processing equipment, and work tables. Each printer must have operational access as well as sufficient clearance to allow maintenance access to the printer. Floors must be level and vibration free with sufficient load

capability for the machine installation. In addition, some of the larger printers may require widened door and elevator openings to move the equipment into the 3D printing lab site. If multiple printers are to be installed, it is important that each printer be oriented such that the exhausts from one printer do not direct air into an adjacent printer. Workflows for operational efficiency should be considered in printer placement in the lab. Any wet benches or sinks used for model cleaning should not be installed in close proximity to the printers. A sample layout for a medium-sized 3D printing lab with a single advanced technology printer and several desktop systems is as shown in Fig. 15.1. The area required for this lab is approximately 900 square feet. When planning space, the proximity to clinical colleagues and OR facilities must also be considered.

Environmental

Most 3D printers can be powered from standard 110 Volt (V) or 240 V single-phase power supplies, while larger systems can require a dedicated 20 Amp-110 V or equivalent circuit. Some of the more complicated systems such as the high volume HP Jet Fusion 4200 require a dedicated 220 V three-phase power supply. Uninterruptible power supplies are recommended to ensure a consistent voltage supply and high quality during printing. While many of the available systems have software that can restart at the printing point where a power failure occurs, these types of software are not fail-safe and will not guarantee a long-running print job that will be successfully completed if interrupted by a power failure.

One common characteristic of 3D printers is the use of heat to cure deposited material. Extruder nozzles, hot build plates, laser, ultraviolet (UV), and infrared light are all prolific heat generators and this heat must be dissipated out of the machine. The amount of heat generated is dependent on machine size and process type. Some typical heat ratings are as shown in Table 15.3.

TABLE 15.2
Selected Representative Printers for a Hospital-Based 3D Printing Lab to Consider.

Technology	Printer Model	Printer Brand	Approximate Cost (USD $)
Material extrusion	S5	Ultimaker (Utrecht, Netherlands)	$5,000
Powder bed fusion	Jet Fusion 4200	HP (Palo Alto, CA)	$200,000
Binder jetting	Projet CJP 660Pro	3D Systems (Rock Hill, SC)	$70,000
Material jetting	J750	Stratasys (Eden Prairie, MN)	$300,000
Vat photopolymerization	Form 3 (SLA)	Formlabs (Cambridge, MA)	$5,000

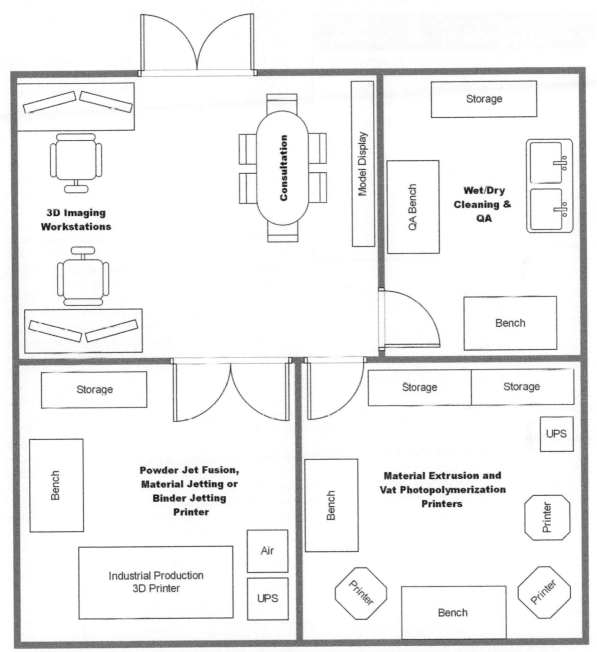

FIG. 15.1 Example layout of an approximately 900 sq ft 3D printing lab including a space for 3D imaging workstations, consultation, industrial production printers, and desktop printers. (Note that UPS = Uninterruptible Power Supply).

Sufficient air conditioning must be provided to extract this heat if expelled within the lab and to maintain a constant temperature in the 20−25°C range with relative humidity 30%−70% noncondensing. The room ventilation system should also provide regular purging of the room air, typically four times per hour.

Modern 3D printers may require cloud connectivity to monitor operation, perform software/firmware

TABLE 15.3
Heat Output for Certain 3D Printing Technologies.

Process	Machine Type	Approximate Heat Output (Watts)
Material extrusion	Ultimaker S5	500
Powder bed fusion	HP Jet Fusion 4200	2600
Binder jetting	3D Systems ProJet CJP 660Pro	1650
Material jetting	Stratasys J750	1485
Vat photopolymerization	Formlabs Form 3	220

updates, download print data, and successfully start prints. Internet access using ethernet or wi-fi is hence required for the 3D printer.

Auxiliary Equipment

Most 3D printers do not require auxiliary equipment to operate, but this is often required for larger, industrial machines. For example, larger systems such as the HP Jet Fusion 4200 and Stratasys J750 system require connection to external venting systems to expel exhaust heat and fumes. In addition, the 4200 system requires compressed air to operate and this air is also needed for an abrasive bead blasting system necessary to clean up finished powder bed fusion models. Another requirement for this type of machine is an explosion-proof vacuum cleaner to clean up powder residue on the model and the machine. Some systems, such as the Projet CLP 660Pro, have an integrated vacuum cleaner inside the build chamber for ease of access for cleaning between model generation. A standard vacuum cleaner would be a useful accessory for all 3D labs to clear any dust or residues within the printer enclosure.

3D Printing Materials

Material types and costs vary depending on the printing technology and printer type (Table 15.4). For 3D printed anatomic models and guides which will be utilized in the OR, models should be printed with biocompatible, sterilizable materials. Although several manufacturers offer sterilizable materials which may come with recommended instructions for use, it is important that the sterilization process is validated by each hospital. In regard to sterilization equipment, common techniques used in

hospitals include autoclave (also known as steam sterilization or moist heat),[22] ethylene oxide gas,[23] and gamma ray ionizing radiation.[24] Since hospitals generally have sterilization facilities which are usually housed close to ORs, it is recommended that these resources are utilized instead of individual 3D printing labs purchasing sterilization equipment.

Material extrusion filaments are readily available and often nonproprietary in a wide range of thermoplastics such as polylactic acid (PLA), acrylonitrile butadiene styrene (ABS), nylon, etc. The filament material is moisture sensitive and needs to be stored in a cool, dry, dark environment. Vacuum sealing helps to keep the filament dry for optimal use. Desiccants (moisture absorbent silica gel) are often used within the vacuum-sealed volume, and dehumidifiers can be used in filament storage areas to maintain a low humidity level and assist with filament life. Properly stored and sealed filament can have a shelf life of at least 1 year and possibly longer.

Powder bed fusion printers such as the HP Jet Fusion 4200 have fusing and detailing agents with a 3−5 L capacity in the standard model. Gloves are recommended when handling agents and proper disposal guidelines must be followed when agent cartridges are depleted. This system also has three printheads which need to be changed when warranted. A printhead cleaning roll is an additional consumable which needs to be replenished on reaching certain build volumes or print layers.

Binder jetting systems print using a core powder material and binding agents. The Projet CJP 660Pro has closed cartridges of these materials for ease of removal and recycling. Parts may be cleaned using Epson salt sprays reducing the need for cutting tools or toxic chemicals. The core power is typically sold in a 14 kg container, while clear and black binders are in 1L cartridges, and CMY (Cyan, Magenta, Yellow) color binding cartridges are provided in 300 mL sizes. Core material and binders need to be stored in a cool, dry, ventilated environment and have a shelf life of 1 year from the date of manufacture.

Material jetting printers use photopolymers or polymers that change properties usually when exposed to UV light. The Stratasys J750 printer can support up to twelve 3.6 kg cartridges of model material and four cartridges of support material. The cartridges should not come into contact with metal or UV radiation. They should be stored in a dry area with adequate ventilation and temperature/humidity control. Cartridge shelf life is limited and is etched on the container.

Vat photopolymerization uses a UV laser focused on the surface of the photopolymer resin which is photochemically solidified to form the 3D object. Proprietary resins are utilized on the Formlabs Form 3 printer; and

TABLE 15.4
Common Material Types and Costs for the Selected Printers.

Machine Type	Material Types	Proprietary	Approximate Cost per L/kg
Ultimaker S5	PLA, ABS	N	$20+/kg
HP Jet Fusion 4200	Nylon	Y	$150/kg
3D Systems ProJet CJP 660Pro	Core powder Clear, black, and color binding cartridges	Y	Core $100/kg Binder $250/L Black $250/L Colors $300/L
Stratasys J750	Photopolymer	Y	$350/kg
Formlabs Form 3	Resin	Y	$150/L

these include standard resins in various colors such as clear, white, black, and gray. Tough and durable, flexible and elastic, biocompatible dental, as well as other resins are also available in 1L cartridges. Resin may be stored in a resin tank for each type of resin. For long-term storage, resin should be poured into a separate, opaque container from the resin tank away from direct sunlight in a dry, cool, and well-ventilated area. Stored resins should be shaken every 2 weeks to keep resins thoroughly mixed.

Health and Safety

It is generally recommended that 3D printers are not located near employee workstations and should be housed in a separate partitioned room with negatively pressured area air flows and a dedicated ventilation system, away from other work areas. The dedicated ventilation system will help prevent migration of 3D printer emissions to other areas.

For material extrusion, which typically uses PLA and ABS thermoplastics to build desired objects, heating of these materials in extrusion nozzles can release ultrafine particles (UFPs) and volatile organic compounds which are harmful to bodily systems. Housing the 3D printer in suitable enclosures (for example, with a fume hood) and ensuring the area is well ventilated and refreshed with HEPA filters will help mitigate this exposure (Fig. 15.2).[25] The Ultimaker S5 can be equipped with an Air Manager that fully encloses the build chamber and creates an inside–out airflow through the filter that removes up to 95% of all UFPs. The Air Manager also acts as a barrier to stop anyone from touching hot or moving parts and interfering with prints, while simultaneously providing a more regulated internal environment for printing.

Powder jet fusion printers such as the Jet Fusion 4200 produce combustible dust within the build

chamber and this must be regularly cleaned using an explosion-protected vacuum cleaner. Again, suitable hand and eye protection must be used during the cleaning process.

3D printers that use UV light for curing, such as the Stratasys J750 and Formlabs Form 3, require the consumption of uncured materials which are considered hazardous in the uncured state and must be handled with care using neoprene or nitrile gloves. Safety glasses may also be required if there is a chance that printing materials will splash into the eyes. Common latex gloves are adequate for handling UV-cured models. The disposal of uncured material must also follow hazardous waste regulations as does liquid waste from the J750 printer.

3D printers contain hot surfaces such as extrusion nozzles, heat blocks, and UV lamps that can also cause skin injury and must be carefully approached. UV lamps and lasers used in curing are a potential eye hazard. Abrasive cleaning of models can also emit particles and sharp objects used in cleaning can produce abrasions and cuts. Chemicals such as sodium hydroxide are often used to clean support materials from models and these can be caustic and cause skin irritation. Care needs to be taken in such cleaning and suitable glove and eye protection needs to be utilized.

Most 3D printers do not emit significant noise, though high volume devices can generate more than 70 dB, which can damage hearing over a long period of time. Printer enclosures can mitigate production noise and hearing protection is advised when noise levels exceed 70 dB, for example, when fine core removal and vacuuming of binder jet printers.

It is important to incorporate 3D printing into standard workplace safety plans, develop standard operating procedures for 3D printers, and train workers on how to safely use and maintain them.

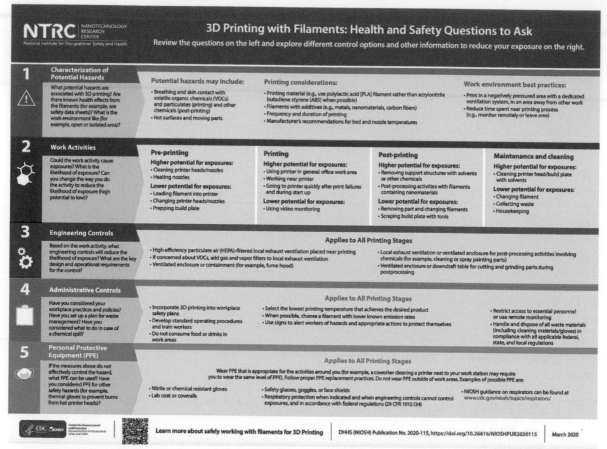

FIG. 15.2 Diagram showing health and safety questions that may be asked for material extrusion. (Reproduced with permission from Reference Glassford EDK, Dunn KH, Hammond D, Tyrawski J. *3D Printing with Filaments: Health and Safety Questions to Ask*. U.S, DHHS (NIOSH) Publication No. 2020-115: Department of Health and Human Services, Centers for Disease Control and Prevention, National Institute for Occupational Safety and Health; 2020. https://www.cdc.gov/niosh/docs/2020-115/pdfs/2020-115.pdf?id=10. 26616/NIOSHPUB2020115. Accessed 4 September 2020.)

Maintenance

All 3D printing technologies deposit and cure material and necessarily produce waste and process residuals. As such they require regular and extensive cleaning to ensure production model quality and efficiency.

Some printers use and deposit support filament during model construction. The support material may be the same as the model material or different depending on the printer type. Regardless, this material must be removed from the build plate prior to a subsequent build and the build plate must be cleaned of debris and any excess adhesive used in the build. The printhead nozzle can also become obstructed over time and may need to be removed and cleaned as

recommended by the printer manufacturer. The inside of the printer must be regularly cleaned using a vacuum and microfiber cloth. On a regular schedule, other mechanical components need to be inspected and lubricated following the manufacturer recommendations.

Printers that deposit powders in the build chamber such as the HP Jet Fusion 4200 and 3D Systems Projet CJP 660Pro require extensive cleaning and vacuuming of excess powders after each build. These systems typically have multiple levels of maintenance with increasing requirements, after every build, weekly, monthly, and yearly. Maintenance contracts are advised as the systems are quite complex and manufacturer-level knowledge and competence is often required. Spare printheads and lamps need to be stocked and cleaning materials are needed such as alcohol swabs, brushes, inspection mirrors, isopropyl alcohol, and cleaning gloves.

In the event that printers need to be idle for long periods of time, periodic maintenance continues to be required to maintain printhead health. Some printers have an away mode that can be set that runs clean and restore cycles on a regular basis. Manual cleaning and inspection can substitute for this.

Remote monitoring of print jobs and printer status is a useful option to implement, particularly in a single-shift operation with small staffing and very long print jobs. Remote web camera and printer status monitoring are embedded in some printer models, and third-party web-based applications are also available as a remote monitoring aid.

Quality Assurance

Radiology departments within hospitals already have established QA programs that make sure that the medical imaging equipment is working properly and that images are interpreted correctly. The same level of QA should be applied to 3D printed medical models being created at the point of care within hospitals. QA is discussed in detail in Chapter 7; however, important points of QA include measures to assure that the image acquisition is being performed appropriately and images are free from major artifacts, image segmentation is accurate, the printers are accurately producing the parts, and post-processing is not affecting the quality of the models. Errors can occur at any point in this process; therefore, it is important that there are check points at every step in the process.

CONCLUSIONS

Personalized patient care is increasingly becoming a reality through technological advancements such as 3D printing. For hospitals, having an in-house 3D printing lab can facilitate the personalization of patient care by making 3D printing more accessible to the end user, allowing for both creative problem solving and faster prototyping of models. Furthermore, combining 3D printing with other methods of advanced image visualization including augmented and virtual reality will further enhance the utility of this technology. Ultimately, including 3D printing in-house at the point of care will enhance best practices, thereby leading to enhanced patient care, increased patient satisfaction, and cost reductions for the healthcare system.

REFERENCES

1. Roser SM, Ramachandra S, Blair H, et al. The accuracy of virtual surgical planning in free fibula mandibular reconstruction: comparison of planned and final results. *J Oral Maxillofac Surg*. 2010;68(11):2824—2832.
2. Helguero CG, Kao I, Komatsu DE, et al. Improving the accuracy of wide resection of bone tumors and enhancing implant fit: a cadaveric study. *J Orthop*. 2015;12(Suppl 2): S188—S194.
3. Sieira Gil R, Roig AM, Obispo CA, Morla A, Pages CM, Perez JL. Surgical planning and microvascular reconstruction of the mandible with a fibular flap using computer-aided design, rapid prototype modelling, and precontoured titanium reconstruction plates: a prospective study. *Br J Oral Maxillofac Surg*. 2015;53(1):49—53.
4. Hanasono MM, Skoracki RJ. Computer-assisted design and rapid prototype modeling in microvascular mandible reconstruction. *Laryngoscope*. 2013;123(3):597—604.
5. Zhang YZ, Chen B, Lu S, et al. Preliminary application of computer-assisted patient-specific acetabular navigational template for total hip arthroplasty in adult single development dysplasia of the hip. *Int J Med Robot*. 2011;7(4): 469—474.
6. Toto JM, Chang EI, Agag R, Devarajan K, Patel SA, Topham NS. Improved operative efficiency of free fibula flap mandible reconstruction with patient-specific, computer-guided preoperative planning. *Head Neck*. 2015;37(11):1660 1664.
7. Ferrara F, Cipriani A, Magarelli N, et al. Implant positioning in TKA: comparison between conventional and patient specific instrumentation. *Orthopedics*. 2015;38(4): e271—280.
8. Itri JN, Tappouni RR, McEachern RO, Pesch AJ, Patel SH. Fundamentals of diagnostic error in imaging. *Radiographics*. 2018;38(6):1845—1865.
9. Wake N, Wysock JS, Bjurlin MA, Chandarana H, Huang WC. "Pin the tumor on the kidney:" an evaluation of how surgeons translate CT and MRI data to 3D models. *Urology*. 2019;131:255—261.
10. Parag P, Hardcastle TC. Interpretation of emergency CT scans in polytrauma: trauma surgeon vs radiologist. *Afr J Emerg Med*. 2020;10(2):90—94.
11. Sakata S, Grove PM, Hill A, Watson MO, Stevenson ARL. Impact of simulated three-dimensional perception on precision of depth judgements, technical performance and perceived workload in laparoscopy. *Br J Surg*. 2017; 104(8):1097—1106.
12. Wake N, Rosenkrantz AB, Huang R, et al. Patient-specific 3D printed and augmented reality kidney and prostate cancer models: impact on patient education. *3D Print Med*. 2019;5(1):4.
13. Ballard DH, Mills P, Duszak Jr R, Weisman JA, Rybicki FJ, Woodard PK. Medical 3D printing cost-savings in orthopedic and maxillofacial surgery: cost analysis of operating

room time saved with 3D printed anatomic models and surgical guides. *Acad Radiol.* 2020;27(8):1103–1113.

14. Wood BC, Sher SR, Mitchell BJ, Oh AK, Rogers GF, Boyajian MJ. Conjoined twin separation: integration of three-dimensional modeling for optimization of surgical planning. *J Craniofac Surg.* 2017;28(1):4–10.

15. Villarreal JA, Yoeli D, Masand PM, Galvan NTN, Olutoye OO, Goss JA. Hepatic separation of conjoined twins: operative technique and review of three-dimensional model utilization. *J Pediatr Surg.* 2020;55(12):2828–2835.

16. Makitie AA, Salmi M, Lindford A, Tuomi J, Lassus P. Three-dimensional printing for restoration of the donor face: a new digital technique tested and used in the first facial allotransplantation patient in Finland. *J Plast Reconstr Aesthetic Surg.* 2016;69(12):1648–1652.

17. Cammarata MJ, Wake N, Kantar RS, et al. Three-dimensional analysis of donor masks for facial transplantation. *Plast Reconstr Surg.* 2019;143(6):1290e–1297e.

18. Clarkson College. *Medical 3D Printing Specialist Certificate;* 2020. https://www.clarksoncollege.edu/radiography-medical-imaging/degree-options/medical-3d-printing-specialist-certificate/index. Accessed August 15, 2020.

19. Chepelev L, Wake N, Ryan J, et al. Radiological Society of North America (RSNA) 3D printing Special Interest Group (SIG): guidelines for medical 3D printing and appropriateness for clinical scenarios. *3D Print Med.* 2018;4(1):11.

20. DICOM. *WG-17 3D.* https://www.dicomstandard.org/wgs/wg-17. Accessed 18 August 2020.

21. Materialise. *Mimics Innovation Suite 23;* 2020. https://www.materialise.com/en/medical/mimics-innovation-suite/23. Accessed September 4, 2020.

22. ISO. *ISO 17665-1:2006 Sterilization of Health Care Products - Moist Heat - Part 1: Requirements for the Development, Validation and Routine Control of a Sterilization Process for Medical Devices;* 2006. https://www.iso.org/standard/43187.html. Accessed August 14, 2020.

23. ISO. *ISO 11135:2014 Sterilization of Health Care Products - Ethylene Oxide -Requirements for the Development, Validation and Routine Control of a Sterilization Process for Medical Devices;* 2014. https://www.iso.org/standard/56137.html. Accessed August 14, 2020.

24. ISO. *ISO 11137-2:2013 Sterilization of Health Care Products - Radiation - Part 2: Establishing the Sterilization Dose;* 2013. https://www.iso.org/standard/62442.html. Accessed August 14, 2020.

25. Glassford EDK, Dunn KH, Hammond D, Tyrawski J. *3D Printing with Filaments: Health and Safety Questions to Ask.* DHHS (NIOSH) Publication No. 2020-115. U.S. Department of Health and Human Services, Centers for Disease Control and Prevention, National Institute for Occupational Safety and Health; 2020. https://www.cdc.gov/niosh/docs/2020-115/pdfs/2020-115.pdf?id=10.26616/NIOSHPUB2020115. Accessed September 4, 2020.

CHAPTER 16

The Future of Medical 3D Printing in Radiology

ADAM E. JAKUS, PHD • YU-HUI HUANG, MD, MS • NICOLE WAKE, PHD

INTRODUCTION

Looking back on the previous 30 years of progress in medical three-dimensional (3D) printing, it is astounding to consider just how far the field has come, with radiology playing a key, central role. Despite the dual infancies of medical imaging and 3D printing technologies in the late 1980s and early 1990s, a few pioneering individuals and organizations endeavored to bring the distinct technologies and communities together, integrating diverse expertise along with new hardware, software, and materials. From anatomic models for medical training and surgical planning, guides to directly assist with surgery, to permanent patient-matched implants, these increasingly deployed applications, in combination with new reimbursement strategies, regulatory involvement and support, as well as new workforce development and education programs in medicine, engineering, and technical support, have all grown from the initial seeds planted 30 years ago (Fig. 16.1).

What about the next 30 years? With so much progress taking place in just the past few decades, let alone the past 5 years, it is no small feat to accurately speculate on what the next 30 years have in store. Using history as a guide, reasonable predictions can be made regarding the technological, clinical, and workforce trajectories of medical 3D printing in radiology. This chapter focuses on what the next 30 years of medical 3D printing might look like and which roles radiology and complimentary disciplines might play. Through the continued adoption and standardization of 3D printing for anatomic models and surgical guides to permanent implants, bioregenerative materials, and even living bioprinted tissues and organs, we can expect

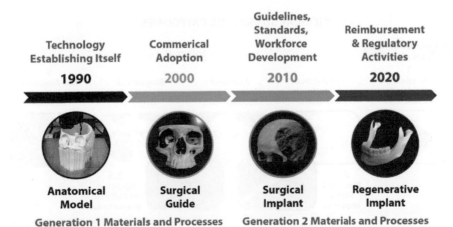

Technology Establishing Itself	Commerical Adoption	Guidelines, Standards, Workforce Development	Reimbursement & Regulatory Activities
1990	**2000**	**2010**	**2020**
Anatomical Model	Surgical Guide	Surgical Implant	Regenerative Implant

Generation 1 Materials and Processes   Generation 2 Materials and Processes

FIG. 16.1 30 years of medical 3D printing, from the introduction and increased adoption of anatomical models, anatomical guides, and patient-matched implants to the emergence of tissue regenerative structures. (*Surgical Implant* photograph from Huang M-T, Juan P-K, Chen S-Y, et al. The potential of the three-dimensional printed titanium mesh implant for cranioplasty surgery applications: biomechanical behaviors and surface properties. *Mater Sci Eng C.* 2019;97:412–419.)

3D Printing for the Radiologist. https://doi.org/10.1016/B978-0-323-77573-1.00013-0

a medical transformation to take place over the next three decades, with radiology at its center. Given the rapid technological advancement and rates of adoption we have witnessed in just the past decade, it is reasonable to divide this discussion into several segments: near term (next 5 years), mid-near term (5—10 years), midterm (10—20 years), and long term (20—30 years).

EMERGING MEDICAL 3D PRINTING TECHNOLOGIES

Prior to delving into the future of medical 3D printing and radiology, it is beneficial to establish a foundational understanding of the emerging medical 3D printing technologies and create a reference system for which to categorize and discuss those technologies and their applications. Generally, medical 3D printing can be divided into five primary groups (Fig. 16.2): educational anatomic models and surgical guides; static, permanent implants; acellular, regenerative biomaterials; cell-containing, living biological/tissue structures for tissue and organ repair, regeneration, and replacement, commonly referred to as "bioprinting"; and synthetic—biological, biomachine interface devices. Numerous intermediate classifications across these groups exist, including coating or modifying static implants with bioactive components; and adding living cells to originally acellular, regenerative biomaterials. It is important to distinguish the various categories of medical 3D printing because they vary with respect to (1) the types

of hardware, software, and materials utilized; specific education and user expertise required; (2) the necessary manufacturing conditions and environment; (3) the existing or still developing standards; regulatory and reimbursement pathways; and (4) their means of use and intended application. It should be noted that acellular regenerative biomaterial and bioprinting are themselves emerging technologies and have not yet been clinically established.

With a longer history than the other medical 3D printing categories, combined with the fact that they are not restricted by criteria and requirements associated with implantation, 3D printed anatomic models and surgical guides are presently the most widely utilized of the five categories. This is demonstrated, in part, by recent activities related to establishing reimbursement pathways for their use. In July 2019, Category III Current Procedural Terminology codes for 3D printed anatomic models and guides were released by the American Medical Association (see Chapter 8); and the joint Radiological Society of North America (RSNA)—American College of Radiology (ACR) 3D Printing Registry was created to track the use of clinical 3D printing. This registry collects anonymized 3D printing case information; clinical indications; model types including which anatomical parts, segmentation, and computer-aided design processing tools, and printing technologies utilized; and intended uses for the models. Information from this registry will be used to determine the Appropriateness Criteria for 3D printing as another

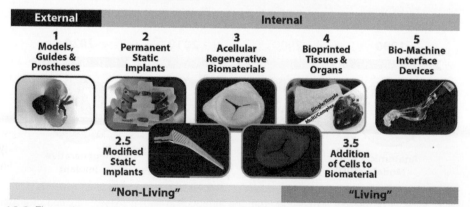

FIG. 16.2 Five major, and two intermediate, categories of medical 3D printing. (Panel 2 photo from Kamel MK, Cheng A, Vaughan B, et al. Sternal reconstruction using customized 3D-printed titanium implants. *Ann Thorac Surg.* 2020;109(6):e411—e414; Panel 2.5 photo from Rivera F, Leonardi F, Maniscalco P, et al. Uncemented fully hydroxyapatite-coated hip stem for intracapsular femoral neck fractures in osteoporotic elderly patients: a multicenter study. *Arthroplast Today.* 2015;1(3):81—84; Panel 5 photo from Jank BJ, Xiong L, Moser PT, et al. Engineered composite tissue as a bioartificial limb graft. *Biomaterials.* 2015;61:246—256.)

modality of visualization. This reimbursement pathway currently only applies to select subcategories of medical 3D printing objects but will ultimately need to be extended to include all five categories of 3D printing as well as possibly integration with augmented and virtual reality technologies.

Current static, permanent implants are primarily employed for bone and hard tissue replacement, providing structural support rather than specific biological activity or function. This encompasses the 3D printed counterparts to many traditionally manufactured implant products made from established, relatively bioinert, yet biocompatible rigid plastics such as polyetheretherketone (PEEK), polyetherketoneketone (PEKK), and polymethylmethacrylate (PMMA) as well as metal alloys such as those based on titanium, stainless steel, or cobalt. Objects in this category are primarily produced via 3D printing methods that rely on heat, such as selective laser sintering/melting (SLS/SLM), electron beam melting (EBM), and more recently material extrusion techniques including fused deposition modeling (FDM) or fused filament fabrication (FFF),[5] and direct ink writing (DIW).[6–8] Although not yet commonly produced in the hospital, there is an increasing abundance of 3D printed static implantable devices that are regulatory cleared.[9] Beyond the standard stock keeping units (SKUs), metal and rigid plastic parts are increasingly being 3D printed into patient-matched implants to treat complex, large-scale tissue resections of the pelvis,[10] spine,[11] rib cage,[12] and skull.[1] Importantly, these implants, although designed to integrate with surrounding tissues, are intended to remain relatively inert and unchanged (static) in the body for years, if not decades after implantation. For the sake of complete discussion, the bioactivity and integration potential of static permanent implants can be enhanced by coating or infusing them with more bioactive/biomimetic materials, such as calcium phosphates.[13]

Acellular, regenerative biomaterial medical 3D printing is arguably the least widely discussed or understood of the first four categories. This lack of awareness derives from the understanding of existing medical materials and their primary purpose within the body—to physically and mechanically support the bioactive components, living cells, and tissues. However, emerging materials can play a strong bioactive role, beyond physical or mechanical support, even without requiring added cells. These objects are usually 3D printed via material extrusion processes, such as FDM and DIW.[14] The biomaterials can be based on synthetically derived polymers, ceramics, and composites; naturally derived

materials, such as collagens, glycosaminoglycans (GAGs), decellularized tissue extracellular matrices (ECM); or mixtures thereof.[15] Several examples include noncell-encapsulating hydrogels,[16] as well as the 3D painted (a variation of DIW) materials such as Hyperelastic Bone (bioceramic based) for hard-tissue repair and regeneration,[17,18] Fluffy-X (Advanced polymer based) for soft-tissue repair and regeneration,[18,19] Tissue Papers for targeted tissue repair and regeneration (Organ ECM based),[20] 3D-Graphene for electrically reliant tissue repair (synthetic based),[21] and mixtures thereof.[22,23] These materials not only have unique compositions but also unique nano/microstructures that, in combination, interact with surrounding tissues and cells to induce new target tissue formation while the implant itself degrades and transforms into natural, healthy tissue. Thus, acellular regenerative biomaterials, unlike static implants, are dynamic in nature and are designed to change and transform after implantation. Although not necessarily required, there is no technical barrier preventing the addition of cells to regenerative biomaterial objects prior to implantation[24,25]—an example of which would be a 3D printed meniscal structure seeded with patient-matched chondrocytes or stem cells immediately prior to implantation;[26] or a gelatin-based 3D printed hydrogel seeded with ovarian-derived follicles (containing oocytes) prior to implantation that restore hormonal and reproductive function.[16]

Cellular medical 3D printing, frequently referred to as "bioprinting" specifically involves 3D printing with live cells or tissue fragments to create structures that are intended to be implanted as is or further conditioned and matured prior to implantation. Being composed of acellular regenerative biomaterials, bioprinted objects are intended to repair and regenerate damaged or missing tissues and, potentially, partial or full organs. The materials in this case, unlike resins, powders, filaments, or particle suspensions, are living cells suspended in a cyto- and biocompatible medium, most often a hydrogel. Like acellular biomaterials, bioprinting processes are primarily material extrusion based (variations of DIW and material jetting),[14] although new cytocompatible vat polymerization materials and processes are emerging.[27] Although hydrogels based on synthetic and/or nonmammalian natural polymers such as polyethylene glycol, alginate, chitosan, cellulose, and others are common in academic research due to their low cost and relative ease of 3D printing, they, unless heavily modified, are not suitable for implantation due to the negative immunological responses they elicit. Mammalian-based hydrogels, such as those comprised of collagen, gelatin (denatured collagen), or decellularized tissue ECM, although more expensive and challenging to 3D print than their non-mammalian counterparts, are more suitable for implantation purposes and are presently the subject of broader, translational biofabrication efforts.

Regardless of the material medium or process used, the comprising cell viability and health is of utmost importance, and can be negatively impacted by a variety of environmental (temperature, pressure, humidity), processing (shear stress from extrusion), and post 3D printing handling, transport, and storage—all of which must be taken into account when 3D printing living cells. Additionally, because these structures contain living cells and lack an immune system, they cannot be terminally sterilized or fend off pathogenic contaminants. Thus, bioprinting living structures for implantation should be done using sterile raw materials, within a sterile environment, using sterile processes. Regarding cell sourcing, there are significant ongoing efforts in academia, government, and industry research labs to establish their sourcing, quality, consistency, and bioactivity whether they be autologous patient primary cells, adult stem cells, induced pluripotent stem cells, or induced pluripotent-derived cells.[28]

Biomachine interface medical 3D printing broadly encompasses technologies and applications that are beyond 3D printing static devices or living tissues and organs. This includes 3D printing of integrated biological-machine structures as well as advanced engineered and augmented tissues and organs. Although presently a collection of ideas with minimal completed proofs of concept, biomachine interface medical 3D printing is a logical technological progression of multi-tissue 3D printing combined with nonmedical 3D printing technologies, including advanced electronics, energy generation, and storage devices. Generally, this category represents the intersection of medical with industrial manufacturing, and although it will still be at least 30 years until even a solid proof of concept is realized, not to mention many more years until broad adoption, this is an area of which current, younger radiologists and medical professionals should be aware.

Despite the stark contrasts among these five categories, they share numerous similarities in the broader context of in-hospital 3D printing. Regardless of application, each of the five approaches requires (or will require) precise and accurate input data, usually derived from the acquisition, interpretation, and segmentation of patient imaging studies, as discussed in previous chapters. Whether that imaging data are derived from CT, MRI, ultrasound, surface scanning, nuclear medicine, other imaging modalities, or combinations thereof, they are the basis for the digital inputs for models, guides, permanent implants, and even future tissue regenerative, bioprinted, and biomachine interface structures. The forms that the digital inputs take may vary substantially between objects created for surgical planning versus bioprinted objects containing a variety of living cells and tissue types. For example, the primary characteristic of surgical models and guides is to emulate the form and architecture of the target tissue/organ based on imaging data. This will hold true for bioprinted structures as well, where the form and architecture will need to be emulated to match the patient. However, in addition to recreating the form factor, possibly down to the vascular level, bioprinted structures will also have to recreate the target tissue/organ's composition and properties. This will not only require digital inputs derived from existing imaging technologies but will also require additional complementary and spatially correlated compositional digital inputs. Thus, the clinical implementation of bioprinting technologies is reliant on the parallel development of imaging technologies that can be used to ascertain biological composition and properties.

It is also important to mention the distinct expertise and knowledge required to pursue each of the five categories. Progressing from models and guides to bioprinted and biomachine structures, there is a gradual transition from pure visualization and image processing to mechanical engineering, materials engineering, tissue engineering, and electrical/systems engineering—all of which are currently distinct disciplines, but share overlaps that may present opportunities for new workforce development and engineering fields in the future.

THE CASE FOR IN-HOSPITAL 3D PRINTING

As of 2020, many hospitals and healthcare institutions throughout the United States and across the world utilize medical 3D printing to create anatomic models and surgical guides in-house for a variety of clinical applications—this is increasingly becoming the norm rather than the exception. However, for organizations that rarely utilize 3D printing for these applications and do not have the required internal equipment or expertise, it is logical to use these third parties, as they have the hardware, software, and know-how (in combination with clinician input). Despite this, there are good reasons why anatomic model and surgical guide 3D printing in the hospital have become much more common. These reasons have been discussed at length in previous chapters but did not take into consideration the added layers of complexity of bringing in-house the other categories of medical 3D printing such as implant 3D printing. Given the differing and added hardware, software, and materials requirements as well as the varying technical know-how, increased risk, and currently uncertain regulatory complexities surrounding in-hospital—fabricated implants, why would anyone want to go through the effort to produce them at the point-of-care rather than relying on external, third-party entities to do so? The answer comes down to four factors: time/cost, availability, logistical practicality, and patient care.

Certainly, the most immediate benefit of producing 3D printed anatomic models and guides onsite is time. If patient data can go from digital imaging data, to physical creation, to use within a day or two, rather than waiting on third-party schedules, manufacturing queues, and shipping, then there is a clear case to be made for efficiency and obvious advantages to the patient. These time benefits are further compounded in the case of 3D printed static, permanent, and acellular regenerative biomaterial implants, where off-the-shelf SKUs simply are not available or do not exist anywhere, and the lead time for receiving a patient-matched implantable device from a third party may be several days to weeks. For patients with critical needs, this period might be the difference between life and death, and for the hospital, will result in added weeks of medical care and increased operating costs. However, the time-saving advantages to producing patient-matched static and acellular regenerative implants in the hospital do not necessarily extend to bioprinted objects, which require large numbers of cells and possible conditioning and maturation times. Acquiring and expanding cells to the sufficient number to 3D print an object that might be required for critical care could take weeks, and conditioning and maturing that structure after printing might take several weeks more. Additionally, since bioprinted objects are living and there are currently no established methods for storing or transporting living tissues without function loss, their postproduction lifetime, like transplanted tissues and organs, is currently limited.

Implant availability, or lack thereof, is another factor that will drive the adoption of in-hospital implant medical 3D printing. As of 2020, the majority of implantable products, regardless of their indicated use or means of production, are mass-produced, and even available in a variety of discrete-sized SKUs. These mass-produced devices and their specific sizes are manufactured in part because there is a large enough demand and patient population to justify their development from a business perspective. However, standard-sized implant products are not appropriate for all patient populations or individual patients. In these instances, three options exist: use whichever implant is available and is the closest fit despite its inappropriateness for the patient, forego the implant and find some other way to treat the patient, or design and manufacture a patient-matched implant. As discussed above, although third-party static implant manufacturing is becoming increasingly available, this still needs to be balanced with time and patient need. For example, a noncritical mandibular implant may be needed for an upcoming surgical procedure—in this case, the time required for a third party to manufacture and ship the implant may be acceptable. In another case, a critical need, specifically designed bronchiotracheal implant may be needed to treat a neonatal infant who may otherwise not survive a week. This latter scenario is an example of compassionate use and is perhaps emblematic of the real value of in-hospital implant medical 3D printing. This logic can be extended to acellular regenerative biomaterials 3D printing and bioprinting as well, although at the moment, these types of implants are not necessarily commercially available from third parties. Regarding bioprinting, it will be unlikely that large supplies of commercially manufactured tissues and organs, compatible with all patient populations, will be readily available for purchase. Thus, like the bronchiotracheal example given previously, they will likely need to be made as needed—and time will play a major factor for their use.

Logistically, it is impractical for a hospital, regardless of its economic status and administrative capabilities, to store and manage an extensive inventory of implantable products of varying SKUs, many of which may never end up being used. This is one of the major factors that will drive adoption of static implant medical 3D printing in the hospital—reduce standing inventory and waste. Although this argument is also possibly applicable to acellular regenerative and bioprinted implants, the logistical concerns surrounding them are more extensive. Currently, shipping live tissues and organs for transplantation is no simple task; it must be done rapidly, with great care, and is still ultimately limited by distance and time. These same challenges will exist for bioprinted tissues and organs as well, with the added complication that, in all likelihood, those tissues and organs will require specific cells from the patient as manufacturing raw material, therefore requiring an additional shipping and handling step. As alluded to previously, until tissue and organ transport and preservation challenges are effectively resolved, such structures will need to be produced near the target patient.

Finally, if it was not believed that patient care could be improved through technological medical advances, then there would ultimately be no major case for in-hospital manufacturing of implants. While obtaining the patient-matched implants from third-party manufacturers will continue to remain a significant part of personalized healthcare, there will remain many instances where patient care can be substantially improved through in-hospital implant manufacturing—and in these instances, radiologists will be the primary facilitator.

A WORD ON STERILIZATION AND QUALITY MANUFACTURING AT THE HOSPITAL

3D printed medical implants, whether they are composed of alloys, plastics, regenerative biomaterials, and/or living cells, must be free of pathogens prior to use and must be manufactured to the necessary level of verifiable and biocompatible quality. Quality and sterilization of static implants have been discussed at length in previous chapters, but it is worth reiterating the importance of ensuring sterility of any 3D printed object that is intended to come into contact with the patient or enter a sterile surgical field. Protocols and standards are currently being developed for sterilization of in-hospital—produced static implant devices, which do not substantially deviate from existing chemical or thermal sterilization methods, but material compatibility must be taken into account before introducing the object to the sterilization procedure. It must also be known whether or not the sterilization process affects the dimension or mechanical properties of the object, as such changes can have downstream adverse influence on the performance of surgical guides and anatomic models.

The characteristic stability that enables static implants to remain relatively unchanged in the body after implantation also permits them to be sterilized using already established methods, such as dry or hot heat (autoclaving), gamma irradiation, ethylene oxide (EtO), hydrogen peroxide (H_2O_2), and others. These processes have an established history, and most hospitals and clinics have some sterilization capabilities. However, these established methods are not readily compatible with acellular regenerative biomaterials. For example, excessive heat or free radical chemical sterilization such as EtO and H_2O_2 will alter if not destroy the base materials. This incompatibility with emerging advanced biomaterials can be addressed through the adoption of novel sterilization techniques, such as peracetic acid liquid/vapor exposure[29] and supercritical CO_2.[30] Fortunately, these emerging processes and hardware are scalable and could be incorporated into hospital environments in a manner analogous to current EtO and autoclaving equipment and processing—allowing for onsite sterilization of in-hospital 3D printed acellular, regenerative implants. However, as of 2020, the FDA still considers these emerging techniques as novel, and they have only been used in conjunction with a few cleared products. Fortunately, the FDA also recognizes the increasing need to reduce reliance on methods such as EtO, and in 2019 launched an Innovation in Sterilization Challenge to work with industry partners to explore and establish novel sterilization techniques for broader use. Ideally, these efforts will establish new approaches to sterilization that are not only compatible with acellular regenerative biomaterials but can also be readily incorporated into existing hospital sterilization infrastructure.

Sterility is further complicated with respect to bioprinted structures, which by their very nature contain microorganisms (human cells) that need to remain viable and functional for the implant to survive and serve its purpose. Thus, sterilization, using traditional or emerging novel methods, is fundamentally not compatible with bioprinted structures. Bioprinted structures intended for implantation, regardless of their complexity, must be manufactured and handled in a fully aseptic and sterile environment and manner. Additionally, raw materials and components used in the bioprinting process, including the cells, media, water, gel materials, plasticware, glassware, metal ware, etc., must all be sterile prior to use. These sterility requirements impart substantial manufacturing, infrastructure, expertise, and practically burden on in-hospital bioprinting, and are the primary reasons why this form of medical 3D printing will not be established within individual hospitals in the near future.

THE NEXT 5 YEARS

In the next 5 years, we can expect to see the continuation of current trends related to medical 3D printing of anatomic models and surgical guides as well as the initial adoption of 3D printing to create static permanent implants (Fig. 16.3). Unlike previous years, where adoption was primarily driven and supported by independent physician activities, hospitals and healthcare institutions will likely begin to provide additional internal support for these activities. This increasing support will be driven by four factors: (1) Hospitals and other healthcare centers are beginning to recognize net positive effect on the long-term bottom-line of medical 3D printing, despite the upfront costs; (2) in an effort to remain competitive with state-of-the-art capabilities, hospitals and medical centers will begin using 3D printing as a means of differentiation and marketing leverage; (3) there are an increasing number of doctors, nurses, engineers, and technicians being exposed to medical 3D printing during their education and training who are entering the healthcare workforce; and (4) related reimbursement pathways for 3D printed surgical models and guides will be increasingly established. Additionally, while the relative costs for SLA,

FDM, and certain material jetting 3D printing hardware and materials are decreasing, their ease of use and accessibility are increasing, reducing the initial technical barrier required to initiate operations.

Beyond the increased utilization of medical 3D printing to create polymeric models and guides, the next 5 years will also see an increase in the in-hospital manufacturing of permanent static implants fabricated from polymers such as PEEK and PEKK, and metal alloys such as Ti64. These materials, although older and more established than many of the polymers and resins used in vat polymerization, FDM, and material jetting 3D printing, have traditionally only been compatible with powder-bed laser or electron-beam–based sintering/fusing/melting 3D printing technologies. Generally, these forms of 3D printing are not only significantly more expensive, in terms of both capital costs and operations, than SLA, FDM, and material jetting 3D printing but are also much more challenging to safely implement and manage in

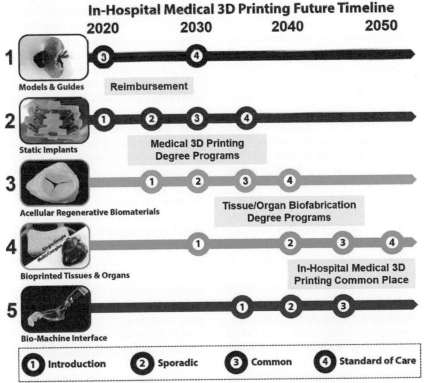

FIG. 16.3 The future of in-hospital medical 3D printing. (Panel 2 photo from Kamel MK, Cheng A, Vaughan B, et al. Sternal reconstruction using customized 3D-printed titanium implants. *Ann Thorac Surg*. 2020;109(6): e411–e414; Panel 5 photo from Jank BJ, Xiong L, Moser PT, et al. Engineered composite tissue as a bioartificial limb graft. *Biomaterials*. 2015;61:246–256.)

a healthcare setting due to the large quantities of loose powder, which presents as health and flammability hazards if handled improperly. On top of the safety and infrastructure challenges, powder-bed fusion technologies generally have a higher threshold for user expertise and skill than SLA, FDM, and material jetting technologies. These cost, technology, safety, and user factors, as well as other factors relating to regulatory and risk management, have until now prevented the broader adoption of in-hospital 3D printing of implants.

Recently, however, the barriers preventing the adoption of in-hospital static implant 3D printing are being challenged by two distinct developments. First, hospitals are beginning to partner with private medical 3D printing companies to bring additive manufacturing of implants in-house as private company owned and operated but colocated manufacturing partners. The partnership between LimaCorporate and New York City's Hospital for Special Surgery is a prime example of this type of approach, where LimaCorporate will operate an implant 3D printing facility onsite with the Hospital for Special Surgery—providing the equipment, expertise, and know-how for patient-matched implant production while also splitting the risk. Partnership models such as this will become more prevalent in the next 5 years and beyond to meet the increasing demand for patient-matched implants, while leveraging the increasing 3D printing expertise of healthcare professionals as well as the established and growing 3D printing companies. One of the concerns with this approach, however, is that the technology and processes brought into the healthcare environment will be restricted to that of the particular private partner, ultimately limiting what can be done onsite. Despite these concerns, these partnership scenarios will not only introduce more patient-matched implant 3D printing to hospitals and healthcare systems but they will also further push the development of the legal, risk, and regulatory frameworks around these types of manufacturing activities.

The second distinct development that will likely begin to emerge over the next 5 years is the increased adoption of extrusion-based, rigid polymer, and metal 3D printing technologies. Unlike the established powder-bed sintering/melting 3D printing processes, material extrusion processes, which can include variants of FDM[31] and DIW, such as 3D painting,[8,17,19,21] are based on relatively simple hardware technologies with

new material compositions that do not employ loose powders, high-energy laser, or electron beams. These characteristics significantly reduce the upfront capital expenditures, safety, and operation infrastructure requirements needed to 3D print mechanically rigid and stable polymers, such as PEEK and PEKK, as well as metals, such as titanium alloys. Polymers used for rigid, permanent implants, such as PEEK, have relatively high melting points, traditionally requiring them to be 3D printed using the powder-bed processes. However, with advances in FDM hardware, capable of reliably operating and extruding at higher temperatures, and new PEEK formulations, implant-grade PEEK filament can now be produced and FDM 3D printed into objects intended for implantation.[31]

FDM metal processes employ metal powder-loaded polymer filaments which are melt extruded in a similar fashion to standard polymer FDM to create a "green body" metal-polymer part. Similarly, DIW processes can employ metallic particle liquid suspensions, which are extruded into 3D "green body" metal-polymer parts. Regardless of the approach, the green body must be sintered at high temperatures in the appropriate gaseous environment, requiring an atmosphere-controlled furnace and supply of the necessary gases. This burns off the polymeric binder, or debinds, and fuses, or sinters, the comprising metal powder together to yield metallic parts. This approach results in final metallic parts being smaller than as-printed green body counterparts, meaning that volume reduction must be considered along with the possibility of warping and/or cracking when originally designing the part and creating the green body. In spite of the final part being metallic, the part's purity and microstructure ultimately dictate its properties and performance. With approximately 30 years of research, development, industrialization, and standard development behind them, powder-bed metal 3D printing processes are presently much more well suited to yield metal parts with the appropriate microstructure and properties; however, FDM and DIW processes, hardware, and material advances are rapidly improving. These advances combined with their increased availability, relatively low cost, ease of operation, small footprint, and growing demand for patient-matched permanent static implants will not only drive the adoption of in-hospital FDM and DIW rigid polymer and metal 3D printing but will also set the stage for in-hospital production of more advanced, tissue regenerative implants.

5–10 YEARS INTO THE FUTURE

From 2025 to 2030, we can expect to see in-hospital 3D printing of patient-matched, static permanent implants at a similar stage of adoption and development as Category 1 is presently (2020). It will be interesting to see which of the two models discussed in the previous section will dominate the in-hospital production of patient-matched, static permanent implants: partnering and colocation of the private implant manufacturer with the hospital, or hospital-led manufacturing using presently emerging FDM and DIW 3D printing technologies. In all likelihood, both approaches will be increasingly common, allowing for more flexible and rapid design and production of rigid polymer and metal patient-matched implants. It is unlikely, however, that the costs of producing patient-matched, static implants will ever be less than the mass-produced, off-the-shelf counterpart (if it exists) of the same material; thus, cost-benefit analyses for in-hospital static implant printing will begin to be established at this time, similar to what is happening with model and guide 3D printing today. More broadly, just as hospitals have been utilizing and growing accustomed to vat polymerization processes and material jetting 3D printing technologies to create the models and guides, the opportunity to create rigid plastic and metal implants through non powder-bed fusion techniques will drive the adoption of advanced FDM and DIW hardware and materials within the hospital. This will set the stage for the initial in-hospital production of acellular regenerative biomaterial implants, which are typically 3D printed using the same technologies.

Just as we expect 2020–2025 to witness the emergence of in-hospital 3D printing of static permanent implants primarily for hard tissue (orthopedic and craniomaxillofacial bone) indications, 2025 and the following years will witness the first cases of in-hospital 3D printing of acellular regenerative biomaterials for tissue regeneration. Prior to 2025, the first off-the-shelf, acellular advanced biomaterial 3D printed products will likely be cleared and made commercially available for a variety of tissue repair indications including bone, cartilage, muscle, ligament, tendon, and nerve, as well as homogeneous soft tissues such as trachea, lung, and liver. The initial regulatory clearance and clinical data derived from the use of these products, in combination with the increasing presence of FDM and DIW hardware and expertise in the hospital, will create the environment for the production of the first in-hospital acellular, regenerative medical 3D printed implants. These implants will be comprised of new synthetic polymer, gel, bioceramic, composite materials, and/or biologically derived,

extracellular matrix proteins and GAGs such as collagens and hyaluronates. Additionally, as a result of autologous primary and stem cell isolation and culture procedures simultaneously becoming more common, as well as rapidly developing induced pluripotent stem cell technologies, 2025–2030 will also likely witness the first in-hospital production of cell-seeded regenerative biomaterial implants, 3D printed advanced biomaterials seeded or incorporated with a patient's own cells prior to implantation. This will set the stage for the in-hospital production of patient-matched bioprinted simple tissues and possibly organs.

By 2025–2030, several initial medical 3D printing postgraduate engineering and technical programs will be in place around the world, and it is likely that some medical school programs will be regularly incorporating medical 3D printing into their curricula as well as residency and fellowship training. With this increased education, hospitals will have access to an increasingly consistent and abundant medical 3D printing workforce, greatly accelerating the adoption of model, guide, and static implant 3D printing activities. One big question that remains regarding in-hospital static and acellular regenerative implant 3D printing is what will the regulatory framework and guidance look like in 2025 or 2030? This is perhaps the most difficult element to predict. However, using history as a guide, it is likely that, at the very least, guidance documents will be in place for in-hospital static implant 3D printing based in part on what is currently being established for in-hospital model and guide 3D printing. Such guidance will likely make use of the existing FDA guidance for *Technical Considerations for Additive Manufactured Medical Devices*[32] and *Framework for the Regulation of Regenerative Medicine Products*.[33]

10–20 YEARS INTO THE FUTURE

With an increasingly large, educated, and skilled medical, engineering, and technical 3D printing workforce, commercially established, off-the-shelf tissue reparative and regenerative products, first demonstrations of successful in-hospital use of 3D printed acellular and post-3D printing cell-seeded regenerative biomaterial structures, and the establishment of regulatory and reimbursement frameworks, 2030–2040 promises to be the period in which the potential of 3D printing in medicine is realized. With anatomic model, surgical guide, and static implant medical 3D printing well established in hospitals, and regenerative biomaterials 3D printing being increasingly utilized for patient-matched tissue and organ repair, bioprinted living tissues and organs, will begin to be established in select hospitals and regions. Additionally, the first commercially produced and clinically utilized 3D printed synthetic–biological interface devices will become commercially available.

The infrastructure surrounding acellular regenerative biomaterial 3D printing is roughly similar to FDM and DIW static implant 3D printing; therefore, it is likely that the production of patient-matched acellular, tissue regenerative biomaterials will follow a similar path to static implants. Private companies will colocate with hospitals to direct and manage implant production in parallel with hospitals taking on the necessary responsibilities, infrastructure, and risk themselves. Although both scenarios will take place, large, established medical manufacturing companies are inherently slow to enter new technology areas with indeterminate risks. Furthermore, acellular regenerative biomaterial 3D printing technologies are not dependent on infrastructure-heavy powder-bed technologies, and therefore are readily amenable to existing hospital infrastructure. Consequently, it is expected that hospital-led acellular, regenerative biomaterial 3D printing activities will likely be more prevalent than colocated private company-led efforts.

Bioprinted tissues and organs will likely be in use at this time, particularly simple musculoskeletal tissues, such as vascularized bone, cartilage, fat, ligaments, tendons, muscle, nerve, skin, and composite tissues thereof. Additionally, bioprinted lung, bronchiotracheal, bladder, liver, and other tissues will have been clinically demonstrated by this time and, although likely not yet standard of care, will be in clinical use in select hospitals for select patient populations. However, numerous questions remain that are difficult to presently gauge: Who is producing these tissues? Where are they producing them? How are they transporting them to the patient? Who is paying for the tissue and organ fabrication? And what is the regulatory environment surrounding tissue and organ fabrication and use, let alone in-hospital production of said living implants? Due to the level of infrastructure required for live tissue fabrication and maturation, which must all be done under highly sterile and controlled conditions, it is likely that individual hospitals will not be broadly producing their own living bioprinted tissues and organs by 2040. Conversely, industry-led production of tissues and organs faces the substantial logistical challenges, not to mention the challenge of establishing a business case for patient-matched organ fabrication. With these challenges in mind, biofabrication will likely take place at regional facilities operated as government-public-private partnerships with surrounding hospital systems. With this approach, not only can the economic

burden required for establishing and maintaining such a facility be shared by multiple interested parties but also the regulatory monitoring required to ensure safety can be concentrated in several select sites, rather than dozens or hundreds of distinct hospitals. This approach can adequately address the logistical challenges surrounding tissue and organ transport and handling and will also give resource-strapped hospital systems and low-population areas, that could normally not justify such an investment, access to the advanced bioprinting technologies. The success of this scenario, however, depends on the capacity for government, private industry, and hospital systems (public, private, and government) to work closely together for the betterment of patient and population health.

Up until this point, patient-matched implants have been almost exclusively characterized by their structure, with comprising material generally selected for the specific medical intent—such as titanium alloys for boney structural implants, or regenerative biomaterials, like Hyperelastic Bone, for boney regeneration—essentially, "off-the-shelf materials" regardless of how advanced they are today, to create patient-matched structures. By 2040, however, not only will the anatomic structure of medical 3D printed implants be matched to the patient but also will the material composition and microstructure will also be patient-matched materials. Extending the prior bone tissue example, bone composition and properties vary significantly not only between sexes and across age populations but can also vary substantially across individuals within the same medical demographic depending on a wide variety of extrinsic and intrinsic biological factors, including age, health, sex, and genetic makeup.[34] Thus, a patient-matched implant comprised of an off-the-shelf material, in one person will perform differently than the same or similar sized patient-matched implant comprised of the same off-the-shelf-material in another. The combination of patient-matched structures, afforded by the continuing advancement of 3D printing and imaging technologies, as well as patient-matched materials, enabled by the continuing advancement of materials design as well as imaging technologies, will yield implants that are not only macroscopically matched to the patient but also compositionally and microstructurally matched as well. It is worth noting that the marriage of patient-matched structures and patient-matched materials is very much dependent on the advances in medical imaging capabilities as well as data interpretation, processing, and digital modeling across length scales (nano/micrometers—centimeters)—a skillset that is uniquely suited to the radiology expertise.

20–30 YEARS INTO THE FUTURE

Between 2040 and 2050, not only will static, acellular, and bioprinted implant medical 3D printing become common place in industry and in hospitals, but also the fields will have advanced to the point where medical 3D printing and biofabrication have established themselves as their own distinct disciplines, with their own educational and training programs, standards organizations, insurance reimbursement pathways, and regulatory programs. It would not be too speculative to state that by 2040 or 2050, complex, large-scale complex tissues, such as entire limbs, and multicomponent organs, such as the heart and kidney, will be able to be created using 3D printing in combination with other manufacturing and bioconditioning technologies. However, with the emergence of biomachine interface 3D printing during this time, it may turn out that creating bioelectronic–mechanical interface devices to replace full limbs or full organs is more effective and cost-efficient than creating the fully biological tissue or organ. Regardless of the details, patient-matched tissue and organ fabrication will likely become well established by 2050, transforming healthcare possibilities for those who can afford and obtain the biofabricated structures. This is where the greatest future uncertainty lies—access.

RADIOLOGY OF THE FUTURE

The ongoing implementation of 3D printed anatomic models and surgical guides in hospitals has resulted in the development of new types of engineers and technical staff with specialties that did not exist 20 years ago. Similarly, as discussed in previous chapters, radiologists are now beginning to receive additional 3D printing education and training. However, moving from anatomic models and surgical guides to living bioprinted implants, new knowledge and skillsets will be required to attain successful outcomes. Due to this complexity, it is unlikely that the necessary knowledge and skills will be in the hands of just one or two people. Radiologists, along with referring physicians as well as engineers and support staff of various disciplines, will all need to collaborate and work together to be able to create safe, functional patient-specific implants, whether they be titanium alloy or living functioning tissue.

Although the radiologists may be leading the hospital 3D printing activities and teams, it is mostly the referring clinicians interfacing with the patients who are ultimately submitting the printing requests to the radiologists and their 3D printing teams. Thus, it is imperative that the referring clinicians have adequate knowledge about the technologies and know what is and is not feasible in order to make informed decisions and requests. Currently, at some institutions with a centralized 3D printing lab, clinicians are able to order 3D printed models as if they were ordering any other medical imaging study with built-in imaging protocols for optimal acquisition. It would be essential for the clinician to communicate their needs and use for the 3D printed object to determine the appropriateness of the order. This includes informed imaging requests, manufacturing requests, and even, in the case of implants, material compositions, or at least communication regarding the specific material needs and requirements. As far as imaging is concerned, the existing American College of Radiology (ACR) Appropriateness Criteria provides evidence-based guidelines to assist referring physicians and other providers in making the most appropriate imaging decision for a specific clinical condition. For example, a patient with acute moderate, severe or penetrating head trauma, the most appropriate initial study is a CT head without IV contrast which has the Appropriateness Criteria rating of "Usually Appropriate" due to CT's sensitivity for depicting acute intracranial hemorrhage, intracranial mass effect, ventricular size, and bone injuries, whereas a MRI head without IV contrast is rated as "Usually Not Appropriate". Similar Appropriateness Criteria will need to be developed around implant characteristics and requests, and referring clinicians will need to be adequately informed and educated in order for those criteria to have reasonable effect.

From imaging, segmentation and interpretation, digital model creation and design, material selection to 3D printing and postprocessing, the entire medical 3D printing process is complex and benefits greatly from the skills of a variety of existing engineering specialties—with no single specialty having the complete range of required skillsets. This will need to change for in-hospital implant 3D printing to become common place. Traditionally, medical imaging and processing has been the expertise of radiologic technologists and biomedical engineers; digital design and file creation, the expertise of mechanical engineers; and materials selection, design, and processing, the expertise of materials engineers. From an economic or managerial standpoint, it would not be practical to have a team of engineers, each with his/her own narrow area of expertise relating to imaging and 3D printing, at each hospital that wants to 3D print implants. Thus, it would be most effective to begin to develop engineering programs specifically around biofabrication, which would cover the knowledge and skills around static, acellular regenerative, and bioprinted implants, pulling knowledge and course work from other engineering disciplines, and creating new courses and bodies of knowledge specifically related to 3D printing technologies, advanced imaging and image processing, biomaterials design and selection, tissue and organ design, cell and tissue culture, and quality management. With these specific skillsets, it is possible to train a Biofabrication Engineer workforce that will be able work with the leading radiologists, who will also have additional 3D printing training, to manage and run the in-hospital 3D printing centers of the future.

While still relatively new, automated deep learning techniques are likely to replace traditional methods for image segmentation including thresholding, edge detection, and region-based approaches which are typically performed by domain experts and can be time-consuming. Deep learning algorithms are good at automatically discovering intricate features from data for object identification and segmentation. These algorithms will continue to improve and evolve, eventually maturing into artificial intelligence capable of identifying anything on any study on any modality with perfect accuracy in seconds translating to nearly automated segmentation for 3D printing. Machine learning and artificial intelligence is already shifting the practice of radiology to be more effective at promoting appropriate care, creating actionable reports and products that are accessible and intelligible to all providers and patients while improving the patient experience by empowering and educating patient about the role of imaging and 3D printing in their care. Menial tasks, such as identifying and segmenting every pulmonary nodule on a CT scan of the chest, will be performed more quickly and accurately by machines than by humans. This will allow radiologists to focus on higher-order tasks, such as identifying a cohesive diagnosis from a litany of imaging findings, history and physical exam findings and assisting referring physicians with treatment plans such as 3D printing acellular biomaterials and bioprinting, as well as ensuring tissue integration and regeneration through ongoing imaging monitoring similar to present-day imaging surveillance for cancer treatment.

As previously discussed in Chapter 10, 3D printing will continue to be incorporated into the radiology residency training and more 3D printing fellowships will continue to emerge to advance the field of 3D printing for clinical applications such as patient-matched anatomic model, surgical guide, and implant fabrication to provide personalized care and improve patient outcome. Specific imaging protocols for various imaging modalities and equipment are already being developed and implemented to optimize 3D printing. Institutions such as Mayo Clinic and Montefiore Medical Center have already integrated a 3D printing ordering set into their electronic medical record as well as storing the virtual 3D models on their Picture Archiving and Communication System to ensure compliance with the Health Insurance Portability and Accountability Act. In addition, Digital Imaging and Communications in Medicine (DICOM) Working Group 17 is actively working to extend the use of DICOM for the creation, storage, and management of 3D printing file types such as stereolithography and mixed reality models into the healthcare setting.[35] This will allow these 3D models to be stored in a manner that allows both direct association with the patient information and any information including the source imaging from which the 3D content was derived. Furthermore, with a future where biofabrication becomes more feasible and accessible in the hospital, radiology will need to further evolve to ensure anatomic accuracy not just at the gross anatomic level but also down to the cellular and molecular architecture. Radiologists familiar with the principles and language of tissue engineering and molecular biology will lead the way in interpreting the emerging high-resolution imaging exams and applying them for biofabrication. With developing selective contrast agents and probes for cellular and molecular imaging, visualization of angiogenesis and ongoing tissue formation can be achieved and monitored to ensure safe integration of biofabrication and optimize patient outcome.

THE RADIOLOGIST OF THE FUTURE

Analogous to the introduction and rapid clinical adoption of X-ray radiographic imaging in the early 20th century, medical 3D printing has similarly and rapidly progressed from being an intriguing curiosity to becoming increasingly utilized across numerous medical specialties. As 3D printed anatomic models and surgical guides become common place, and 3D printing technologies and materials improve and become more accessible, the broader adoption of in-hospital, patient-matched 3D printed implants, both permanent and regenerative, is not far behind. Regardless of their composition and intended use, these 3D printed objects are enabled and made possible by the collection, interpretation, and digital-to-physical translation of complex imaging data—this is the home and core of radiology. As a result, the future of both medical 3D printing and radiology will become increasingly intertwined, and it will likely not be uncommon in 30 years to see radiologists leading teams of technical specialists in creating not only models and guides but also patient-matched, living tissues and organs as well as biomachine interface devices. This future, however, is dependent on continued technology development; but perhaps more importantly, continued education and increased communication and collaboration between radiologists, primary care providers, engineers, and others (Fig. 16.3).

REFERENCES

1. Huang M-T, Juan P-K, Chen S-Y, et al. The potential of the three-dimensional printed titanium mesh implant for cranioplasty surgery applications: biomechanical behaviors and surface properties. *Mater Sci Eng C.* 2019;97:412−419.
2. Kamel MK, Cheng A, Vaughan B, et al. Sternal reconstruction using customized 3D-printed titanium implants. *Ann Thorac Surg.* 2020;109(6):e411−e414.
3. Rivera F, Leonardi F, Maniscalco P, et al. Uncemented fully hydroxyapatite-coated hip stem for intracapsular femoral neck fractures in osteoporotic elderly patients: a multicenter study. *Arthroplast Today.* 2015;1(3):81−84.
4. Jank BJ, Xiong L, Moser PT, et al. Engineered composite tissue as a bioartificial limb graft. *Biomaterials.* 2015;61: 246−256.
5. Gibson MA, Mykulowycz NM, Shim J, et al. 3D printing metals like thermoplastics: fused filament fabrication of metallic glasses. *Mater Today.* 2018;21(7):697−702.
6. Taylor SL, Jakus AE, Shah RN, Dunand DC. Iron and nickel cellular structures by sintering of 3D-printed oxide or metallic particle inks. *Adv Eng Mater.* 2017;19(11): 1600365.
7. Taylor SL, Ibeh AJ, Jakus AE, Shah RN, Dunand DC. NiTi-Nb micro-trusses fabricated via extrusion-based 3D-printing of powders and transient-liquid-phase sintering. *Acta Biomater.* 2018;76.
8. Jakus AE, Taylor SL, Geisendorfer NR, Dunand DC, Shah RN. Metallic architectures from 3D-printed powder-based liquid inks. *Adv Funct Mater.* 2015;25(45): 6985−6995.
9. Di Prima M, Coburn J, Hwang D, Kelly J, Khairuzzaman A, Ricles L. Additively manufactured medical products − the FDA perspective. *3D Print Med.* 2016;2(1):1.
10. Wong KC, Kumta SM, Geel NV, Demol J. One-step reconstruction with a 3D-printed, biomechanically evaluated custom implant after complex pelvic tumor resection. *Comput Aided Surg.* 2015;20(1):14−23.
11. Siu TL, Rogers JM, Lin K, Thompson R, Owbridge M. Custom-made titanium 3-dimensional printed interbody cages for treatment of osteoporotic fracture−related spinal deformity. *World Neurosurg.* 2018;111:1−5.
12. Thompson RG. 3.2 − Anatomics 3D-printed titanium implants from head to heel. In: Froes FH, Qian M, eds.

13. *Titanium in Medical and Dental Applications.* Woodhead Publishing; 2018:225−237.
13. Qin J, Yang D, Maher S, et al. Micro- and nano-structured 3D printed titanium implants with a hydroxyapatite coating for improved osseointegration. *J Mater Chem B.* 2018;6(19):3136−3144.
14. Jakus AE, Rutz AL, Shah RN. Advancing the field of 3D biomaterial printing. *Biomed Mater.* 2016;11(1):014102.
15. Rutz AL, Hyland KE, Jakus AE, Burghardt WR, Shah RN. A multimaterial bioink method for 3D printing tunable, cell-compatible hydrogels. *Adv Mater.* 2015;27(9): 1607−1614.
16. Laronda MM, Rutz AL, Xiao S, et al. A bioprosthetic ovary created using 3D printed microporous scaffolds restores ovarian function in sterilized mice. *Nat Commun.* 2017; 8(1):15261.
17. Jakus AE, Rutz AL, Jordan SW, et al. Hyperelastic "bone": a highly versatile, growth factor−free, osteoregenerative, scalable, and surgically friendly biomaterial. *Sci Transl Med.* 2016;8(358):358ra127.
18. Huang YH, Jakus AE, Jordan SW, et al. 3D-printed "hyperelastic bone" scaffolds accelerate bone regeneration in critical-sized calvarial bone defects. *Plast Reconstr Surg.* 2019; 143(5).
19. Jakus AE, Geisendorfer NR, Lewis PL, Shah RN. 3D-Printing porosity: a new approach to creating elevated porosity materials and structures. *Acta Biomater.* 2018;72.
20. Jakus AE, Laronda MM, Rashedi AS, et al. "Tissue Papers" from organ-specific decellularized extracellular matrices. *Adv Funct Mater.* 2017;27(34):1700992.
21. Jakus AE, Secor EB, Rutz AL, Jordan SW, Hersam MC, Shah RN. Three-dimensional printing of high-content graphene scaffolds for electronic and biomedical applications. *ACS Nano.* 2015;9(4):4636−4648.
22. Jakus AE, Shah RN. Multi and mixed 3D-printing of graphene-hydroxyapatite hybrid materials for complex tissue engineering. *J Biomed Mater Res.* 2017;105(1): 274−283.
23. Driscoll JA, Lubbe R, Jakus AE, et al. 3D-printed ceramic-demineralized bone matrix hyperelastic bone composite scaffolds for spinal fusion. *Tissue Engg Part A.* 2019.
24. Liu X, Jakus AE, Kural M, et al. Vascularization of natural and synthetic bone scaffolds. *Cell Trans.* 2018; 27(8).
25. Alluri R, Jakus A, Bougioukli S, et al. 3D printed hyperelastic "bone" scaffolds and regional gene therapy: a novel approach to bone healing. *J Biomed Mater Res.* 2018; 106(4):1104−1110.
26. Ghodbane SA, Brzezinski A, Patel JM, et al. Partial meniscus replacement with a collagen-Hyaluronan infused three-dimensional printed polymeric scaffold. *Tissue Eng A.* 2019;25(5−6):379−389.
27. Ng WL, Lee JM, Zhou M, et al. Vat polymerization-based bioprinting—process, materials, applications and regulatory challenges. *Biofabrication.* 2020;12(2):022001.
28. Haake K, Ackermann M, Lachmann N. Concise review: towards the clinical translation of induced pluripotent stem cell-derived blood cells—ready for take-off. *Stem Cell Transl Med.* 2019;8(4):332−339.

29. Pellegata AF, Bottagisio M, Boschetti F, et al. Terminal sterilization of equine-derived decellularized tendons for clinical use. *Mater Sci Eng C.* 2017;75:43−49.

30. Hennessy RS, Jana S, Tefft BJ, et al. Supercritical carbon dioxide−based sterilization of decellularized heart valves. *J Am Coll Cardiol.* 2017;2(1):71−84.

31. Basgul C, Yu T, MacDonald DW, Siskey R, Marcolongo M, Kurtz SM. Structure-property relationships for 3D printed PEEK intervertebral lumbar cages produced using fused filament fabrication. *J Mater Res.* 2018;33(14): 2040−2051.

32. *Technical Considerations for Additive Manufactured Medical Devices. Guidance Document Website.* https://www.fda.gov/ regulatory-information/search-fda-guidance documents/ technical-considerations-additive-manufactured-medical-devices. Published 2017. Accessed 2020.

33. *Framework for the Regulation of Regenerative Medicine Products.* https://www.fda.gov/vaccines-blood-biologics/cellular-gen e-therapy-products/framework   regulation-regenerative-medicine-products. Accessed 2020.

34. Riggs BL, Melton III LJ, Robb RA, et al. Population-based study of age and sex differences in bone volumetric density, size, geometry, and structure at different skeletal sites. *J Bone Miner Res.* 2004;19(12):1945−1954.

35. DICOM Working Group Minutes. *WG-17 3D.* https:// www.dicomstandard.org/wgs/wg-17/. Accessed 2020.

Reference Index

'*Note*: Page numbers followed by "*t*" indicate tables.'

Subject Index

'*Note*: Page numbers followed by "f" indicate figures and "t" indicate tables.'

CPI Antony Rowe
Eastbourne, UK
May 28, 2021